Cardiovascular Care

made

Incredibly Easy!®

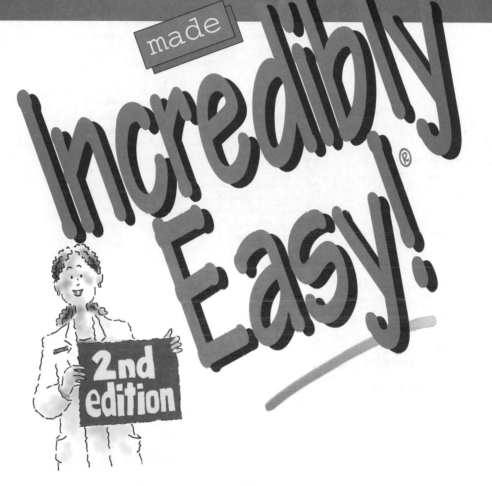

2nd edition

 Wolters Kluwer | Lippincott Williams & Wilkins
Health

Philadelphia · Baltimore · New York · London
Buenos Aires · Hong Kong · Sydney · Tokyo

Staff

Executive Publisher
Judith A. Schilling McCann, RN, MSN

Editorial Director
David Moreau

Clinical Director
Joan M. Robinson, RN, MSN

Art Director
Mary Ludwicki

Senior Managing Editor
Jaime Stockslager Buss, MSPH, ELS

Clinical Project Manager
Lorraine M. Hallowell, RN, BSN, RVS

Editors
Diane Labus, Liz Schaeffer

Copy Editors
Kimberly Bilotta (supervisor), Scotti Cohn,
Dorothy P. Terry, Pamela Wingrod

Designers
Lynn Foulk, Georg Purvis

Illustrator
Bot Roda

Digital Composition Services
Diane Paluba (manager), Joyce Rossi Biletz

Associate Manufacturing Manager
Beth J. Welsh

Editorial Assistants
Karen J. Kirk, Jeri O'Shea, Linda K. Ruhf

Indexer
Karen C. Comerford

Library of Congress Cataloging-in-Publication Data

Cardiovascular care made incredibly easy!.–2nd ed.
      p. ; cm.
Includes bibliographical references and index.
1. Heart–Diseases–Nursing–Outlines, syllabi, etc. 2.
Heart–Diseases–Nursing–Examinations, questions,
etc. I. Lippincott Williams & Wilkins.
[DNLM: 1. Cardiovascular Diseases–nursing. WY
152.5 C26743 2009]
RC674.C3585 2009
616.1'20231–dc22
ISBN-13: 978-0-7817-8824-3 (alk. paper)
ISBN-10: 0-7817-8824-2 (alk. paper)   2008003553

Contents

Contributors and consultants

Helen Christina Ballestas, RN, MSN, CRRN
Nursing Faculty
New York Institute of Technology
Old Westbury

Margaret T. Bowers, RN, MSN, APRN-BC
Assistant Clinical Professor and Nurse Practitioner
Duke University School of Nursing
Durham, N.C.

Sara L. Clutter, RN, MSN
Assistant Professor of Nursing
Waynesburg (Pa.) College

Shelley Yerger Hawkins, APRN-BC, DSN, FNP, GNP, FAANP
Post Doctoral Fellow
University of North Carolina
Chapel Hill

Fiona Johnson, RN, MSN, CCRN
Clinical Education Specialist
Memorial Health University Medical Center
Savannah, Ga.

Gary R. Jones, FNP-C, MSN
Family Nurse Practitioner
St. Johns Heart Center
Joplin, Mo.

Colleen Lad, BSN
Clinical Educator
Saint Luke's Mid America Heart Institute
Kansas City, Mo.

Theresa M. Leonard, RN, BSN, CCRN
Unit Educator, Invasive Cardiology
Stony Brook (N.Y.) University Medical Center

Susan Sample, RN, MSN, CRNP
Director of Nursing
Lancaster (Pa.) General Hospital

Cindy R. Schuch, RN, BSN, MS
RN Administrator
Sanford Health Network
Sioux Falls, S.D.

Rita M. Wick, RN, BSN
Education Specialist
Berkshire Health Systems
Pittsfield, Mass.

Not another boring foreword

If you're like me, you're too busy to wade through a foreword that uses pretentious terms and umpteen dull paragraphs to get to the point. So let's cut right to the chase! Here's why this book is so terrific:

It will teach you all the important things you need to know about cardiovascular care. (And it will leave out all the fluff that wastes your time.)

It will help you remember what you've learned.

It will make you smile as it enhances your knowledge and skills.

Don't believe me? Try these recurring logos on for size:

Advice from the experts—tips and tricks from other cardiovascular care nurses on how to best perform cardiovascular care

Peak technique—clear, concise explanations about the best ways to perform cardiovascular procedures

Now I get it!—simplified explanations of difficult concepts related to the cardiovascular system

No place like home—key information about adapting care to a home environment

Memory joggers—acronyms and other mnemonics that aid recall of important information.

See? I told you! And that's not all. Look for me and my friends in the margins throughout this book. We'll be there to explain key concepts, provide important care reminders, and offer reassurance. Oh, and if you don't mind, we'll be spicing up the pages with a bit of humor along the way, to teach and entertain in a way that no other resource can.

I hope you find this book helpful. Best of luck throughout your career!

Joy

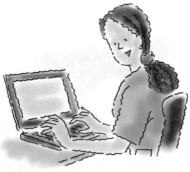

1

Anatomy and physiology

Just the facts

In this chapter, you'll learn:

♦ components of the heart

♦ the way in which the heart contracts

♦ the heart's role in blood flow.

A look at the cardiovascular system

The cardiovascular system (sometimes called the *circulatory system*) consists of the heart, blood vessels, and lymphatics. This network brings life-sustaining oxygen and nutrients to the body's cells, removes metabolic waste products, and carries hormones from one part of the body to another.

Right to the lungs...and left to the body

The heart consists of two separate pumps: The right side pumps the blood to the lungs, and the left side pumps the blood to the rest of the body.

Where the heart lies

About the size of a closed fist, the heart lies beneath the sternum in the mediastinum (the cavity between the lungs), between the second and sixth ribs. In most people, the heart rests obliquely, with its right side below and almost in front of the left. Because of its oblique angle, the heart's broad part (base) is at its upper right, and its pointed end (apex) is at its lower left. The apex is the point of maximal impulse, where heart sounds are the loudest.

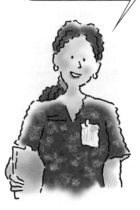

Talk about networking! The cardiovascular system is a complex network that helps sustain life.

Heart structure

Surrounded by a sac called the *pericardium*, the heart has a wall made up of three layers: the myocardium, endocardium, and epicardium. Within the heart lie four chambers (two atria and two ventricles) and four valves (two atrioventricular [AV] and two semilunar valves). (See *Inside the heart.*)

Inside the heart

Within the heart lie four chambers (two atria and two ventricles) and four valves (two atrioventricular and two semilunar valves). A system of blood vessels carries blood to and from the heart, as shown below.

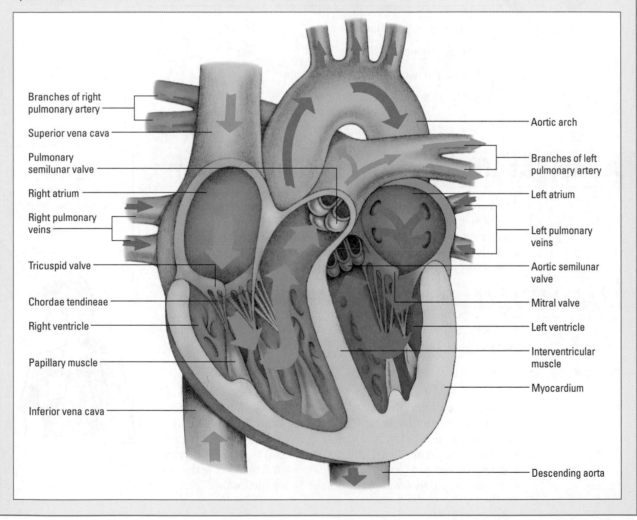

Branches of right pulmonary artery

Superior vena cava

Pulmonary semilunar valve

Right atrium

Right pulmonary veins

Tricuspid valve

Chordae tendineae

Right ventricle

Papillary muscle

Inferior vena cava

Aortic arch

Branches of left pulmonary artery

Left atrium

Left pulmonary veins

Aortic semilunar valve

Mitral valve

Left ventricle

Interventricular muscle

Myocardium

Descending aorta

The pericardium

The pericardium is a fibroserous sac that surrounds the heart and the roots of the great vessels (those vessels that enter and leave the heart). It consists of the fibrous pericardium and the serous pericardium.

Fibrous fits freely

The fibrous pericardium, composed of tough, white fibrous tissue, fits loosely around the heart, protecting it.

Serous is smooth

The serous pericardium, the thin, smooth inner portion, has two layers:
- The parietal layer lines the inside of the fibrous pericardium.
- The visceral layer adheres to the surface of the heart.

And fluid in between

Between the fibrous and serous pericardium is the pericardial space. This space contains pericardial fluid, which lubricates the surfaces of the space and allows the heart to move easily during contraction.

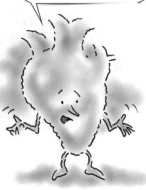

Sure, I have a wall up, but my myocardial layer helps me to contract.

The wall

The wall of the heart consists of three layers:

The *epicardium*, the outer layer (and the visceral layer of the serous pericardium), is made up of squamous epithelial cells overlying connective tissue.

The *myocardium*, the middle layer, forms most of the heart wall. It has striated muscle fibers that cause the heart to contract.

The *endocardium*, the heart's inner layer, consists of endothelial tissue with small blood vessels and bundles of smooth muscle.

The chambers

The heart contains four hollow chambers: two atria and two ventricles.

Upstairs...

The atria, the upper chambers, are separated by the interatrial septum. They receive blood returning to the heart and pump blood to the ventricles.

...where the blood comes in

The right atrium receives blood from the superior and inferior venae cavae. The left atrium, which is smaller but has thicker walls than the right atrium, forms the uppermost part of the heart's left border. It receives blood from the two pulmonary veins.

Downstairs...

The right and left ventricles, which are separated by the interventricular septum, make up the two lower chambers. The ventricles receive blood from the atria. Composed of highly developed musculature, the ventricles are larger and have thicker walls than the atria.

...where the blood goes out

The right ventricle pumps blood to the lungs. The left ventricle, which is larger than the right, pumps blood through all other vessels of the body.

Memory jogger

If you can remember that there are two distinct heart sounds, you can recall that there are two sets of heart valves. Closure of the atrioventricular valves makes the first heart sound, the *lub*; closure of the semilunar valves makes the second heart sound, the *dub*.

The valves

The heart contains four valves: two AV valves and two semilunar valves.

Forward flow only

The valves allow forward flow of blood through the heart and prevent backward flow. They open and close in response to pressure changes caused by ventricular contraction and blood ejection. The two AV valves separate the atria from the ventricles. The tricuspid valve, or right AV valve, prevents backflow from the right ventricle into the right atrium. The mitral valve, or left AV valve, prevents backflow from the left ventricle into the left atrium. One of the two semilunar valves is the pulmonic valve, which prevents backflow from the pulmonary artery into the right ventricle. The other semilunar valve is the aortic valve, which prevents backflow from the aorta into the left ventricle.

On the cusps

The tricuspid valve has three triangular cusps, or leaflets. The mitral, or bicuspid, valve contains two cusps, a large anterior and a smaller posterior. Chordae tendineae (tendinous cords) attach the cusps of the AV valves to papillary muscles in the ventricles. The semilunar valves have three cusps that are shaped like half-moons. (See *Heart valves*.)

The semilunar valves, which prevent blood backflow into the ventricles, are shaped like half-moons.

Heart valves

The four valves of the heart are illustrated below. Note the number of cusps in each valve.

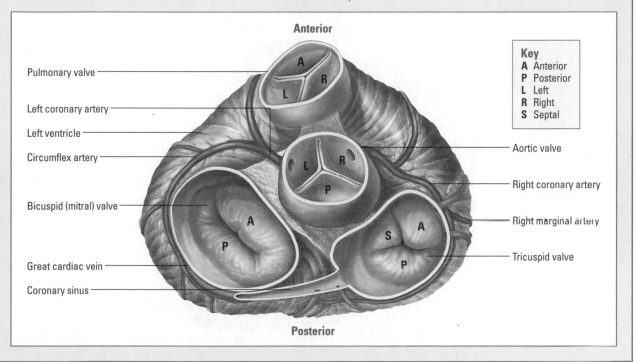

Anterior

Pulmonary valve

Left coronary artery

Left ventricle

Circumflex artery

Bicuspid (mitral) valve

Great cardiac vein

Coronary sinus

Key
A Anterior
P Posterior
L Left
R Right
S Septal

Aortic valve

Right coronary artery

Right marginal artery

Tricuspid valve

Posterior

Conduction system

The heart's conduction system causes it to contract, moving blood throughout the body. For this system to work properly, the heart requires electrical stimulation as well as a mechanical response. (See *The cardiac conduction system*, page 6.)

We have the qualities a properly functioning heart is looking for in pacemaker cells...

Automaticity, conductivity, and contractility.

Electrical stimulation

The conduction system contains pacemaker cells, which have three unique characteristics:

☝ automaticity, the ability to generate an electrical impulse automatically

✌ conductivity, the ability to pass the impulse to the next cell

🤟 contractility, the ability to shorten the fibers in the heart when receiving the impulse.

The cardiac conduction system

Specialized fibers propagate electrical impulses throughout the heart's cells, causing the heart to contract. This illustration shows the elements of the cardiac conduction system.

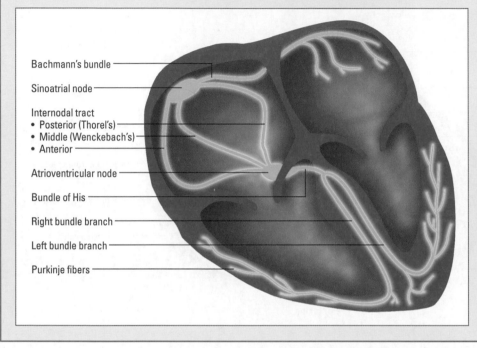

Bachmann's bundle

Sinoatrial node

Internodal tract
• Posterior (Thorel's)
• Middle (Wenckebach's)
• Anterior

Atrioventricular node

Bundle of His

Right bundle branch

Left bundle branch

Purkinje fibers

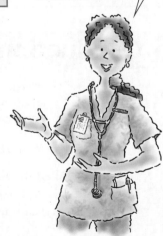

You might say that the heart has a firing squad. If the SA node doesn't fire, the AV node fires. If the SA node and the AV node fail, the ventricles fire their own impulse.

Start with a bang

The sinoatrial (SA) node, located on the endocardial surface of the right atrium, near the superior vena cava, is the normal pacemaker of the heart, generating an impulse between 60 and 100 times per minute. The SA node's firing spreads an impulse throughout the right and left atria, resulting in atrial contraction.

Slow and fill

The AV node, situated low in the septal wall of the right atrium, slows impulse conduction between the atria and ventricles. This "resistor" node allows the contracting atria to fill the ventricles with blood before the lower chambers contract.

Impulsive signal

From the AV node, the impulse travels to the bundle of His (modified muscle fibers), which branches off to the right and left bundles. Finally, the impulse travels to the Purkinje fibers, the distal portions of the left and right bundle branches. These fibers fan across the surface of the ventricles from the endocardium to the myocardium. As the impulse spreads, it signals the blood-filled ventricles to contract.

Just in case

The conduction system has two built-in safety mechanisms. If the SA node fails to fire, the AV node generates an impulse between 40 and 60 times per minute. If the SA node and the AV node fail, the ventricles can generate their own impulse between 20 and 40 times per minute.

> The cardiac cycle lasts from the start of one heartbeat all the way to the start of the next.

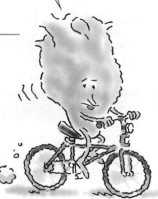

Mechanical events

Following electrical stimulation, mechanical events must occur in the proper sequence and to the proper degree to provide adequate blood flow to all body parts. These events are collectively known as the *cardiac cycle*, which consists of the period from the one heartbeat to the beginning of the next. The cardiac cycle has two phases—systole and diastole. (See *Events of the cardiac cycle*, page 8.)

Contract...

At the beginning of systole, the ventricles contract. Increasing blood pressure in the ventricles forces the AV valves (mitral and tricuspid) to close and the semilunar valves (pulmonic and aortic) to open. As the ventricles contract, ventricular blood pressure builds until it exceeds the pressure in the pulmonary artery and the aorta. Then the semilunar valves open, and the ventricles eject blood into the aorta and the pulmonary artery.

...and release

When the ventricles empty and relax, ventricular pressure falls below the pressure in the pulmonary artery and the aorta. At the beginning of diastole, the semilunar valves close to prevent the backflow of blood into the ventricles, and the mitral and tricuspid valves open, allowing blood to flow into the ventricles from the atria.

Events of the cardiac cycle

The cardiac cycle consists of the following five events.

Isovolumetric ventricular contraction

In response to ventricular depolarization, tension in the ventricles increases. This rise in pressure within the ventricles leads to closure of the mitral and tricuspid valves. The pulmonic and aortic valves stay closed during the entire phase.

Atrial systole

Known as the *atrial kick,* atrial systole (coinciding with late ventricular diastole) supplies the ventricles with the remaining 30% of the blood for each heartbeat.

Ventricular ejection

When ventricular pressure exceeds aortic and pulmonary arterial pressure, the aortic and pulmonic valves open and the ventricles eject blood.

Isovolumetric relaxation

When ventricular pressure falls below the pressure in the aorta and pulmonary artery, the aortic and pulmonic valves close. All valves are closed during this phase. Atrial diastole occurs as blood fills the atria.

Ventricular filling

Atrial pressure exceeds ventricular pressure, which causes the mitral and tricuspid valves to open. Blood then flows passively into the ventricles. About 70% of ventricular filling takes place during this phase.

When the ventricles become full, near the end of this phase, the atria contract to send the remaining blood to the ventricles. Then a new cardiac cycle begins as the heart enters systole again.

Output = rate x volume

Cardiac output refers to the amount of blood the heart pumps in 1 minute. It's equal to the heart rate multiplied by the stroke volume, the amount of blood ejected with each heartbeat. Stroke volume, in turn, depends on three major factors: preload, contractility, and afterload. (See *Understanding preload, contractility, and afterload.*)

Understanding preload, contractility, and afterload

If you think of the heart as a balloon, it can help you understand stroke volume.

Blowing up the balloon

Preload is the stretching of muscle fibers in the ventricles. This stretching results from blood volume in the ventricles at end diastole. According to *Starling's law,* the more the heart muscles stretch during diastole, the more forcefully they contract during systole. Think of preload as the balloon stretching as air is blown into it. The more air being blown, the greater the stretch.

The balloon's stretch

Contractility refers to the inherent ability of the myocardium to contract normally. Contractility is influenced by preload. The greater the stretch the more forceful the contraction—or, the more air in the balloon, the greater the stretch, and the farther the balloon will fly when air is allowed to expel.

The knot that ties the balloon

Afterload refers to the pressure that the ventricular muscles must generate to overcome the higher pressure in the aorta to get the blood out of the heart. *Resistance* is the knot on the end of the balloon, which the balloon has to work against to get the air out.

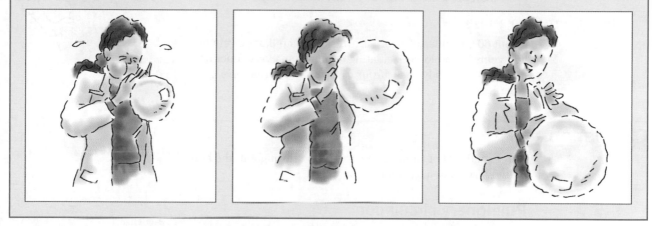

Blood flow

Blood flows through the body in five types of vessels, involving three methods of circulation.

Blood vessels

The five distinct types of blood vessels are:
- arteries
- arterioles
- capillaries
- venules
- veins.

The structure of each type of vessel differs according to its function in the cardiovascular system and the pressure exerted by the volume of blood at various sites within the system.

Built for high speed...

Arteries have thick, muscular walls to accommodate the flow of blood at high speeds and pressures. *Arterioles* have thinner walls than arteries. They constrict or dilate to control blood flow to the *capillaries*, which (being microscopic) have walls composed of only a single layer of endothelial cells.

...and low pressure

Venules gather blood from the capillaries; their walls are thinner than those of arterioles. *Veins* have thinner walls than arteries but have larger diameters because of the low blood pressure of venous return to the heart.

Frequent flyer miles

About 60,000 miles of arteries, arterioles, capillaries, venules, and veins keep blood circulating to and from every functioning cell in the body. (See *Major arteries* and *Major veins*, page 12.)

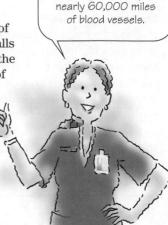

Combined, the arterioles, venules, and capillaries equal nearly 60,000 miles of blood vessels.

Circulation

Three methods of circulation carry blood throughout the body: pulmonary, systemic, and coronary.

Pulmonary circulation

In pulmonary circulation, blood travels to the lungs to pick up oxygen and release carbon dioxide.

Returns and exchanges

As blood moves from the heart to the lungs and back again, it proceeds as follows:
• Unoxygenated blood travels from the right ventricle through the pulmonic valve into the pulmonary arteries.
• Blood passes through progressively smaller arteries and arterioles into the capillaries of the lungs.
• Blood reaches the alveoli and exchanges carbon dioxide for oxygen.
• Oxygenated blood then returns via venules and veins to the pulmonary veins, which carry it back to the heart's left atrium.

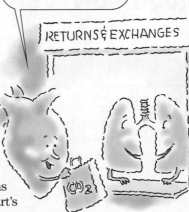

I'd like to exchange this for some oxygen, please.

RETURNS & EXCHANGES

CO_2

Major arteries

This illustration shows the body's major arteries.

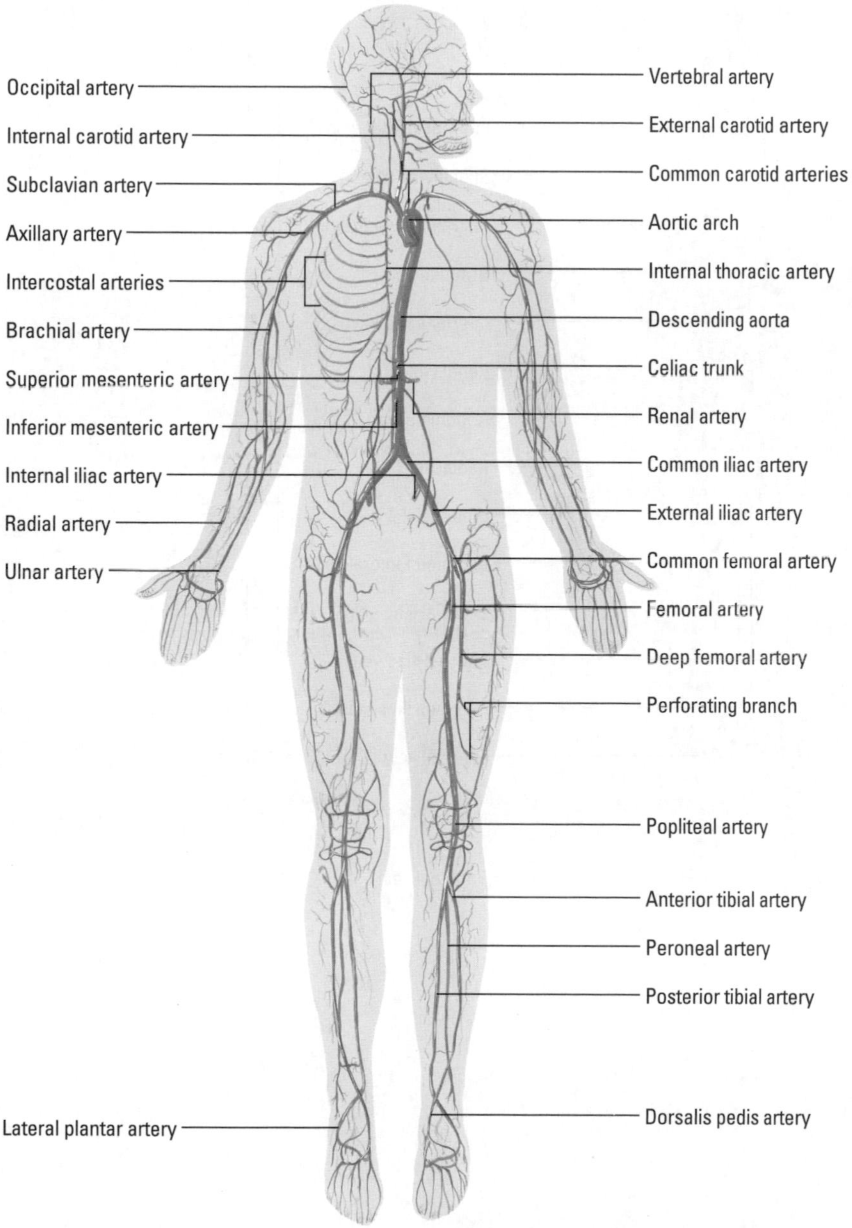

Occipital artery

Internal carotid artery

Subclavian artery

Axillary artery

Intercostal arteries

Brachial artery

Superior mesenteric artery

Inferior mesenteric artery

Internal iliac artery

Radial artery

Ulnar artery

Lateral plantar artery

Vertebral artery

External carotid artery

Common carotid arteries

Aortic arch

Internal thoracic artery

Descending aorta

Celiac trunk

Renal artery

Common iliac artery

External iliac artery

Common femoral artery

Femoral artery

Deep femoral artery

Perforating branch

Popliteal artery

Anterior tibial artery

Peroneal artery

Posterior tibial artery

Dorsalis pedis artery

Major veins

This illustration shows the body's major veins.

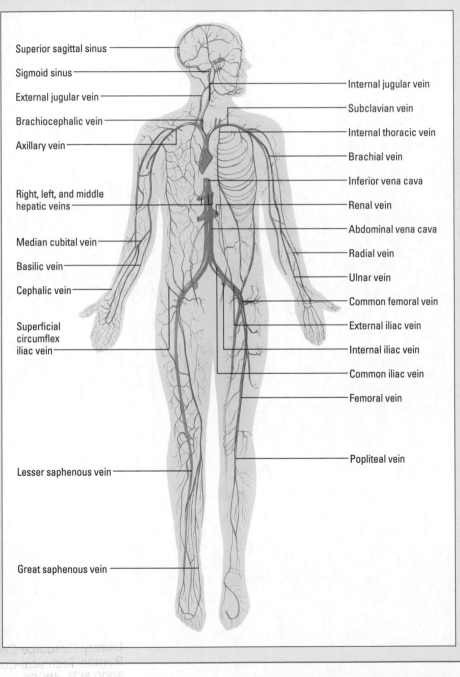

Superior sagittal sinus

Sigmoid sinus

External jugular vein

Brachiocephalic vein

Axillary vein

Right, left, and middle hepatic veins

Median cubital vein

Basilic vein

Cephalic vein

Superficial circumflex iliac vein

Lesser saphenous vein

Great saphenous vein

Internal jugular vein

Subclavian vein

Internal thoracic vein

Brachial vein

Inferior vena cava

Renal vein

Abdominal vena cava

Radial vein

Ulnar vein

Common femoral vein

External iliac vein

Internal iliac vein

Common iliac vein

Femoral vein

Popliteal vein

Systemic circulation

Systemic circulation begins when blood pumped from the left ventricle carries oxygen and other nutrients to body cells. This same circulation also transports waste products for excretion.

Branching out

The major artery, the aorta, branches into vessels that supply specific organs and areas of the body. As it arches out of the top of the heart and down to the abdomen, three arteries branch off the top of the arch to supply the upper body with blood:
• The left common carotid artery supplies blood to the brain.
• The left subclavian artery supplies the left arm.
• The innominate, or brachiocephalic, artery branches into the right common carotid artery (which supplies blood to the brain) and the right subclavian artery (which supplies blood to the right arm).
• The right innominate, right subclavian, and left subclavian arteries supply blood to the chest wall.

As the aorta descends through the thorax and abdomen, its branches supply the organs of the GI and genitourinary systems, spinal column, and lower chest and abdominal muscles. Then the aorta divides into the iliac arteries, which further divide into femoral arteries.

Division = addition = perfusion

As the arteries divide into smaller units, the number of vessels increases dramatically, thereby increasing the area of tissue to which blood flows (the *area of perfusion*).

Dilation is another part of the equation

At the ends of the arterioles and the beginnings of the capillaries, strong sphincters control blood flow into the tissues. These sphincters dilate to permit more flow when needed, close to shunt blood to other areas, or constrict to increase blood pressure.

A large area of low pressure

Although the capillary bed contains the tiniest vessels, it supplies blood to the largest number of cells. Capillary pressure is extremely low to allow for the exchange of nutrients, oxygen, and carbon dioxide with body cells. From the capillaries, blood flows into venules and, eventually, into veins.

No backflow

Valves in the veins prevent blood backflow. Pooled blood in each valved segment is moved toward the heart by pressure from the moving volume of blood from below.

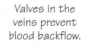

Valves in the veins prevent blood backflow.

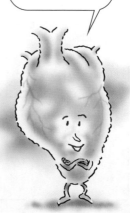

Vessels that supply the heart

Coronary circulation involves the arterial system of blood vessels that supplies oxygenated blood to the heart and the venous system that removes oxygen-depleted blood from it.

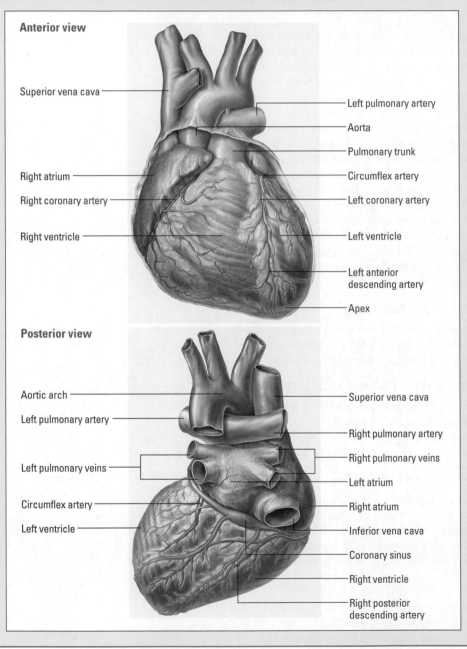

Anterior view

Superior vena cava

Left pulmonary artery

Aorta

Pulmonary trunk

Right atrium

Circumflex artery

Right coronary artery

Left coronary artery

Right ventricle

Left ventricle

Left anterior descending artery

Apex

Posterior view

Aortic arch

Superior vena cava

Left pulmonary artery

Right pulmonary artery

Right pulmonary veins

Left pulmonary veins

Left atrium

Circumflex artery

Right atrium

Left ventricle

Inferior vena cava

Coronary sinus

Right ventricle

Right posterior descending artery

The veins merge until they form two main branches, the superior vena cava and inferior vena cava, that return blood to the right atrium.

Coronary circulation

The heart relies on the coronary arteries and their branches for its supply of oxygenated blood. It also depends on the cardiac veins to remove oxygen-depleted blood. (See *Vessels that supply the heart.*)

The heart gets its part

During left ventricular systole, blood is ejected into the aorta. During diastole, blood flows out of the heart and then through the coronary arteries to nourish the heart muscle.

From the right...

The right coronary artery supplies blood to the right atrium, part of the left atrium, most of the right ventricle, and the inferior part of the left ventricle.

...and from the left

The left coronary artery, which splits into the anterior descending artery and circumflex artery, supplies blood to the left atrium, most of the left ventricle, and most of the interventricular septum.

Superficially speaking

The cardiac veins lie superficial to the arteries. The largest vein, the coronary sinus, opens into the right atrium. Most of the major cardiac veins empty into the coronary sinus; the anterior cardiac veins, however, empty into the right atrium.

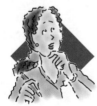

Quick quiz

1. During systole the ventricles contract. This causes:
   A. all four heart valves to close.
   B. all four heart valves to open.
   C. the AV valves to close and the semilunar valves to open.
   D. the AV valves to open and the semilunar valves to close.

Answer: C. During systole the pressure is greater in the ventricles than in the atria, causing the AV valves (the tricuspid and mitral valves) to close. The pressure in the ventricles is also greater than the pressure in the aorta and pulmonary artery, forcing the semilunar valves (the pulmonic and aortic valves) to open.

2. The normal pacemaker of the heart is:
   A.   the SA node.
   B.   the AV node.
   C.   the bundle of His.
   D.   the ventricles.

Answer: A. Normally, the SA node is the heart's pacemaker, generating 60 to 100 impulses per minute. The AV node is the secondary pacemaker of the heart (40 to 60 beats/minute). The ventricles are the last line of defense (20 to 40 beats/minute). The bundle of His isn't a pacemaker of the heart; it sends impulses to the Purkinje fibers.

3. The pressure the ventricular muscle must generate to overcome the higher pressure in the aorta refers to:
   A.   stroke volume.
   B.   contractility.
   C.   preload.
   D.   afterload.

Answer: D. Afterload is the pressure the ventricular muscle must generate to overcome the higher pressure in the aorta to get the blood out of the heart.

4. The vessels that carry oxygenated blood back to the heart and left atrium are the:
   A.   capillaries.
   B.   pulmonary veins.
   C.   pulmonary arteries.
   D.   pulmonary arterioles.

Answer: B. Oxygenated blood returns by way of venules and veins to the pulmonary veins, which carry it back to the heart's left atrium.

5. The layer of the heart responsible for contraction is the:
   A.   myocardium.
   B.   pericardium.
   C.   endocardium.
   D.   epicardium.

Answer: A. The myocardium has striated muscle fibers that cause the heart to contract.

Scoring

☆☆☆   If you answered all five questions correctly, super! Your knowledge is circulating smoothly.

☆☆   If you answered four questions correctly, great! You have a handle on the heart of things.

☆   If you answered fewer than four questions correctly, don't worry! You're sure to jump on the cardiac cycle next chapter.

Assessment

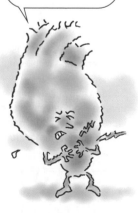

Just the facts

In this chapter, you'll learn:

♦ methods to obtain a cardiovascular health history

♦ techniques used in a physical examination of the cardio-vascular system

♦ normal and abnormal cardiovascular findings.

Obtaining a health history

The first step in assessing the cardiovascular system is to obtain a health history. Begin by introducing yourself and explaining what will occur first during the health history and later during the physical examination. Then ask about the patient's chief complaint. Also, be sure to ask about the patient's personal *and* family health history.

> The pain I'm experiencing is sudden, radiating, steady, acute, and sharp. Does that help?

Chief complaint

You'll find that patients with cardiovascular problems typically cite specific complaints, such as chest pain, palpitations, syncope, intermittent claudication, and peripheral edema. Let's take a closer look at each of these chief complaints as well as some other common signs and symptoms.

Chest pain

Many patients with cardiovascular problems complain at some point of chest pain. Chest pain can arise suddenly or gradually and can radiate to the arms, neck, jaw, or back. It can be steady or intermittent, mild or acute, and it can range in character from a sharp, shooting sensation to a feeling of heaviness, fullness, or even indigestion.

A full menu of causes

The cause of chest pain may be difficult to determine at first. Chest pain can be provoked or aggravated by stress, anxiety, exertion, deep breathing, or eating certain foods. (See *Understanding chest pain.*)

Understanding chest pain

Use this table to help you more accurately assess chest pain and its possible causes.

What it feels like	Where it's located	What makes it worse	What causes it	What makes it better
Aching, squeezing, pressure, heaviness, burning pain; usually subsides within 10 minutes	Substernal; may radiate to jaw, neck, arms, and back	Eating, physical effort, smoking, cold weather, stress, anger, hunger, lying down	Angina pectoris	Rest, nitroglycerin (*Note:* Unstable angina appears even at rest.)
Tightness or pressure; burning, aching pain; possibly accompanied by shortness of breath, diaphoresis, weakness, anxiety, or nausea; sudden onset; lasts ½ to 2 hours	Typically across chest but may radiate to jaw, neck, arms, and back	Exertion, anxiety	Acute myocardial infarction	Opioid analgesics such as morphine
Sharp and continuous pain; may be accompanied by friction rub; sudden onset	Substernal; may radiate to neck and left arm	Deep breathing, supine position	Pericarditis	Sitting up, leaning forward, anti-inflammatory drugs
Excruciating, tearing pain; may be accompanied by blood pressure difference between right and left arm; sudden onset	Retrosternal, upper abdominal, or epigastric; may radiate to back, neck, and shoulders	Not applicable	Dissecting aortic aneurysm	Analgesics, surgery
Sudden, stabbing pain; may be accompanied by cyanosis, dyspnea, or cough with hemoptysis	Over lung area	Inspiration	Pulmonary embolus	Analgesics
Sudden and severe pain; sometimes accompanied by dyspnea, increased pulse rate, decreased breath sounds, or deviated trachea	Lateral thorax	Normal respiration	Pneumothorax	Analgesics, chest tube insertion

Understanding chest pain (continued)

What it feels like	Where it's located	What makes it worse	What causes it	What makes it better
Dull, pressurelike, squeezing pain	Substernal, epigastric areas	Food, cold liquids, exercise	Esophageal spasm	Nitroglycerin, calcium channel blockers
Sharp, severe pain	Lower chest or upper abdomen	Eating a heavy meal, bending, lying down	Hiatal hernia	Antacids, walking, semi-Fowler's position
Burning feeling after eating; sometimes accompanied by hematemesis or tarry stools; sudden onset that generally subsides within 15 to 20 minutes	Epigastric area	Lack of food, eating highly acidic foods	Peptic ulcer	Food, antacids
Gripping, sharp pain; may be accompanied by nausea and vomiting	Right epigastric or abdominal areas; may radiate to shoulders	Eating fatty foods, lying down	Cholecystitis	Rest and analgesics, surgery
Continuous or intermittent sharp pain; possibly tender to touch; gradual or sudden onset	Anywhere in chest	Movement, palpation	Chest-wall syndrome	Time, analgesics, heat applications
Dull or stabbing pain; usually accompanied by hyperventilation or breathlessness; sudden onset; can last less than a minute or as long as several days	Anywhere in chest	Increased respiratory rate, stress, anxiety	Acute anxiety	Slowing of respiratory rate, stress relief

Pinpointing pain

If the patient's chest pain isn't severe, proceed with the history. Ask if the patient feels diffuse pain or can point to the painful area. Ask whether he has any discomfort that radiates to his neck, jaw, arms, or back. If he does, ask him to describe it. Is it a dull, aching, pressurelike sensation? A sharp, stabbing, knifelike pain? Does he feel it on the surface or deep inside? Ask him to rate the pain on a scale of 1 to 10, in which 1 means negligible and 10 means the worst imaginable.

Going steady?

Then find out whether the pain is constant or intermittent. If it's intermittent, how long does it last? Ask if movement, exertion, breathing, position changes, or eating certain foods worsens or helps relieve the pain. Does anything in particular seem to bring it on? Find out what medications the patient is taking, if any, and ask about recent dosage or schedule changes.

Palpitations

Defined as a conscious awareness of one's heartbeat, palpitations are usually felt over the precordium or in the throat or neck. The patient may describe them as pounding, jumping, turning, fluttering, or flopping. He may also describe a sensation of missed or skipped beats. Palpitations may be regular or irregular, fast or slow, paroxysmal or sustained.

A racing rhythm that suddenly stops can mean paroxysmal atrial tachycardia. No slamming on the brakes for me!

Don't skip this beat

To help characterize the palpitations, ask the patient to simulate their rhythm by tapping his finger on a hard surface. An irregular "skipped beat" rhythm points to premature ventricular contractions, whereas an episodic racing rhythm that ends abruptly suggests paroxysmal atrial tachycardia (brief periods of tachycardia alternating with normal sinus rhythm).

Maybe it was that triple shot of espresso

Next, ask if the patient has a history of hypertension or if he has recently started digoxin therapy. Be sure to obtain a drug history, and ask about caffeine, tobacco, and alcohol consumption and use of illicit drugs or herbal supplements. Palpitations may accompany use of these substances.

No big deal—unless...

Palpitations are typically insignificant and are relatively common. However, they can be caused by such cardiovascular disorders as arrhythmias, hypertension, mitral prolapse, and mitral stenosis.

Syncope

Syncope is a brief loss of consciousness caused by a lack of blood to the brain. It usually occurs abruptly and lasts for seconds to minutes. It may result from such cardiovascular disorders as aortic arch syndrome, aortic stenosis, and arrhythmias.

Barely breathing

When syncope occurs, the patient typically lies motionless, with his skeletal muscles relaxed. The depth of unconsciousness varies—some patients can hear voices or see blurred outlines;

others are unaware of their surroundings. The patient is strikingly pale with a slow, weak pulse, hypotension, and almost imperceptible breathing.

Fainting facts

If the patient reports a fainting episode, gather information about the episode from him and his family. Did he feel weak, light-headed, nauseous, or sweaty just before he fainted? Did he get up quickly from a chair or from lying down? During the fainting episode, did he have muscle spasms or incontinence? How long was he unconscious? When he regained consciousness, was he alert or confused? Did he have a headache? Has he fainted before? If so, how often do the episodes occur?

Intermittent claudication

Intermittent claudication is cramping limb pain that's brought on by exercise and relieved by 1 or 2 minutes of rest. It most commonly occurs in the legs. This pain may be acute or chronic. When pain is acute and not relieved by rest, it may signal acute arterial occlusion.

Midlife crisis

Intermittent claudication is most common in men ages 50 to 60 who have a history of diabetes mellitus, hyperlipidemia, hypertension, or tobacco use. It typically results from such cardiovascular disorders as aortic arteriosclerotic occlusive disease, acute arterial occlusion, or arteriosclerosis obliterans.

Claudication interrogation

If the legs are affected, ask the patient how far he can walk before pain occurs and how long he must rest before it subsides. Can he walk as far as he could before, or does he need to rest longer? Does the pain-rest pattern vary? Is the pain in one leg or both? Where is the pain located? Has the pain affected his lifestyle?

Peripheral edema

Peripheral edema results from excess interstitial fluid in the arms or legs. It may be unilateral or bilateral, slight or dramatic, pitting or nonpitting.

In your face (and arm and leg)

Arm and facial edema may be caused by superior vena cava syndrome or thrombophlebitis. Leg edema is an early sign of right-sided heart failure, especially if it's bilateral. It can also signal thrombophlebitis and chronic venous insufficiency.

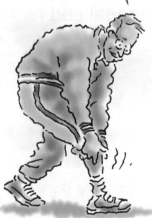

Intermittent claudication really cramps my lifestyle.

Since when?

Ask the patient how long he has had the edema. Did it develop suddenly or gradually? Does the edema decrease if the patient elevates his arms or legs? Is it worse in the mornings, or does it get progressively worse during the day? Did the patient recently injure the affected extremities or have surgery or an illness that may have immobilized him? Does he have a history of any cardiovascular disease? Is he taking medications? Which drugs has he taken in the past?

Other signs and symptoms

Other common signs and symptoms to ask the patient about include:
- shortness of breath on exertion, when lying down, or at night
- cough
- cyanosis or pallor
- weakness
- fatigue
- unexplained weight change
- dizziness
- headache
- high or low blood pressure
- peripheral skin changes, such as decreased hair distribution, skin color changes, or a thin, shiny appearance to the skin.

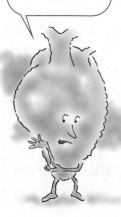

Yeah, yeah. Blame me. Shortness of breath and coughing can be heart-related.

Personal and family health

After you've asked about the patient's chief complaint, then inquire about his family history and past medical history, including heart disease, diabetes, and chronic lung, kidney, or liver disease. (See *Recognizing cardio risk.*)

All in the family

Ask if any family members have had heart disease, a history of myocardial infarction (MI), or an unexplained, sudden death. Find out at what age the MIs occurred.

Getting personal

In addition to obtaining information about the patient's family history, be sure to ask the patient about his:
- stress level and coping mechanisms
- current health habits, such as smoking and exercise habits, alcohol and caffeine intake, and dietary intake of fat and sodium
- drug use, including over-the-counter drugs, illicit drugs, and herbal supplements

Recognizing cardio risk

As you analyze a patient's condition, remember that age, sex, and race are important considerations in identifying patients at risk for cardiovascular disorders.

Most common

For example, coronary artery disease most commonly affects white men between ages 40 and 60. Hypertension is most common in blacks.

Also at risk

Women are also vulnerable to heart disease. Postmenopausal women and those with diabetes mellitus are at particular risk and are more likely to present with atypical symptoms.

We aren't getting any younger

Overall, elderly people have a higher incidence of cardiovascular disease than do younger people. Many elderly people have increased systolic blood pressure because blood vessel walls become increasingly rigid with age.

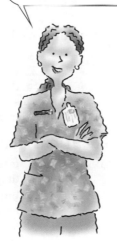

Be sure to ask about a patient's occupational risks. Standing for long periods at work can be problematic.

- previous operations
- environmental or occupational hazards
- activities of daily living.

Also related

Also ask the patient these questions:
- Are you ever short of breath? If so, what activities cause you to be short of breath?
- How many pillows do you use for sleep?
- Do you feel dizzy or fatigued?
- Do your rings or shoes feel tight?
- Do your ankles swell?
- Have you noticed changes in color or sensation in your legs? If so, what are those changes?
- If you have sores or ulcers, how quickly do they heal?
- Do you stand or sit in one place for long periods at work?

Performing a physical assessment

The key to accurate assessment is regular practice, which helps improve technique and efficiency. A consistent, methodical approach to your assessment can help you identify abnormalities.

Shopping list

For the physical assessment, you'll need a stethoscope with a bell and a diaphragm, an appropriate-sized blood pressure cuff, a ruler, and a penlight or other flexible light source. Make sure the room is quiet.

Dressed down

Ask the patient to remove all clothing except his underwear and to put on an examination gown. Have the patient lie on his back, with the head of the examination table at a 30 to 45 degree angle. Stand on the patient's right side if you're right-handed or his left side if you're left-handed so you can auscultate more easily.

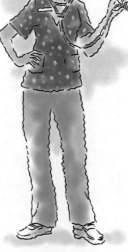

I have my stethoscope. Now all I need is a patient!

Assessing the heart

During your assessment, inspect, palpate, percuss, and auscultate the heart.

Inspection

First, take a moment to assess the patient's general appearance. Is he overly thin? Obese? Alert? Anxious? Note his skin color, temperature, turgor, and texture. Are his fingers clubbed? If the patient is dark-skinned, inspect his mucous membranes for pallor.

Checking out the chest

Next, inspect the chest. Note landmarks you can use to describe your findings and to identify structures underlying the chest wall. (See *Identifying cardiovascular landmarks*.) Also, look for pulsations, symmetry of movement, retractions, or heaves (a strong outward thrust of the chest wall that occurs during systole).

Location, location

Position a light source, such as a flashlight or gooseneck lamp, so that it casts a shadow on the patient's chest. Note the location of the apical impulse. You should find it in the fifth intercostal space, medial to the left midclavicular line. Because it corresponds to the apex of the heart, the apical pulse helps indicate how well the left ventricle is working. The apical pulse is usually the point of maximal impulse.

Remember, though, that the apical impulse can be seen only in about 50% of adults. You'll notice it more easily in children and in patients with thin chest walls. To find the apical impulse in a woman with large breasts, displace the breasts during the examination.

Palpation

Maintain a gentle touch when you palpate so that you don't obscure pulsations or similar findings. Using the ball of your hand, then your fingertips, palpate over the precordium to find the api-

Memory jogger

To remember the order in which you should perform assessment of the cardiovascular system, just think, "I'll Properly Perform Assessment":

Inspection

Palpation

Percussion

Auscultation.

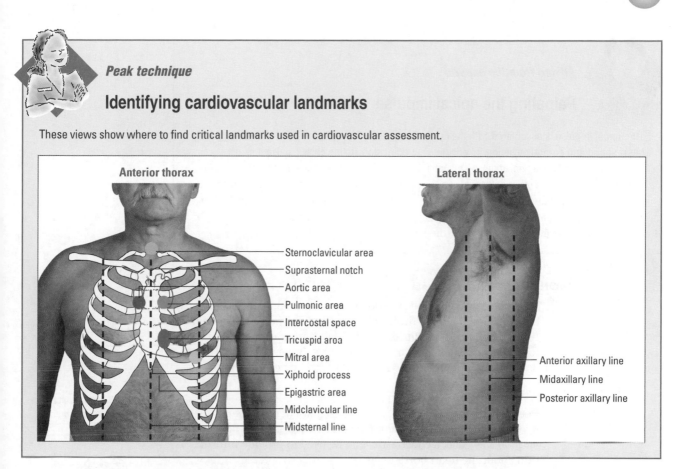

Peak technique

Identifying cardiovascular landmarks

These views show where to find critical landmarks used in cardiovascular assessment.

Anterior thorax

- Sternoclavicular area
- Suprasternal notch
- Aortic area
- Pulmonic area
- Intercostal space
- Tricuspid area
- Mitral area
- Xiphoid process
- Epigastric area
- Midclavicular line
- Midsternal line

Lateral thorax

- Anterior axillary line
- Midaxillary line
- Posterior axillary line

cal impulse. Note heaves or thrills (fine vibrations that feel like the purring of a cat). (See *Palpating the apical impulse*, page 26.)

The apical impulse may be difficult to palpate in an obese or pregnant patient and in a patient with a thick chest wall. If it's difficult to palpate with the patient lying on his back, have him lie on his left side or sit upright. It may also be helpful to have the patient exhale completely and hold his breath for a few seconds.

Not normally there

Palpate the sternoclavicular, aortic, pulmonic, tricuspid, and epigastric areas for pulsations, which normally aren't felt in those areas. In a thin patient, though, an aortic arch pulsation in the sternoclavicular area or an abdominal aorta pulsation in the epigastric area may be a normal finding.

Percussion

Although percussion isn't as useful as other assessment techniques, it may help you locate cardiac borders.

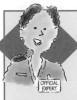

Advice from the experts

Palpating the apical impulse

The apical impulse is associated with the first heart sound and carotid pulsation. To ensure that you're feeling the apical impulse and not a muscle spasm or some other pulsation, use one hand to palpate the patient's carotid artery and the other to palpate the apical impulse. Then compare the timing and regularity of the impulses. The apical impulse should roughly coincide with the carotid pulsation.

Note the amplitude, size, intensity, location, and duration of the apical impulse. You should feel a gentle pulsation in an area about ½″ to ¾″ (1.5 to 2 cm) in diameter.

From resonance to dullness

Begin percussing at the anterior axillary line, and percuss toward the sternum along the fifth intercostal space. The sound changes from resonance to dullness over the left border of the heart, normally at the midclavicular line. The right border of the heart is usually aligned with the sternum and can't be percussed.

Borderline trouble

Percussion may be difficult in an obese patient (because of the fat overlying the chest) or in a female patient (because of breast tissue). In this case, a chest X-ray can be used to provide information about the heart border.

Auscultation

You can learn a great deal about the heart by auscultating for heart sounds. Cardiac auscultation requires a methodical approach and lots of practice. Begin by warming the stethoscope in your hands, and then identify the sites where you'll auscultate: over the four cardiac valves and at Erb's point, the third intercostal space at the left sternal border. Use the bell to hear low-pitched sounds and the diaphragm to hear high-pitched sounds. (See *Sites for heart sounds*.)

Have a plan

Auscultate for heart sounds with the patient in three positions: lying on his back with the head of the bed raised 30 to 45 degrees, sitting up, and lying on his left side. You can start at the base and work downward, or start at the apex and work upward. Whichever approach you use, be consistent. (See *Auscultation tips*, page 28.)

> Now hear this: Auscultation is one of the most important—and difficult—parts of the assessment.

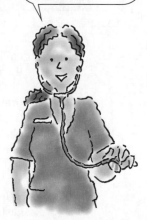

Sites for heart sounds

When auscultating for heart sounds, place the stethoscope over the four different sites illustrated at right.

Normal heart sounds indicate events in the cardiac cycle, such as the closing of heart valves, and are reflected to specific areas of the chest wall. Auscultation sites are identified by the names of heart valves but aren't located directly over the valves. Rather, these sites are located along the pathway blood takes as it flows through the heart's chambers and valves.

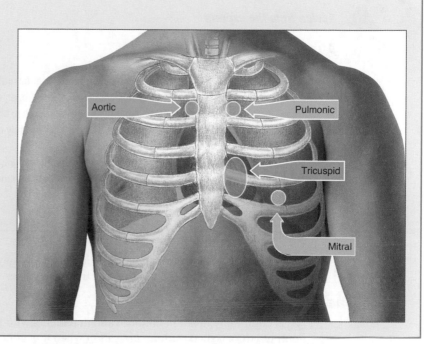

Aortic

Pulmonic

Tricuspid

Mitral

Use the diaphragm to listen as you go in one direction; use the bell as you come back in the other direction. Be sure to listen over the entire precordium, not just over the valves.

Determine the *dub*

As you proceed, note heart rate and rhythm. Always identify normal heart sounds (S_1 and S_2) and then listen for adventitious sounds, such as third and fourth heart sounds (S_3 and S_4), murmurs, and rubs.

Start auscultating at the aortic area where S_2 is loudest. S_2 is best heard at the base of the heart at the end of ventricular systole. This sound corresponds to closure of the pulmonic and aortic valves and is generally described as sounding like "dub." It's a shorter, higher-pitched, louder sound than S_1. When the pulmonic valve closes later than the aortic valve during inspiration, you'll hear a split S_2.

Listen for the *lub*

From the base of the heart, move to the pulmonic area and then down to the tricuspid area. Next, move to the mitral area, where S_1 is loudest. S_1 is best heard at the apex of the heart. This sound corresponds to closure of the mitral and tricuspid valves and is generally described as sounding like "lub." Low-pitched and dull,

S_3 and S_4 sounds predict trouble.

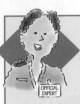

Advice from the experts

Auscultation tips

Follow these tips when you auscultate a patient's heart:
• Concentrate as you listen for each sound.
• Avoid auscultating through clothing or wound dressings because they can block sound.
• Avoid picking up extraneous sounds by keeping the stethoscope tubing off the patient's body and other surfaces.

• Until you gain proficiency at auscultation and can examine a patient quickly, explain to him that even though you may listen to his chest for a long period, it doesn't necessarily mean anything is wrong.
• Ask the patient to breathe normally and to hold his breath periodically to enhance sounds that may be difficult to hear.

S_1 occurs at the beginning of ventricular systole. It may be split if the mitral valve closes just before the tricuspid valve.

S_3: Classic sign of heart failure

S_3 is commonly heard in children and in patients with high cardiac output (CO). Called *ventricular gallop* when it occurs in adults, S_3 may be a cardinal sign of heart failure.

S_3 is best heard at the apex when the patient is lying on his left side. Often compared to the y sound in "Ken-tuck-y," S_3 is low-pitched and occurs when the ventricles fill rapidly. It follows S_2 in early ventricular diastole and probably results from vibrations caused by abrupt ventricular distention and resistance to filling. In addition to heart failure, S_3 may also be associated with such conditions as pulmonary edema, atrial septal defect, and acute MI. It may also be heard during the last trimester of pregnancy.

> Don't worry. An S_3 is common in children.

S_4: An MI aftereffect

Also called an *atrial gallop*, S_4 is an adventitious heart sound that's heard over the tricuspid or mitral area when the patient is on his left side. You may hear an S_4 in patients who are elderly or those with hypertension, aortic stenosis, or history of MI.

S_4, commonly described as sounding like "Ten-nes-see," occurs just before S_1, after atrial contraction. The S_4 sound indicates increased resistance to ventricular filling. It results from vibrations caused by forceful atrial ejection of blood into ventricles that don't move or expand as much as they should.

Auscultating for murmurs

Murmurs occur when structural defects in the heart's chambers or valves cause turbulent blood flow. Turbulence may also be caused by changes in the viscosity of blood or the speed of blood flow. Listen for murmurs over the same precordial areas used in auscultation for heart sounds.

> Whoa! A murmur is turbulent blood flow, caused by a structural defect in the heart.

Making the grade

Murmurs can occur during systole or diastole and are described by several criteria. (See *Tips for describing murmurs*.) Their pitch can be high, medium, or low. They can vary in intensity, growing louder or softer. (See *Grading murmurs*.) They can vary by location, sound pattern (blowing, harsh, or musical), radiation (to the neck or axillae), and period during which they occur in the cardiac cycle (pansystolic or midsystolic).

For more information, see "Murmurs," page 36.

Sit up, please

The best way to hear murmurs is with the patient sitting up and leaning forward. You can also have him lie on his left side. (See *Positioning the patient for auscultation*, page 30.)

Auscultating for pericardial friction rub

Listening for a pericardial friction rub is also an important part of your assessment. To do this, have the patient sit upright, lean forward, and exhale. Listen with the diaphragm of the stethoscope over the third intercostal space on the left side of the chest. A pericardial friction rub has a scratchy, rubbing quality. If you suspect a rub but have trouble hearing one, ask the patient to hold his breath.

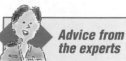

Advice from the experts

Tips for describing murmurs

Describing murmurs can be tricky. After you've auscultated a murmur, list the terms you would use to describe it. Then check the patient's chart to see how others have described it or ask an experienced colleague to listen and describe the murmur. Compare the descriptions and then auscultate for the murmur again, if necessary, to confirm the description.

Grading murmurs

Use the system outlined below to describe the intensity of a murmur. When recording your findings, use Roman numerals as part of a fraction, always with VI as the denominator. For instance, a grade III murmur would be recorded as "grade III/VI."
- Grade I is a barely audible murmur.
- Grade II is audible but quiet and soft.

- Grade III is moderately loud, without a thrust or thrill.
- Grade IV is loud, with a thrill.
- Grade V is very loud, with a thrust or a thrill.
- Grade VI is loud enough to be heard before the stethoscope comes into contact with the chest.

Peak technique

Positioning the patient for auscultation

If heart sounds are faint or undetectable, try listening to them with the patient seated and leaning forward or lying on his left side, which brings the heart closer to the surface of the chest. These illustrations show how to position the patient for high- and low-pitched sounds.

Forward leaning

The forward-leaning position is best suited for hearing high-pitched sounds related to semilunar valve problems, such as aortic and pulmonic valve murmurs. To auscultate for these sounds, place the diaphragm of the stethoscope over the aortic and pulmonic areas in the right and left second intercostal spaces, as shown at right.

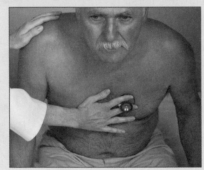

Left lateral recumbent

The left lateral recumbent position is best suited for hearing low-pitched sounds, such as mitral valve murmurs and extra heart sounds. To hear these sounds, place the bell of the stethoscope over the apical area, as shown at right.

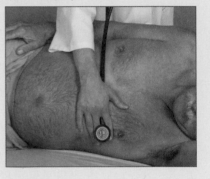

Assessing the vascular system

Assessing the vascular system is important because it can reveal arterial and venous disorders. Examine the patient's arms when you take his vital signs. Check the legs later during the physical examination, when the patient is lying on his back. Remember to evaluate leg veins when the patient is standing.

Inspection

Start your assessment of the vascular system the same way you start an assessment of the cardiac system—by making general observations. Are the arms equal in size? Are the legs symmetrical?

Inspect the skin color. Note how body hair is distributed. Also note lesions, scars, clubbing, and edema of the extremities. If the patient is confined to bed, check the sacrum for swelling. Examine the fingernails and toenails for abnormalities.

Start at the top

Next, move on to a closer inspection. Start by observing the vessels in the patient's neck. Inspection of these vessels can provide information about blood volume and pressure in the right side of the heart.

The carotid artery should appear to have a brisk, localized pulsation. This pulsation doesn't decrease when the patient is upright, when he inhales, or when you palpate the carotid. Note whether the pulsations are weak or bounding.

Inspect the jugular veins. The internal jugular vein has a softer, undulating pulsation. Unlike the pulsation of the carotid artery, pulsation of the internal jugular vein changes in response to position, breathing, and palpation. The vein normally protrudes when the patient is lying down and lies flat when he stands.

Take this lying down

To check the jugular venous pulse, have the patient lie on his back. Elevate the head of the bed 30 to 45 degrees, and turn the patient's head slightly away from you. Normally, the highest pulsation occurs no more than 1½″ (about 4 cm) above the sternal notch. Pulsations above that point indicate central venous pressure elevation and jugular vein distention.

Palpation

The first step in palpation is to assess the patient's skin temperature, texture, and turgor. Palpate the patient's arms and legs for temperature and edema. Edema is graded on a four-point scale. If your finger leaves a slight imprint, the edema is recorded as +1. If your finger leaves a deep imprint that only slowly returns to normal, the edema is recorded as +4.

Then check capillary refill by assessing the nail beds on the fingers and toes. Refill time should be no more than 3 seconds, or the time it takes to say "capillary refill."

Artery check!

Palpate for arterial pulses by gently pressing with the pads of your index and middle fingers. Start at the top of the patient's body with the temporal artery, and work your way down. Check the carotid, brachial, radial, femoral, popliteal, posterior tibial, and dorsalis pedis pulses on each side of the body, comparing pulse volume and symmetry. *Don't palpate both carotid arteries at the same time or press too firmly. If you do, the patient may faint or become bradycardic.* If you haven't put on gloves for the examination, do so before you palpate the femoral arteries.

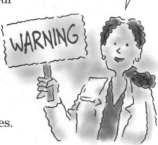

Pressing too firmly on the carotid artery may make the patient faint.

WARNING

The pulses get pluses

All pulses should be regular in rhythm and equal in strength. Pulses are graded on the following scale: 4+ is bounding, 3+ is increased, 2+ is normal, 1+ is weak, and 0 is absent. (See *Assessing arterial pulses*, page 32.)

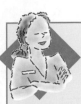

Peak technique

Assessing arterial pulses

To assess arterial pulses, apply pressure with your index and middle fingers. The following illustrations show where to position your fingers when palpating various pulses.

Carotid pulse
Lightly place your fingers just medial to the trachea and below the jaw angle. *Never* palpate both carotid arteries at the same time.

Radial pulse
Apply gentle pressure to the medial and ventral side of the wrist, just below the base of the thumb.

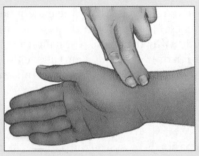

Popliteal pulse
Press firmly in the popliteal fossa at the back of the knee.

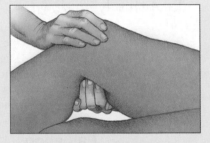

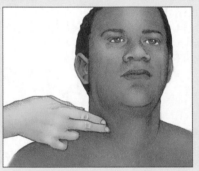

Posterior tibial pulse
Apply pressure behind and slightly below the malleolus of the ankle.

Femoral pulse
Press relatively hard at a point inferior to the inguinal ligament. For an obese patient, palpate in the crease of the groin, halfway between the pubic bone and the hip bone.

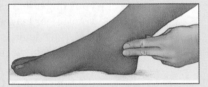

Brachial pulse
Position your fingers medial to the biceps tendon.

Dorsalis pedis pulse
Place your fingers on the medial dorsum of the foot while the patient points his toes down. The pulse is difficult to palpate here and may appear absent in healthy patients.

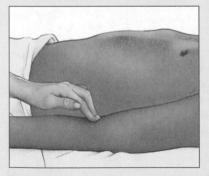

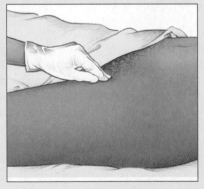

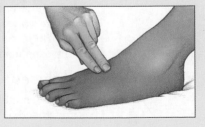

Auscultation

After you palpate, use the bell of the stethoscope to begin auscultation. Following the palpation sequence, listen over each artery. If necessary, ask the patient to momentarily stop breathing so you can clearly hear abnormal sounds. You shouldn't hear sounds over the carotid arteries. A hum, or bruit, sounds like buzzing, blowing, or high-pitched, musical sound and could indicate arteriosclerotic obstruction. (For more information, see "Bruits," page 38.)

Moving on up

Assess the upper abdomen for abnormal pulsations, which could indicate the presence of an abdominal aortic aneurysm. Finally, auscultate the femoral and popliteal pulses, checking for a bruit or other abnormal sounds.

Recognizing abnormal findings

This section outlines some common abnormal cardiovascular system assessment findings and their causes.

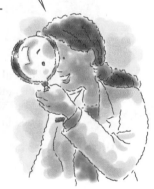

Hmmm...no body hair on the arms or legs. Could be a problem with arterial blood flow.

Abnormal skin and hair findings

Cyanosis, pallor, or cool or cold skin may indicate poor CO and tissue perfusion. Conditions causing fever or increased CO may make the skin warmer than normal. Absence of body hair on the arms or legs may indicate diminished arterial blood flow to those areas. Clubbing of fingers is a sign of chronic hypoxia caused by a lengthy cardiovascular or respiratory disorder. (See *Findings in arterial and venous insufficiency*, page 34.)

How swell!

Swelling, or edema, may indicate heart failure or venous insufficiency. It may also be caused by varicosities or thrombophlebitis.

Chronic right-sided heart failure may cause ascites and generalized edema. If the patient has vein compression in a specific area, he may have localized swelling along the path of the compressed vessel. Right-sided heart failure may cause swelling in the lower legs.

Abnormal pulsations

A displaced apical impulse may indicate an enlarged left ventricle, which can be caused by heart failure or hypertension. A forceful

Findings in arterial and venous insufficiency

Assessment findings differ in patients with arterial insufficiency and those with chronic venous insufficiency. These illustrations show those differences.

Arterial insufficiency

In a patient with arterial insufficiency, pulses may be decreased or absent. His skin will be cool, pale, and shiny, and he may have pain in his legs and feet. Ulcerations typically occur in the area around the toes and heel, and the foot usually turns deep red when dependent. Nails may be thick and ridged.

Chronic venous insufficiency

In a patient with chronic venous insufficiency, check for ulcerations around the ankle. Pulses are present but may be difficult to find because of edema. The foot may become cyanotic when dependent.

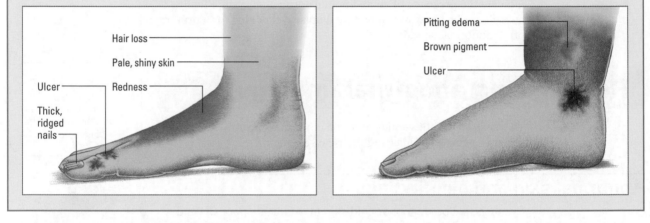

apical impulse, or one lasting longer than a third of the cardiac cycle, may point to increased CO. If you find a pulsation in the patient's aortic, pulmonic, or tricuspid area, his heart chamber may be enlarged or he may have valvular disease.

Pulses here, there, everywhere

Increased CO or an aortic aneurysm may also produce pulsations in the aortic area. A patient with an epigastric pulsation may have early heart failure or an aortic aneurysm. A pulsation in the sternoclavicular area suggests an aortic aneurysm. A patient with anemia, anxiety, increased CO, or a thin chest wall might have slight pulsations to the right and left of the sternum.

Weak ones, strong ones

A weak arterial pulse may indicate decreased CO or increased peripheral vascular resistance, both of which point to arterial atherosclerotic disease. Many elderly patients have weak pedal pulses.

Able to increase cardiac output in a single bound!

Pulse waveforms

To identify abnormal arterial pulses, check the waveforms below and see which one matches your patient's peripheral pulse.

Weak pulse
A weak pulse has a decreased amplitude with a slower upstroke and downstroke. Possible causes of a weak pulse include increased peripheral vascular resistance, as sometimes occurs in response to cold temperatures or with severe heart failure, and decreased stroke volume, as occurs with hypovolemia or aortic stenosis.

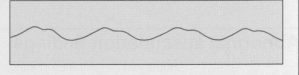

Bounding pulse
A bounding pulse has a sharp upstroke and downstroke with a pointed peak. The amplitude is elevated. Possible causes of a bounding pulse include increased stroke volume, as with aortic insufficiency, or stiffness of arterial walls, as with aging.

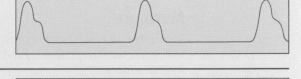

Pulsus alternans
Pulsus alternans has a regular, alternating pattern of a weak and strong pulse. This pulse is associated with left-sided heart failure.

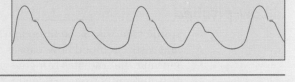

Pulsus bigeminus
Pulsus bigeminus is similar to pulsus alternans but occurs at irregular intervals. This pulse is caused by premature atrial or ventricular beats.

Pulsus paradoxus
Pulsus paradoxus has increases and decreases in amplitude associated with the respiratory cycle. Marked decreases occur when the patient inhales. Pulsus paradoxus is associated with pericardial tamponade, advanced heart failure, and constrictive pericarditis.

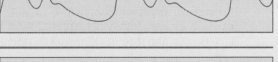

Inspiration   Expiration

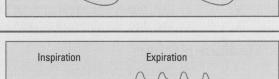

Pulsus biferiens
Pulsus biferiens shows an initial upstroke, a subsequent downstroke, and then another upstroke during systole. Pulsus biferiens is caused by aortic stenosis and aortic insufficiency.

Strong or bounding pulsations usually occur in patients with conditions that cause increased CO, such as hypertension, hypoxia, anemia, exercise, or anxiety. (See *Pulse waveforms*.)

Heave ho! What a thrill!

A heave, lifting of the chest wall felt during palpation, along the left sternal border may mean right ventricular hypertrophy; over the left ventricular area, a ventricular aneurysm. A thrill, which is a palpable vibration, usually suggests valvular dysfunction.

Abnormal auscultation findings

Abnormal auscultation findings include abnormal heart sounds (previously discussed), heart murmurs, and bruits. (See *Recognizing abnormal heart sounds*.)

Murmurs

Murmurs can result from several conditions and have widely varied characteristics. Here's a rundown on some of the more common murmurs.

Low-pitched

Aortic stenosis, a condition in which the aortic valve has calcified and restricts blood flow, causes a midsystolic, low-pitched, harsh murmur that radiates from the valve to the carotid artery. The murmur shifts from crescendo to decrescendo and back.

Crescendo describes a murmur that increases in intensity; a *decrescendo* murmur decreases in intensity. The crescendo-decrescendo murmur of aortic stenosis results from the turbulent, highly pressured flow of blood across stiffened leaflets and through a narrowed opening.

Medium-pitched

During auscultation, listen for a murmur near the pulmonic valve. This murmur might indicate pulmonic stenosis, a condition in which the pulmonic valve has calcified and interferes with the flow of blood out of the right ventricle. The murmur is medium-pitched, systolic, and harsh and shifts from crescendo to decrescendo and back. The murmur is caused by turbulent blood flow across a stiffened, narrowed valve.

High-pitched

In a patient with aortic insufficiency, blood flows backward through the aortic valve and causes a high-pitched, blowing, decrescendo, diastolic murmur. The murmur radiates from the aortic valve area to the left sternal border.

> Crescendo is the term for a murmur that increases in intensity. La-la-LA!

Recognizing abnormal heart sounds

Whenever auscultation reveals an abnormal heart sound, try to identify the sound and its timing in the cardiac cycle. Knowing those characteristics can help you identify the possible cause for the sound. Use this chart to put all that information together.

Abnormal heart sound	Timing	Possible causes
Accentuated S_1	Beginning of systole	• Mitral stenosis • Fever
Diminished S_1	Beginning of systole	• Mitral insufficiency • Heart block • Severe mitral insufficiency with a calcified, immobile valve
Split S_1	Beginning of systole	• Right bundle-branch block • Premature ventricular contractions
Accentuated S_2	End of systole	• Pulmonary or systemic hypertension
Diminished or inaudible S_2	End of systole	• Aortic or pulmonic stenosis
Persistent S_2 split	End of systole	• Delayed closure of the pulmonic valve, usually from overfilling of the right ventricle, causing prolonged systolic ejection time
Reversed or paradoxical S_2 split that appears during expiration and disappears during inspiration	End of systole	• Delayed ventricular stimulation • Left bundle-branch block • Prolonged left ventricular ejection time
S_3 (ventricular gallop)	Early diastole	• Overdistention of the ventricles during the rapid-filling segment of diastole or mitral insufficiency of ventricular failure (normal in children and young adults)
S_4 (atrial or presystolic gallop)	Late diastole	• Pulmonic stenosis • Hypertension • Coronary artery disease • Aortic stenosis • Forceful atrial concentration due to resistance to ventricular filling late in diastole (resulting from left ventricular hypertrophy)
Pericardial friction rub (grating or leathery sound at the left sternal border, usually muffled, high-pitched, and transient)	Throughout systole and diastole	• Pericardial inflammation

In a patient with pulmonic insufficiency, blood flows backward through the pulmonic valve, causing a blowing, diastolic, decrescendo murmur at Erb's point (at the left sternal border of the third intercostal space). If the patient has a higher than normal pulmonary pressure, the murmur is high-pitched. If not, it's low-pitched.

High-pitched and blowing

In a patient with mitral insufficiency, blood regurgitates into the left atrium. This regurgitation produces a high-pitched, blowing murmur throughout systole (pansystolic or holosystolic). The murmur may radiate from the mitral area to the left axillary line. You can hear it best at the apex.

In a patient with tricuspid insufficiency, blood regurgitates into the right atrium. This backflow of blood through the valve also causes a high-pitched, blowing murmur, this time throughout systole in the tricuspid area. The murmur becomes louder when the patient inhales.

Low-pitched and rumbling

Mitral stenosis is a condition in which the mitral valve has calcified and is blocking blood flow out of the left atrium. Listen for a low-pitched, rumbling, crescendo-decrescendo murmur in the mitral valve area. This murmur results from turbulent blood flow across the stiffened, narrowed valve.

Tricuspid stenosis is a condition in which the tricuspid valve has calcified and is blocking blood flow through the valve from the right atrium. Listen for a low, rumbling, crescendo-decrescendo murmur in the tricuspid area. The murmur results from turbulent blood flow across the stiffened, narrowed valvular leaflets.

Bruits

A murmurlike sound of vascular (rather than cardiac) origin is called a *bruit*. If you hear a bruit during arterial auscultation, the patient may have occlusive arterial disease or an arteriovenous fistula. Various high CO conditions—such as anemia, hyperthyroidism, and pheochromocytoma—may also cause bruits.

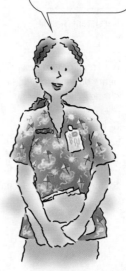

Bruits are of vascular, not cardiac origin.

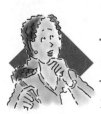

Quick quiz

1. When listening to heart sounds, you can best hear S_1 at the:
A. base of the heart.
B. apex of the heart.
C. aortic area.
D. second intercostal space to the right of the sternum.

Answer: B. S_1 is best heard at the apex of the heart.

2. You're auscultating for heart sounds in a 3-year-old girl and hear an S_3. You assess this sound to be:
A. a normal finding.
B. a probable sign of heart failure.
C. a possible sign of atrial septal defect.
D. a probable sign of mitral stenosis.

Answer: A. Although an S_3 can indicate heart failure in an adult, it's a normal finding in a child.

3. When grading arterial pulses, a 1+ grade indicates:
A. bounding pulse.
B. increased pulse.
C. weak pulse.
D. absent pulse.

Answer: C. A 1+ pulse indicates weak pulses and is associated with diminished cardiac perfusion.

4. When assessing a patient for jugular vein distention, you should position him:
A. sitting upright.
B. lying flat on his back.
C. lying on his back, with the head of the bed elevated 30 to 45 degrees.
D. lying on his left side.

Answer: C. Assessing jugular vein distention should be done when the patient is in semi-Fowler's position (head of the bed elevated 30 to 45 degrees). If the patient lies flat, his veins will be more distended; if he sits upright, the veins will be flat.

5. Capillary refill time is normally:
   A.   less than 15 seconds.
   B.   7 to 10 seconds.
   C.   4 to 6 seconds.
   D.   1 to 3 seconds.

Answer: D. Capillary refill time that lasts longer than 3 seconds is considered delayed and indicates decreased perfusion.

Scoring

☆☆☆   If you answered all five questions correctly, feel pumped! You've been assessed a success!

☆☆   If you answered four questions correctly, sensational! You've passed this inspection.

☆   If you answered fewer than four questions correctly, keep at it! Remember, good assessment involves practice, practice, and more practice.

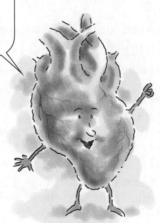

Way to go! Keep reading to find out about other matters of the heart.

3

Prevention and risk reduction

Just the facts

In this chapter, you'll learn:

♦ the incidence of cardiovascular disease in the United States

♦ modifiable and nonmodifiable risk factors for cardiovascular disease

♦ strategies for preventing cardiovascular disease.

Understanding cardiovascular disease

Cardiovascular disease (CVD) is a term used to describe various conditions that affect the structure and function of the heart and blood vessels. Common types of cardiovascular disease include:
• coronary artery disease (CAD)
• heart failure
• cerebrovascular disease
• peripheral artery disease.

Heart-breaking numbers

CVD is the leading cause of mortality and morbidity among men and women in the United States. Estimates indicate that more than 58 million people in the United States have CVD, costing the nation more than $274 billion each year.

Hocus focus

Prevention and risk reduction strategies for CVD tend to focus on atherosclerotic disease, or atherosclerosis. Atherosclerosis occurs when lipid deposits, thrombi, or calcifications cause inflammation and arterial wall changes.

Risk assessment

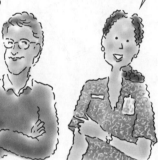

Find out your patient's risk score. The more you know about a patient's risk, the more you can do to prevent disease from developing.

Atherosclerotic disease, which includes CAD, used to be considered a normal, inevitable part of the aging process. However, the Framingham Heart Study—which followed 5,209 healthy men and women for several years in search of characteristics shared by those who eventually developed CAD—identified factors to help assess a patient's risk of CAD. Now, a Framingham Risk Score is an important part of caring for patients who have or are at risk for CAD. Knowing a patient's risk can guide health care providers to plan interventions that may help prevent or reduce the patient's risk of developing atherosclerotic disease.

What's the score?

The Framingham Risk Score estimates a patient's risk of developing CAD by assigning a score to these patient factors:
- age
- total cholesterol level
- high-density lipoprotein (HDL) level
- low-density lipoprotein (LDL) level
- blood pressure
- presence or absence of diabetes mellitus
- smoking status.

Individual risk factor scores differ for men and women and may be based on total cholesterol level or LDL cholesterol level. A patient's total score (the sum of the individual risk factor scores) determines his 10-year risk of developing CAD. (See *Sample score sheet for estimating coronary heart disease risk.*) The patient's relative risk of developing disease can then be determined by comparing the patient's score with the total scores of individuals of the same sex and age whose risk of CAD is average or low.

Other applications

Researchers hope that ongoing research will provide evidence to support using the Framingham Risk Score for risk assessment of other atherosclerotic diseases, such as peripheral vascular arterial disease (associated with major limb loss) and cerebrovascular arterial disease.

Sample score sheet for estimating coronary heart disease risk

This example from the National Heart, Lung, and Blood Institute (NHLBI) illustrates a sample score sheet for a 55-year-old man with a total cholesterol level of 250 mg/dl, a high-density lipoprotein cholesterol level of 39 mg/dl, and a blood pressure of 146/88 mm Hg. The patient also has diabetes and is a nonsmoker.

According to the NHLBI, practitioners should use the Total Cholesterol Score Sheet to determine coronary heart disease (CHD) risk when total cholesterol and HDL cholesterol levels are known; they should use the LDL Cholesterol Score Sheet when LDL cholesterol and HDL cholesterol levels are known.

Step	Factor	Points
1	Age = 55 years	4
2	*Total cholesterol = 250 mg/dl	2
3	HDL cholesterol = 39 mg/dl	1
4	Blood pressure = 146/88 mm Hg	2
5	Diabetic − yes	2
6	Cigarette smoker = no	0
7	Point total	11
8	Estimated 10-year CHD risk	31%
9	Low 10-year CHD risk	7%
	Relative risk (step 8 divided by step 9)	31 ÷ 7 = 4.4

This score is the patient's 10-year risk of developing CHD.

This score represents the CHD risk of a man who is the same age as the patient but is in optimal health (has a low risk profile).

This score is the patient's relative risk. It means that the patient is more than four times as likely to develop CHD than a man of the same age with a low risk profile.

* Use of the LDL cholesterol approach in the score sheets is appropriate when fasting LDL cholesterol estimates are available. This approach is analogous to that shown for total cholesterol categories.

Source: National Heart, Lung, and Blood Institute, National Institute of Health. National Heart Lung and Blood Institute, National Institutes of Health. "Sample Score Sheet for Estimating Coronary Heart Disease Risk." Available at http://www.nhlbi.nih.gov/about/framingham/risksamp.htm

Risk factors

Understanding the risk factors associated with CVD helps patients and health care providers develop strategies for prevention and risk reduction. Risk factors may be *modifiable* (controllable) or *nonmodifiable* (not controllable).

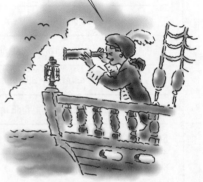

If I discover the fountain of youth, does that mean age becomes a modifiable risk factor?

Nonmodifiable risk factors

Nonmodifiable risk factors for CVD include:
- advanced age
- sex
- heredity.

Advanced age

Although specific age-related changes may vary from person to person, individuals generally become more vulnerable to CVD with age. Complex organ systems start to decline, so other systems are forced to compensate.

With every beat of my heart

Age-related heart changes include:
- thickening and stiffening of the left ventricle
- fibrotic changes in the valves
- valve calcification
- increased reliance on atrial contractions to maintain cardiac output
- increased sensitivity to hypovolemia
- fibrotic changes in the bundle branches (a common cause of bundle branch block in people older than age 65).

Vascular variations

Changes in the vascular system that tend to be age-related include:
- thickened intimal and medial layers of the arteries
- decreased arterial diameter
- stiffer, less elastic arterial walls due to calcium and lipid deposits.

These changes cause hypertension to develop.

Sex

Research has shown that men are at greater risk for developing CAD at a younger age than women. In men, risk increases beginning at age 45, whereas the risk in women increases after menopause (around age 55). Additionally, the lifetime risk of developing CAD is 1 in 2 for men and 1 in 3 for women.

Hormones: Helpful or hurtful?

Hormone replacement therapy for postmenopausal women was once thought to protect women from CVD. However, studies have shown that the risk of stroke, myocardial infarction (MI), and deep vein thrombosis increases with hormone replacement therapy.

> When assessing a postmenopausal woman's risk of CVD, ask if she's receiving hormone replacement therapy. She may be at risk for MI.

Heredity

Researchers' understanding of the complex relationship between genes and environmental factors in the development of CVD is in its infancy. However, many researchers believe that one-half of CVD cases can be attributed to genetic causes.

Genes on the scene

For example, some individuals with familial hypercholesterolemia (an inherited metabolic disorder affecting LDL receptors) carry a genetic mutation that makes it difficult for their cells to remove LDL from their blood. Patients with familial hypercholesterolemia have high serum cholesterol levels and are at risk for developing atherosclerosis.

History lesson

Obtaining a patient's family history helps to identify patterns of early CVD and familial risk factors. For example, a patient has a higher risk of developing early CVD if he has a first-degree male relative who was diagnosed with CVD before age 55 or a female first-degree relative who was diagnosed with CVD before age 65.

Modifiable risk factors

Unfortunately, early development of CVD is commonly the result of lifestyle choices involving modifiable risk factors. Risk reduction strategies aim to reduce or eliminate the impact of these factors.

Modifiable risk factors include:
- smoking
- dyslipidemia
- hypertension
- diabetes mellitus
- obesity
- sedentary lifestyle.

Smoking

Smoking is the most common modifiable risk factor for CVD. In the United States, smoking causes almost as many deaths from heart disease as it does from lung cancer. The more a patient smokes and the longer he smokes, the higher his risk of CVD.

The damage done

Nicotine stimulates the sympathetic nervous system to constrict the arteries, which causes arterial wall damage. This damage promotes the formation of atherosclerotic plaque, causing tissues to become starved for oxygen.

Stuck on you

Smoking also makes platelets stickier, making them more likely to adhere to artery walls.

Quitters wanted

All patients should be encouraged to quit smoking. Health care providers should educate patients about the risks of smoking and help develop an action plan for quitting. The best formal smoking cessation programs combine:
• behavioral modification therapies
• medications such as antidepressants
• nicotine replacement strategies, such as nicotine patches or gum.

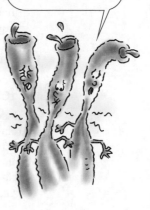

No wonder we're so constricted. Here comes that nicotine again!

Dyslipidemia

Dyslipidemia refers to abnormal lipoprotein levels in the blood. Lipoproteins, which are compounds that have proteins on the outside and lipids (fats) on the inside, carry cholesterol in the bloodstream.

High is good, low is bad

Types of lipoproteins include:
• LDL—considered the "bad cholesterol" because it carries cholesterol into the tissues
• HDL—considered the "good cholesterol" because it removes cholesterol from tissues and returns it to the liver.

Therefore, the risk of developing CVD increases when a patient has:
• increased LDL levels
• decreased HDL levels
• abnormal lipid metabolism.

Tri this on for size

Triglycerides are lipids produced by the liver. They're also found in food. Elevated triglyceride levels increase the risk of CVD and

may also lead to pancreatitis. Factors that contribute to elevated triglyceride levels include:
• obesity
• smoking
• excess alcohol consumption.

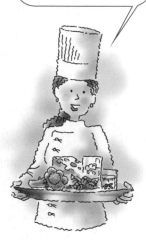

Diet plays a big role in modifying such risk factors as dyslipidemia, diabetes, and obesity.

Take it down a notch

Addressing dyslipidemia by reducing serum LDL levels helps prevent or slow the progression of atherosclerotic disease. Strategies for reducing serum LDL levels include:
• dietary changes, such as following a Mediterranean-style diet that replaces saturated fats with polyunsaturated fats (particularly omega-3 fatty acids) and avoiding trans fats, which increase LDL levels
• drug therapy if necessary (see *Drugs that lower cholesterol*).

Track progress (or lack thereof)

The National Cholesterol Program recommends obtaining a patient's lipid profiles every 5 years starting at age 20.

Hypertension

Hypertension (increased blood pressure) tends to be discovered incidentally because patients usually don't experience symptoms.

Drugs that lower cholesterol

Drugs that lower cholesterol include various statins, the antilipemic ezetimibe (Zetia), bile acid resins, nicotinic acid, and fibrates.

Statins
Examples of statins include lovastatin (Advicor), pravastatin (Pravachol), simvastatin (Zocor), fluvastatin (Lescol), atorvastatin (Lipitor), and rosuvastatin (Crestor). These drugs inhibit the action of an enzyme that controls the rate at which the body produces cholesterol. They also lower triglyceride levels and raise high-density lipoprotein (HDL) levels. Statins are more effective in lowering low-density lipoprotein (LDL) levels than other types of drugs.

Ezetimibe
Ezetimibe reduces the amount of cholesterol absorbed by the body. It's sometimes used in combination with a statin to further reduce LDL levels.

Bile acid resins
Bile acid resins bind with cholesterol-containing bile acids in the intestines. The cholesterol is then eliminated from the body when the drug is excreted in the stool.

Nicotinic acid
Also called *niacin,* this water-soluble B vitamin improves levels of total cholesterol, LDLs, triglycerides, and HDLs when taken in doses above the recommended daily allowance.

Fibrates
Fibrates lower triglycerides and, to a lesser degree, raise HDL levels. Fibrates are less effective in lowering LDL levels.

A diagnosis of hypertension is confirmed when two or more elevated blood pressure readings are obtained on separate occasions. (See *Classifying blood pressure.*)

Dangerous deposits

Hypertension causes inflammation and damages the lining of the arteries. This damage increases fat deposits, which lead to atherosclerosis. In addition, plaque deposits become unstable, leading to thromboses and emboli. Damage to the small, fragile arteries of the organs can lead to heart attacks, retinopathies, stroke, peripheral artery disease, and kidney failure.

Taking control

Treating hypertension includes:
• lifestyle modifications, such as smoking cessation and dietary changes
• medications to control blood pressure, such as beta-adrenergic blockers.

DASH into a proper diet

Following the Dietary Approaches to Stop Hypertension (DASH) diet plan can significantly improve blood pressure. This plan involves eating a diet that's low in sodium (2,400 mg/day or less) but high in fruits, vegetables, and low-fat dairy. (See *Tips for reducing sodium intake.*)

Classifying blood pressure

The *Seventh Report of the Joint National Committee on Prevention, Detection, Evaluation, and Treatment of High Blood Pressure* outlines these classifications for blood pressure.

Category	Systolic blood pressure (mm Hg)		Diastolic blood pressure (mm Hg)
Normal	< 120	and	< 80
Prehypertension	120 to 139	or	80 to 89
Hypertension, stage 1	140 to 159	or	90 to 99
Hypertension, stage 2	≥ 160	or	≥ 100

Adapted from *Seventh Report of the Joint National Committee on Prevention, Detection, Evaluation, and Treatment of High Blood Pressure.* NIH Publication No. 03-5231. Bethesda, Md.: National Institutes of Health; National Heart, Lung, and Blood Institute; National High Blood Pressure Education Program, May 2003.

No place like home

Tips for reducing sodium intake

Only a small amount of sodium occurs naturally in foods. Most sodium is added to foods during processing. To help your patient cut down on sodium intake, offer these suggestions.

Read those labels
• Read food labels to determine sodium content.
• Use food products with reduced sodium or no added salt.
• Be aware that soy sauce, broth, and foods that are pickled or cured have high sodium contents.

Now you're cookin'
• Instead of cooking with salt, use herbs, spices, cooking wines, lemon, lime, or vinegar to enhance food flavors.
• Cook pasta and rice without salt.
• Rinse canned foods, such as tuna, to remove some sodium.

• Avoid adding salt to foods, especially at the table.
• Avoid condiments such as soy and teriyaki sauces and monosodium glutamate (MSG)—or use lower-sodium versions.

You are what you eat
• Eat fresh poultry, fish, and lean meat rather than canned, smoked, or processed versions (which typically contain a lot of sodium).
• Whenever possible, eat fresh foods rather than canned or convenience foods.
• Limit intake of cured foods (such as bacon and ham), foods packed in brine (pickles, olives, and sauerkraut) and condiments (mustard, ketchup, horseradish, and Worcestershire sauce).
• When dining out, ask how food is prepared. Ask that your food be prepared without added salt or MSG.

Mighty meds

Drugs used to help reduce blood pressure include:
• thiazide diuretics such as hydrochlorothiazide (HydroDIURIL), which increase sodium, chloride, and water excretion by the kidneys
• atenolol (Tenormin), which decreases the heart's excitability, cardiac output, and oxygen consumption and decreases the release of renin from the kidney
• angiotensin-converting enzyme inhibitors such as lisinopril (Zestril), which block the conversion of angiotensin I to angiotensin II (a potent vasoconstrictor).

It's cool to comply

Because the patient may not experience symptoms of his hypertension, he may have difficulty understanding why drug therapy is necessary. Stress to the patient the importance of complying with drug therapy to control blood pressure. Also advise him to report adverse effects such as fatigue.

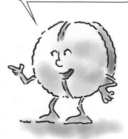

Remind patients that, even though they may not feel the symptoms of hypertension, they may need medications to treat it.

Diabetes mellitus

Diabetes mellitus is a chronic disease in which the body has trouble producing or using insulin (the hormone that enables the body to use glucose).

What's your type?

With type 1 diabetes, the body can't produce enough insulin. With type 2 diabetes, the body can't use insulin efficiently. Type 2 diabetes accounts for 90% of all diabetes cases.

Diabetic disturbances

Diabetes causes disturbances in protein and fat metabolism, which can lead to weight problems. As a result, most patients with type 2 diabetes are overweight or obese. Maintaining a normal weight through diet and exercise and taking prescribed medications are crucial to maintaining adequate blood sugar control.

Diabetes also damages small- and medium-size arteries, which can lead to heart attack, stroke, renal failure, and peripheral artery disease. It also accelerates the development of atherosclerosis. Diabetes is also a contributing factor in 50% of heart attacks.

Obesity

Obesity is defined as a body mass index (BMI) of 30 or greater. It develops, in part, as a result of dietary habits and a sedentary lifestyle. Basically, if an individual eats more calories than his body uses, the excess calories are stored in the body as adipose tissue (fat). Patients who have a larger waist measurement than hip measurement are at greater risk for developing CVD.

Putting a number on it

Researchers estimate that a man with a BMI of 45 in early adulthood may have a reduced life expectancy of up to 13 years. A woman with a BMI of 45 may have a life expectancy reduced by 8 years.

Obesity outcomes

Obesity increases the risk of CVD by causing the heart to have to work harder, which leads to increased blood pressure. It also increases LDL levels and decreases HDL levels.

Nothing to snore at

Obesity is also a major contributing factor in sleep apnea, which impacts the heart. With sleep apnea, a person experiences multiple cycles during sleep in which he stops breathing, partially wakes, and then begins breathing again. These periods of apnea cause the oxygen level in the blood to drop, putting strain on the

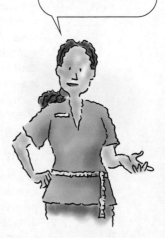

Is your patient's waist bigger than his hips? Then he's at risk for CVD.

heart. This strain can lead to right-sided heart failure and pulmonary hypertension.

Sedentary lifestyle

Patients with sedentary lifestyles are more likely to be overweight or obese. Encouraging physical activity can help patients achieve and maintain target weight goals, thus decreasing the risk of CVD. The recommended amount of exercise is 30 minutes of moderate physical activity per day on most days of the week.

Reasons to move

Cardiovascular benefits of exercise include:
- improved lipid metabolism
- decreased blood pressure
- enhanced insulin sensitivity
- utilization of excess calories, which prevents them from being stored as fat.

> Phew! That was quite a workout. I can feel my lipid metabolism improving as we speak!

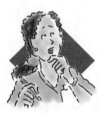

Quick quiz

1. Prehypertension is indicated by a systolic blood pressure range of:

    A. 100 to 120 mm Hg.
    B. 110 to 130 mm Hg.
    C. 120 to 139 mm Hg.
    D. 140 to 159 mm Hg.

Answer: C. According to the *Seventh Report of the Joint National Committee on Prevention, Detection, Evaluation, and Treatment of High Blood Pressure,* prehypertension is classified as a systolic blood pressure ranging from 120 to 139 mm Hg or a diastolic blood pressure of 80 to 89 mm Hg.

2. The recommended maximum daily dietary sodium intake is:

    A. 2,400 mg per day.
    B. 3,300 mg per day.
    C. 4,000 mg per day.
    D. 5,000 mg per day.

Answer: A. Sodium intake should be limited to 2,400 mg per day.

3. Which risk factors are used to calculate the Framingham Risk Score?

    A. Race, age, weight, smoking status, and LDL level

    B. Gender, age, LDL level, HDL level, smoking status, and diabetes status

    C. Gender, weight, race, age, smoking status, and diabetes status

    D. Race, age, smoking status, diabetes status, and HDL level

Answer: B. The Framingham Risk Score is calculated based on gender, age, LDL level, HDL level, smoking status, and the presence of diabetes.

4. What's the recommended amount of exercise for decreasing the risk of CVD?

    A. 30 minutes of moderate physical activity 1 day per week

    B. 1 hour of low-impact activity 2 days per week

    C. 30 minutes of moderate physical activity 3 days per week

    D. 30 minutes of moderate physical activity most days of the week

Answer: D. Engaging in moderate physical activity for at least 30 minutes per day on most days of the week decreases the risk of developing CVD and also lessens the risk of developing hypertension and diabetes.

5. The National Cholesterol Program recommends routine screenings for abnormal lipid levels:

    A. every 5 years beginning at age 40.

    B. every 5 years beginning at age 20.

    C. every 10 years beginning at age 30.

    D. every 10 years beginning at age 20.

Answer: B. The National Cholesterol Program recommends screening for abnormal lipid levels every 5 years beginning at age 20.

Scoring

☆☆☆ If you answered all five questions correctly, fantastic! You put your whole heart into studying this chapter.

☆☆ If you answered four questions correctly, nice work! There's no preventing you from reducing CVD risk.

☆ If you answered fewer than four questions correctly, no worries. Now that you've assessed your risk, you can go back and review.

4

Diagnostic tests and procedures

Just the facts

In this chapter, you'll learn:

♦ normal and abnormal laboratory findings

♦ tests for diagnosing cardiovascular disorders

♦ procedures used in cardiovascular care

♦ monitoring techniques for patients with cardiovascular disorders.

A look at diagnostic tests and procedures

Advances in diagnostic testing allow for earlier and easier diagnosis and treatment of cardiovascular disorders. For example, in some patients, echocardiography—a noninvasive and risk-free test—can provide as much diagnostic information about valvular heart disease as can cardiac catheterization—an invasive and high-risk test. Monitoring and testing also help guide and evaluate treatment, as well as identify complications. Before the patient undergoes testing, explain the procedure in terms he can easily understand. Make sure an informed consent form is signed, if necessary. These tests may cause anxiety, so be sure to provide emotional support.

Cardiac tests range from the relatively simple (analyzing the patient's blood for cardiac enzymes, proteins, and clotting time) to the very sophisticated (imaging and radiographic tests which reveal a detailed image of the heart). Other cardiac tests include various forms of electrocardiography and hemodynamic monitoring.

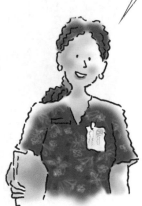

Confirm that informed consent is obtained for tests that require it.

Cardiac enzymes and proteins

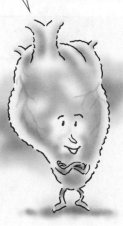

Levels of cardiac enzymes and proteins typically rise when I'm damaged.

Analyzing cardiac enzymes and proteins (markers) is an important step in diagnosing acute myocardial infarction (MI) and in evaluating other cardiac disorders. After an MI, damaged cardiac tissue releases significant amounts of enzymes and proteins into the blood. Specific blood tests help reveal the extent of cardiac damage and help monitor healing progress. (See *Cardiac enzyme and protein patterns*.)

Cardiac markers to monitor include:
- creatine kinase (CK)
- myoglobin
- troponin I and troponin T
- homocysteine
- C-reactive protein (CRP)
- B-type natriuretic peptide (BNP).

Creatine kinase

CK is present in heart muscle, skeletal muscle, and brain tissue. Its isoenzyme CK-MB is found specifically in the heart muscle.

Old reliable

Elevated levels of CK-MB reliably indicate acute MI. Generally, CK-MB levels rise about 6 hours after the onset of acute MI, peak after about 18 hours, and may remain elevated for up to 72 hours. Normal CK levels are 38 to 190 units/L for men and 10 to 150 units/L for women.

Nursing considerations

- Explain to the patient that the test will help confirm or rule out MI.
- Inform him that blood samples will be drawn at timed intervals.
- Be aware that muscle trauma caused by I.M. injections can raise CK levels.
- Handle the collection tube gently to prevent hemolysis, and send the sample to the laboratory immediately.
- If a hematoma develops at the venipuncture site, apply warm soaks to help ease discomfort.

Myoglobin

Myoglobin, which is normally found in skeletal and cardiac muscle, functions as an oxygen-bonding muscle protein. It's released

Cardiac enzyme and protein patterns

Because they're released by damaged tissue, serum proteins and isoenzymes (catalytic proteins that vary in concentration in specific organs) can help identify the compromised organ and assess the extent of damage. After acute myocardial infarction, cardiac enzymes and proteins rise and fall in a characteristic pattern, as shown in the graph below.

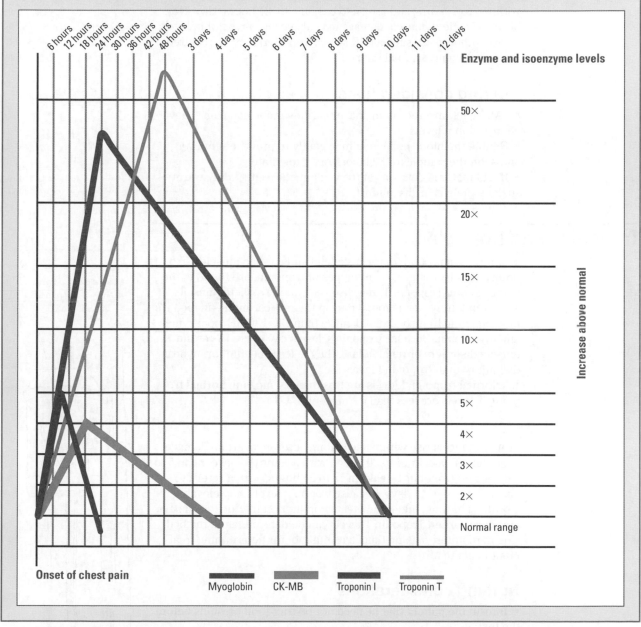

into the bloodstream when ischemia, trauma, and inflammation of the muscle occur. Normal myoglobin values are 0 to 0.09 mcg/ml.

First, but not as reliable

Rising myoglobin levels may be the first marker of cardiac injury after acute MI. Levels may rise within 30 minutes to 4 hours, peak within 6 to 7 hours, and return to baseline by 24 hours. However, because skeletal muscle damage may also cause myoglobin levels to rise, other tests (such as CK-MB or troponin) may be required to determine myocardial injury.

Nursing considerations

• I.M. injections, recent angina, or cardioversion can cause elevated myoglobin levels.
• Handle the blood collection tube gently to prevent hemolysis, and send the sample to the laboratory immediately.
• If a hematoma develops at the venipuncture site, apply warm soaks to help ease discomfort.

Troponin I and troponin T

Troponin is a protein found in skeletal and cardiac muscles. Troponin I and troponin T, two isotypes of troponin, are found in the myocardium. Troponin T may also be found in skeletal muscle. Troponin I, however, is found only in the myocardium—in fact, it's more specific to myocardial damage than CK, CK-MB isoenzymes, and myoglobin. Because troponin T levels can occur in certain muscle disorders or renal failure, they're less specific for myocardial injury than troponin I levels are.

Normal troponin I levels are less than 0.4 mcg/ml; normal troponin T levels are less than 0.1 mcg/ml.

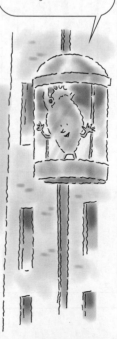

Troponin levels stay elevated even if the MI happened days before.

Up for days

Troponin levels rise within 3 to 6 hours after myocardial damage. Troponin I peaks in 14 to 20 hours, with a return to baseline in 5 to 7 days, and troponin T peaks in 12 to 24 hours, with a return to baseline in 10 to 15 days. Because troponin levels stay elevated for a prolonged time, they can detect an infarction that occurred several days earlier. Troponin T levels can be determined at the bedside in minutes, making them a useful tool for determining treatment in acute MI.

Nursing considerations

• Inform the patient that he need not restrict food or fluids before the test.

- Tell him that multiple blood samples may be drawn.
- Sustained vigorous exercise, cardiotoxic drugs such as doxorubicin (Adriamycin), renal disease, and certain surgical procedures can cause elevated troponin T levels.
- Handle the collection tube gently to prevent hemolysis, and send the sample to the laboratory immediately.
- If a hematoma develops at the venipuncture site, apply warm soaks to help ease discomfort.

Homocysteine

Homocysteine is an amino acid that's produced by the body. High homocysteine levels can irritate blood vessels, leading to atherosclerosis. High levels can also raise low-density lipoprotein (LDL) levels and make blood clot more easily, increasing the risk of blood vessel blockages. Normal homocysteine levels are less than or equal to 13 µmol/L.

Nursing considerations

- Perform a venipuncture; collect the sample in a 5-ml tube containing EDTA.
- Send the sample to the laboratory immediately to be frozen in a plastic vial on dry ice.
- If a hematoma develops at the venipuncture site, apply warm soaks to help ease discomfort.

C-reactive protein

CRP is a substance produced by the liver. A high CRP level indicates that inflammation exists at some location in the body. Other diagnostic tests are needed to determine the location of the inflammation and its cause. Elevated CRP levels can indicate such conditions as MI, angina, systemic lupus erythematosus, postoperative infection, trauma, and heatstroke. Recent studies have also shown a correlation between CRP levels and coronary artery disease (CAD).

An elevated CRP level indicates that inflammation exists somewhere in the body.

Nursing considerations

- Perform a venipuncture, and collect the sample in a 5-ml nonanticoagulated tube.
- If a hematoma develops at the venipuncture site, apply warm soaks to help ease discomfort.

B-type natriuretic peptide

BNP is a hormone polypeptide secreted by ventricular tissues in the heart. The substance is secreted as a response to the increased ventricular volume and pressure that occur when a patient is in heart failure.

A grade for heart failure

A BNP test helps accurately diagnose and grade the severity of heart failure. A quick diagnosis of heart failure in patients who present with dyspnea is important in order to begin appropriate treatment early.

Nursing considerations

• Perform a venipuncture, and collect the sample in a 5-ml tube containing EDTA.
• If a hematoma develops at the venipuncture site, apply warm soaks to help ease discomfort.

Lipid studies

Lipid studies include triglycerides, total cholesterol, and lipoprotein fractionation. They measure lipid levels in the body and help evaluate the risk of CAD.

Triglycerides

Triglycerides are the main storage form of lipids and constitute about 95% of fatty tissue. Monitoring triglyceride levels in the blood helps with early identification of hyperlipidemia and identification of patients at risk for CAD.

What's normal?

Triglyceride values less than 150 mg/dl are widely accepted as normal.

What's abnormal?

Triglyceride levels between 150 and 199 mg/dl are considered borderline high. Levels between 200 and 499 mg/dl are considered high. Levels greater than 500 mg/dl are very high.

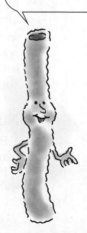

Lipid studies can tell you if arteries are becoming clogged.

One test leads to another

Measuring cholesterol may also be necessary, because cholesterol and triglyceride levels vary independently. If both triglyceride and cholesterol levels are high, the patient is at risk for CAD.

Nursing considerations

• Because triglycerides are highly affected by a fat-containing meal, with levels rising and peaking 4 hours after ingesting a meal, tell the patient that he should abstain from food for 9 to 12 hours before the test and from alcohol for 24 hours before the test. The patient may drink water.
• Perform a venipuncture, collect a sample in a 7-ml tube containing EDTA, and send the sample to the laboratory immediately.
• Avoid prolonged venous occlusion. Remove the tourniquet within 1 minute of application.

Total cholesterol

The total serum cholesterol test measures the circulating levels of the two forms in which cholesterol appears in the body—free cholesterol and cholesterol esters.

What's your level?

For adults, a desirable cholesterol level is less than 200 mg/dl. Levels are considered borderline high if they're between 200 and 240 mg/dl, and high if they're greater than 240 mg/dl.

For children ages 12 to 18, desirable levels are less than 170 mg/dl. Levels are considered high if they're greater than 200 mg/dl.

Nursing considerations

• Fasting isn't needed for isolated cholesterol checks or screening, but fasting is required if total cholesterol is part of a lipid profile. If fasting is required, instruct the patient to abstain from food and drink for 12 hours before the test.
• Perform a venipuncture, and collect the sample in a 7-ml tube containing EDTA. The patient should be in a sitting position for 5 minutes before the blood is drawn. Fingersticks can also be used for initial screening when using an automated analyzer.
• Document any drugs the patient is taking.
• Send the sample to the laboratory immediately.

A desirable total cholesterol level is less than 200 mg/dl.

Lipoprotein fractionation

Lipoprotein fractionation tests are used to isolate and measure the two types of cholesterol in blood: high-density lipoproteins (HDLs) and low-density lipoproteins (LDLs).

This is good

HDL level is inversely related to the risk of CAD—that is, the higher the HDL level, the lower the incidence of CAD. For males, normal HDL values range from 37 to 70 mg/dl; in females, from 40 to 85 mg/dl.

This isn't

Conversely, the higher the LDL level, the higher the incidence of CAD. For individuals who don't have CAD, desirable LDL levels are less than 130 mg/dl, borderline high levels are in the range of 130 to 159 mg/dl, and high levels are more than 160 mg/dl. For individuals who have CAD, optimal levels are less than 100 mg/dl, and higher than optimal levels are more than 100 mg/dl.

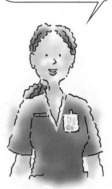

A high HDL level means a lower incidence of CAD, but a high LDL level means a higher incidence of CAD.

Nursing considerations

• Tell the patient to maintain a normal diet for 2 weeks before the test.
• Tell him to abstain from alcohol for 24 hours before the test.
• As ordered, tell the patient to discontinue use of thyroid hormone, hormonal contraceptives, and antilipemic agents until after the test because they alter results.
• Perform a venipuncture, and collect the sample in a 7-ml tube containing EDTA.
• Send the sample to the laboratory immediately to avoid spontaneous redistributions among the lipoproteins. If the sample can't be transported immediately, refrigerate it but don't allow it to freeze.

Coagulation tests

Partial thromboplastin time (PTT), prothrombin time (PT), and activated clotting time are tests that measure clotting time. They're used to measure response to treatment as well as to screen for clotting disorders.

Partial thromboplastin time

The PTT test evaluates all the clotting factors of the intrinsic pathway, except platelets. It's done by measuring the time it takes a clot to form after adding calcium and phospholipid emulsion to a plasma sample. Normally, a clot forms 21 to 35 seconds after the reagents are added.

The PTT test also helps monitor a patient's response to heparin therapy. For a patient on anticoagulant therapy, check with the attending doctor to find out what PTT test results to expect.

Nursing considerations

- Tell the patient receiving heparin therapy that this test may be repeated at regular intervals to assess response to treatment.
- Perform a venipuncture, and collect the sample in a 7-ml tube containing sodium citrate.
- Completely fill the collection tube, invert it gently several times, and send it to the laboratory on ice.
- For a patient on anticoagulant therapy, additional pressure may be needed at the venipuncture site to control bleeding.

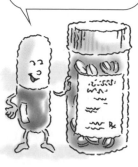

I do declare! A clot should form 21 to 35 seconds after beginning the PTT test.

Prothrombin time

Prothrombin, or factor II, is a plasma protein produced by the liver. The PT test (also known as *pro time*) measures the time required for a clot to form in a citrated plasma sample after the addition of calcium ions and tissue thromboplastin (factor III).

Excellent choice, sir!

The PT test is an excellent screening procedure for overall evaluation of extrinsic coagulation factors V, VII, and X and of prothrombin and fibrinogen. It's also the test of choice for monitoring oral anticoagulant therapy.

Count to 10 (or more)

Normally, PT ranges from 10 to 14 seconds. In a patient receiving warfarin (Coumadin) therapy, the goal of treatment is to attain a PT level 1.5 to 2 times the normal control value—for example, a level of 15 to 20 seconds. (See *Understanding the INR*, page 62.)

Nursing considerations

- Check the patient's history for use of medications that may affect test results, such as vitamin K or antibiotics.

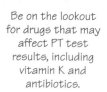

Be on the lookout for drugs that may affect PT test results, including vitamin K and antibiotics.

Advice from the experts

Understanding the INR

The International Normalized Ratio (INR) system is generally viewed as the best means of standardizing measurement of prothrombin time to monitor oral anticoagulant therapy.

Guidelines for patients receiving warfarin (Coumadin) therapy recommend an INR result of 2.0 to 3.0. For patients with mechanical prosthetic heart valves, an INR result of 2.5 to 3.5 is recommended.

What's the problem?
Increased INR values may indicate disseminated intravascular coagulation, cirrhosis, hepatitis, vitamin K deficiency, salicylate intoxication, uncontrolled oral anticoagulation, or massive blood transfusion.

• Perform a venipuncture, and collect the sample in a 7-ml siliconized tube.
• Completely fill the collection tube, and invert it gently several times to adequately mix the sample and anticoagulant. If the tube isn't filled to the correct volume, an excess of citrate appears in the sample.

Activated clotting time

Activated clotting time, or automated coagulation time, measures the time it takes whole blood to clot.

Out-of-body experiences

This test is commonly performed during procedures that require extracorporeal (occurring outside the body) circulation, such as cardiopulmonary bypass, ultrafiltration, hemodialysis, and extracorporeal membrane oxygenation.

Nursing considerations

• Explain to the patient that the test requires a blood sample that's usually drawn from an existing vascular access site; therefore, no venipuncture is necessary.
• Explain that two samples will be drawn. The first one will be discarded so that heparin in the tubing doesn't interfere with the results.

On your mark! Get set! Clot!

• If the sample is drawn from a line with a continuous infusion, stop the infusion before drawing the sample.
• Withdraw 5 to 10 ml of blood from the line and discard it.
• Withdraw a clean sample of blood into the special tube containing the celite provided with the activated clotting time unit.
• Turn on the activated clotting time unit, and wait for the signal to insert the tube.
• Flush the vascular access site according to your facility's protocol.

Electrocardiography

The heart's electrical conduction system can be recorded numerous ways, but the most common methods are a 12-lead electrocardiogram (ECG), continuous cardiac monitoring, an exercise ECG, Holter monitoring, and electrophysiology studies (EPS). (See *How to read any ECG: An 8-step guide*, pages 64 and 65.)

ECG is a valuable and commonly used tool, so take a systematic approach and look for changes from the patient's previous results.

12-lead electrocardiogram

The 12-lead ECG measures the heart's electrical activity and records it as waveforms. It's one of the most valuable and commonly used diagnostic tools.

A test with 12 views

The standard 12-lead ECG uses a series of electrodes placed on the patient's extremities and chest wall to assess the heart from 12 different views (leads). The 12 leads include three bipolar limb leads (I, II, and III), three unipolar augmented limb leads (aV_R, aV_L, and aV_F), and six unipolar precordial limb leads (V_1 to V_6). The limb leads and augmented leads show the heart from the frontal plane. The precordial leads show the heart from the horizontal plane.

ECG can be used to identify myocardial ischemia and infarction, rhythm and conduction disturbances, chamber enlargement, electrolyte imbalances, and drug toxicity.

Nursing considerations

• Use a systematic approach to interpret the ECG recording. (See *Normal ECG waveforms*, page 66.) Compare the patient's previous ECG with the current one, if available. Doing so will help you identify changes.

(Text continues on page 66.)

How to read any ECG: An 8-step guide

An electrocardiogram (ECG) waveform has three basic elements: a P wave, a QRS complex, and a T wave. They're joined by five other useful diagnostic elements: the PR interval, the U wave, the ST segment, the J point, and the QT interval. The diagram to the right shows how these elements are related.

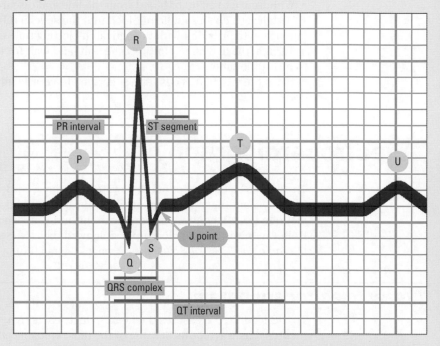

Getting in step

This 8-step guide will enable you to read any ECG.

Step 1: Evaluate the P wave

Observe the P wave's size, shape, and location in the waveform. If the P wave consistently precedes the QRS complex, the sinoatrial (SA) node is initiating the electrical impulse, as it should be.

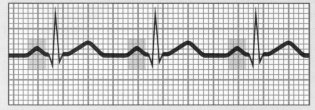

Step 2: Evaluate the atrial rhythm

The P wave should occur at regular intervals, with only small variations associated with respiration. Using a pair of calipers, you can easily measure the interval between P waves—the P-P interval. Compare the P-P intervals in several ECG cycles. Make sure the calipers are set at the same point—at the beginning of

the wave or on its peak. Instead of lifting the calipers, rotate one of its legs to the next P wave, to ensure accurate measurements.

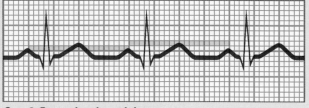

Step 3: Determine the atrial rate

To determine the atrial rate quickly, count the number of P waves in two 3-second segments. Multiply this number by 10. For a more accurate determination, count the number of small squares between two P waves, using either the apex of the wave or the initial upstroke of the wave. Each small square equals 0.04 second; 1,500 squares equal 1 minute ($0.04 \times 1,500 = 60$ seconds). So, divide 1,500 by the number of squares you counted between the

P waves. This calculation gives you the atrial rate—the number of contractions per minute.

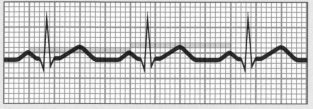

Step 4: Calculate the duration of the PR interval

Count the number of small squares between the beginning of the P wave and the beginning of the QRS complex. Multiply the number of squares by 0.04 second. The normal interval is between 0.12 and 0.20 second, or between 3 and 5 small squares. A wider interval indicates delayed conduction of the impulse through the atrioventricular node to the ventricles. A short PR interval indicates that the impulse originated in an area other than the SA node.

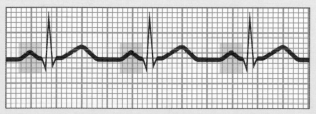

Step 5: Evaluate the ventricular rhythm

Use the calipers to measure the R-R intervals. Remember to place the calipers on the same point of the QRS complex. If the R-R intervals remain consistent, the ventricular rhythm is regular.

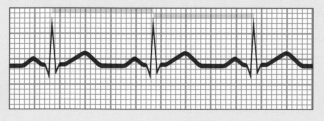

Step 6: Determine the ventricular rate

To determine the ventricular rate, use the same formula as in step 3. In this case, however, count the number of small squares between two R waves to do the calculation. Also, check that the QRS complex is shaped appropriately for the lead you're monitoring.

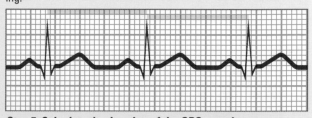

Step 7: Calculate the duration of the QRS complex

Count the number of squares between the beginning and the end of the QRS complex, and multiply by 0.04 second. A normal QRS complex is less than 0.12 second, or less than 3 small squares wide. Some references specify 0.06 to 0.10 second as the normal duration of the QRS complex.

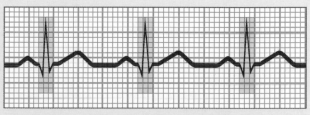

Step 8: Calculate the duration of the QT interval

Count the number of squares from the beginning of the QRS complex to the end of the T wave. Multiply this number by 0.04 second. The normal range is 0.36 to 0.44 second, or 9 to 11 small squares wide.

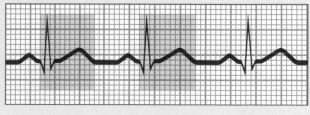

Normal ECG waveforms

Each of the 12 standard leads of an electrocardiogram (ECG) takes a different view of heart activity, and each generates its own characteristic tracing. The tracings shown here represent a normal heart rhythm viewed from each of the 12 leads. Keep in mind:
• An upward (positive) deflection indicates that the wave of depolarization flows toward the positive electrode.

• A downward (negative) deflection indicates that the wave of depolarization flows away from the positive electrode.
• An equally positive and negative (biphasic) deflection indicates that the wave of depolarization flows perpendicularly to the positive electrode.

Each lead represents a picture of a different anatomic area; when you find abnormal tracings, compare information from the different leads to pinpoint areas of cardiac damage.

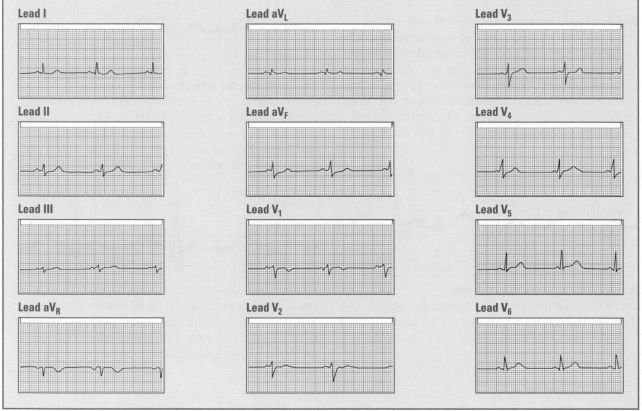

Lead I   Lead aV_L   Lead V_3
Lead II   Lead aV_F   Lead V_4
Lead III   Lead V_1   Lead V_5
Lead aV_R   Lead V_2   Lead V_6

Waves of waves

• P waves should be upright; however, they may be inverted in lead aV_R or biphasic or inverted in leads III, aV_L, and V_1.
• PR intervals should always be constant, like QRS-complex durations.
• QRS-complex deflections vary in different leads. Observe for pathologic Q waves.
• ST segments should be isoelectric or have minimal deviation.

• ST-segment elevation greater than 1 mm above the baseline and ST-segment depression greater than 0.5 mm below the baseline are considered abnormal. Leads facing toward an injured area have ST-segment elevations, and leads facing away show ST-segment depressions.

Don't sound the alarm—yet

• The T wave normally deflects upward in leads I, II, and V_3 through V_6. It's inverted in lead aV_R and variable in the other leads. T-wave changes have many causes and aren't always a reason for alarm. Excessively tall, flat, or inverted T waves occurring with such symptoms as chest pain may indicate ischemia.

• A normal Q wave generally has a duration less than 0.04 second. An abnormal Q wave has a duration of 0.04 second or more, a depth greater than 4 mm, or a height one-fourth of the R wave. Abnormal Q waves indicate myocardial necrosis, developing when depolarization can't follow its normal path because of damaged tissue in the area.

• Remember that aV_R normally has a large Q wave, so disregard this lead when searching for abnormal Q waves.

Continuous cardiac monitoring

Because it allows continuous observation of the heart's electrical activity, cardiac monitoring is used in patients at risk for life-threatening arrhythmias. Like other forms of electrocardiography, cardiac monitoring uses electrodes placed on the patient's chest to transmit electrical signals that are converted into a cardiac rhythm tracing on an oscilloscope. (See *Positioning monitor leads*, page 68.)

Hardwire vs. wireless

Two types of monitoring may be performed: hardwire or telemetry. In *hardwire monitoring*, the patient is connected to a monitor at the bedside. The rhythm display appears at the bedside, or it may be transmitted to a console at a remote location. *Telemetry* uses a small transmitter connected to the ambulatory patient to send electrical signals to another location, where they're displayed on a monitor screen.

Job description

Regardless of the type, cardiac monitors can display the patient's heart rate and rhythm, produce a printed record of cardiac rhythm, and sound an alarm if the heart rate exceeds or falls below specified limits. Monitors also recognize and count abnormal heartbeats as well as changes. (See *Identifying cardiac monitor problems*, page 69.)

Memory jogger

To help you remember where to place electrodes in a five-electrode configuration, think of the phrase "white to the upper right." Then think of snow over trees (white electrode over green electrode) and smoke over fire (black electrode above red electrode). And of course, chocolate (brown electrode) lies close to the heart.

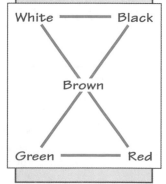

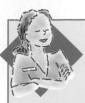

Peak technique

Positioning monitor leads

These illustrations show correct electrode positions for some of the monitoring leads you'll use most often. The abbreviations used are RA, right arm; LA, left arm; RL, right leg; LL, left leg; C, chest; and G, ground. For each lead, you'll see electrode placement for a five-leadwire system and a three-leadwire telemetry system.

One for one
In the five-leadwire system, the electrode position for one lead may be identical to the electrode position for another lead. In this case, simply change the lead selector switch to the setting that corresponds to the lead you want. In some cases, you'll need to reposition the electrodes.

Two for three
In the three-leadwire telemetry system, you can create the same lead with two electrodes that you do with three simply by eliminating the ground electrode.

Five-leadwire system

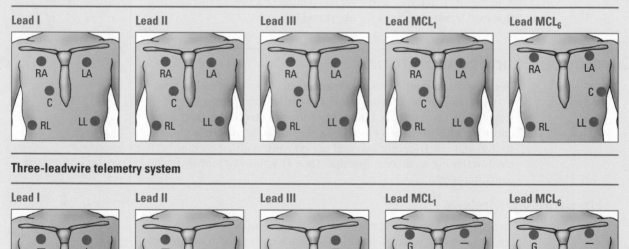

Three-leadwire telemetry system

Nursing considerations

• Make sure all electrical equipment and outlets are grounded to avoid electric shock and interference (artifacts). Also ensure that the patient is clean and dry to prevent electric shock.

• If the patient's skin is very oily, scaly, or diaphoretic, rub the electrode site with a dry 4″ × 4″ gauze pad before applying the electrode, to help reduce interference in the tracing.

Advice from the experts

Identifying cardiac monitor problems

Problem	Possible causes	Solutions
False–high-rate alarm	Monitor interpreting large T waves as QRS complexes, which doubles the rate	• Reposition electrodes to a lead where QRS complexes are taller than T waves.
	Skeletal muscle activity	• Place electrodes away from major muscle masses.
False–low-rate alarm	Shift in electrical axis from patient movement, making QRS complexes too small to register	• Reapply electrodes. Set gain so height of complex is greater than 1 mV.
	Low amplitude of QRS	• Increase gain.
	Poor contact between electrode and skin	• Reapply electrodes.
Artifact (waveform interference)	Patient having seizures, chills, or anxiety	• Notify the doctor and treat the patient as ordered. • Keep the patient warm and reassure him.
	Patient movement	• Help the patient relax.
	Electrodes applied improperly	• Check electrodes and reapply, if necessary.
	Static electricity	• Make sure cables don't have exposed connectors. • Change static-causing bedclothes.
	Electrical short circuit in leadwires or cable	• Replace broken equipment. Use stress loops when applying leadwires.
	Interference from decreased room humidity	• Regulate humidity to 40%.

• Assess skin integrity, and reposition the electrodes every 24 hours or as necessary.
• Document a rhythm strip at least every 8 hours and with any change in the patient's condition (or as stated by your facility's policy).

Exercise electrocardiography

Exercise electrocardiography is a noninvasive test that helps assess cardiovascular response to an increased workload. Commonly known as a *stress test*, it provides diagnostic information that can't be obtained from a resting ECG. This test may also assess response to treatment.

Stop in a hurry

Stop the test if the patient experiences chest pain, fatigue, or other signs and symptoms that reflect exercise intolerance. These findings may include severe dyspnea, claudication, weakness or dizziness, hypotension, pallor or vasoconstriction, disorientation, ataxia, ischemic ECG changes (with or without pain), rhythm disturbances or heart block, and ventricular conduction abnormalities.

Drugs do it, too

If the patient can't perform physical exercise, a stress test can be performed by I.V. injection of a coronary vasodilator, such as dipyridamole (Persantine) or adenosine. Other methods of stressing the heart include dobutamine administration and pacing (in the patient with a pacemaker). During the stress test, nuclear scanning or echocardiography may also be performed. (See *Drug-induced stress tests*.)

> Stop electrocardiography if the patient experiences chest pain, fatigue, or other signs and symptoms that reflect exercise intolerance.

Nursing considerations

- Tell the patient not to eat, drink caffeinated beverages, or smoke cigarettes for 4 hours before the test.
- Explain that he should wear loose, lightweight clothing and snug-fitting but comfortable shoes, and emphasize that he should

---

Now I get it!

Drug-induced stress tests

If a patient can't tolerate physical activity, a drug-induced stress test can be used so that the doctor can measure the reaction of the heart to exertion.

Exercise without the effort

A drug such as dypyridamole (Persantine) or dobutamine is administered to the patient, which causes the heart to react as if the person were exercising, though the patient is actually at rest.

No blood, no tracer

The drug will either dilate the coronary arteries (persantine) or increase the heart rate (dobutamine). The medication is given

through an I.V. access, along with thallium (a radioactive substance known as a tracer). These substances travel through the bloodstream to the heart, where they're picked up by the heart muscle cells. Those areas of the heart muscle that lack an adequate blood supply pick up the tracer very slowly or not at all.

A set of images is recorded, with a second set of images taken 3 to 4 hours later. A cardiologist reads the scan to determine areas of the heart muscle that have diminished blood supply or have suffered permanent damage from a heart attack.

immediately report any chest pain, leg discomfort, breathlessness, or fatigue.
• Check the doctor's orders to determine which cardiac drugs should be administered or withheld before the test. Beta-adrenergic blockers, for example, can limit the patient's ability to raise his heart rate and are generally withheld the day of the test.
• Inform the patient that he may receive an injection of thallium during the test so that the doctor can evaluate coronary blood flow. Reassure him that the injection involves negligible radiation exposure.
• Tell the patient that, after the test, his blood pressure and ECG will be monitored for 10 to 15 minutes.

Holter monitoring

Also called *ambulatory electrocardiography*, Holter monitoring allows recording of heart activity as the patient follows his normal routine. Like exercise electrocardiography, Holter monitoring can provide considerably more diagnostic information than a standard resting ECG. In addition, Holter monitoring can record intermittent arrhythmias.

This test usually lasts about 24 hours (about 100,000 cardiac cycles). The patient wears a small tape recorder connected to bipolar electrodes placed on his chest and keeps a diary of his activities and associated symptoms.

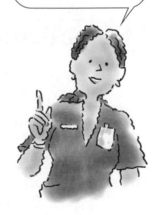

Holter monitoring records the heart's activity for 24 hours while the patient follows a normal routine.

Nursing considerations

• Urge the patient not to tamper with the monitor or disconnect leadwires or electrodes. Demonstrate how to check the recorder for proper function.
• Tell the patient that he can't bathe or shower while wearing the monitor. He also needs to avoid electrical appliances, which can interfere with the monitor's recording.
• Emphasize to the patient the importance of keeping track of his activities, regardless of symptoms.
• Evaluation of the recordings will guide further treatment.

Electrophysiology studies

EPS studies are used to diagnose and treat abnormal heart rhythms. The procedure involves passing two to four temporary electrode catheters into multiple heart chambers. The electrodes are usually positioned in the right atrium, the atrioventricular node, the bundle of His region, and the apex of the right ventricle. The electrodes stimulate (pace) the heart and record the heart's electrical conduction.

Normal conduction intervals in adults are as follows: HV interval, 35 to 55 msec; AH interval, 45 to 150 msec; and PA interval, 20 to 40 msec.

Nursing considerations

• Explain to the patient that EPS studies evaluate the heart's conduction system. Instruct him to restrict food and fluids for at least 6 hours before the test. Inform him that the studies take 1 to 3 hours.
• Have the patient void before the test.
• Monitor the patient's vital signs, as ordered. If they're unstable, check them every 15 minutes and alert the doctor. Observe for shortness of breath, chest pain, pallor, or changes in pulse rate, cardiac rhythm, or blood pressure. Enforce bed rest for 4 to 6 hours.
• Check the catheter insertion site for bleeding; apply a pressure bandage and sandbag to the site until bleeding stops.

EPS studies evaluate my conduction system.

Hemodynamic monitoring

Hemodynamic monitoring is used to assess cardiac function and determine the effectiveness of therapy. Methods include arterial blood pressure monitoring, pulmonary artery pressure (PAP) monitoring, cardiac output monitoring, and cardiac catheterization.

Arterial blood pressure monitoring

In arterial blood pressure monitoring, the doctor inserts a catheter into the radial or femoral artery to measure blood pressure or obtain samples for arterial blood gas studies.

Making waves

A transducer transforms the flow of blood during systole and diastole into a waveform, which appears on an oscilloscope.

Nursing considerations

• Explain the procedure to the patient and his family, including the purpose of arterial pressure monitoring.
• After catheter insertion, observe the pressure waveform to assess arterial pressure.

• Assess the insertion site for signs of infection, such as redness and swelling. Notify the doctor immediately if you note such signs.

• Carefully assess the neurovascular status of the extremity distal to the catheter insertion. Notify the doctor of diminished pulses; pale, cool skin; and decreased movement. Also notify the doctor if the patient reports numbness or tingling in that area.

• Document the date, time, and site of catheter insertion; type of flush solution used; type of dressing applied; and the patient's tolerance of the procedure.

Pulmonary artery pressure monitoring

Continuous PAP and intermittent pulmonary artery wedge pressure (PAWP) measurements provide important information about left ventricular function and preload. Use this information for monitoring and for aiding diagnosis, refining assessment, guiding interventions, and projecting patient outcomes.

Many ports, many uses

The procedure uses a pulmonary artery (PA) catheter, which contains several lumen ports:

• The balloon inflation lumen inflates the balloon at the distal tip of the catheter for PAWP measurement.

• A distal lumen measures PAP when connected to a transducer and measures PAWP during balloon inflation. Blood samples may also be obtained from this port.

• A proximal lumen measures right atrial pressure (central venous pressure).

• The thermistor connector lumen contains temperature-sensitive wires, which feed information into a computer for cardiac output calculation.

• Another lumen may provide a port for pacemaker electrodes or measurement of mixed venous oxygen saturation. (See *Normal PA waveforms*, page 74.)

What can I say? A PA catheter has many uses.

What are you reading?

Normal results from PAP monitoring are:

• right atrial pressure—1 to 6 mm Hg
• systolic right ventricular pressure—20 to 30 mm Hg
• end-diastolic right ventricular pressure—less than 5 mm Hg
• systolic PAP—20 to 30 mm Hg
• diastolic PAP—10 to 15 mm Hg
• mean PAP—less than 20 mm Hg
• PAWP—6 to 12 mm Hg
• left atrial pressure—about 10 mm Hg.

Now I get it!

Normal PA waveforms

During pulmonary artery (PA) catheter insertion, the waveforms on the monitor change as the catheter advances through the heart.

Right atrium

When the catheter tip enters the right atrium, the first heart chamber on its route, a waveform like the one show below appears on the monitor. Note the two small upright waves. The *a* waves represent the right ventricular end-diastolic pressure; the *v* waves, right atrial filling.

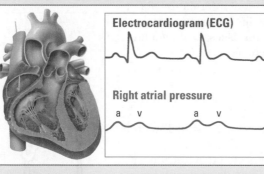

Right ventricle

As the catheter tip reaches the right ventricle, you'll see a waveform with sharp systolic upstrokes and lower diastolic dips, as shown below.

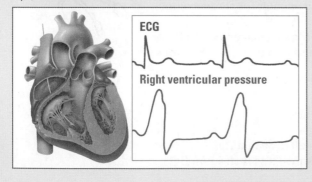

Pulmonary artery

The catheter then floats into the pulmonary artery, causing a pulmonary artery pressure (PAP) waveform such as the one shown below. Note that the upstroke is smoother than on the right ventricle waveform. The dicrotic notch indicates pulmonic valve closure.

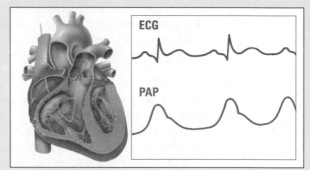

PAWP

Floating into a distal branch of the pulmonary artery, the balloon wedges where the vessel becomes too narrow for it to pass. The monitor now shows a pulmonary artery wedge pressure (PAWP) waveform, with two small upright waves, as shown below. The *a* wave represents left ventricular end-diastolic pressure; the *v* wave, left atrial filling. The balloon is then deflated, and the catheter is left in the pulmonary artery.

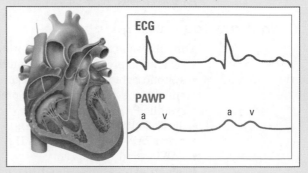

Potential PAP patients

PAP monitoring is indicated for patients who are hemodynamically unstable, need fluid management or continuous cardiopulmonary assessment, or are receiving multiple or frequently administered cardioactive drugs.

PAP monitoring is also crucial for patients experiencing shock, trauma, pulmonary or cardiac disease, or multiple organ dysfunction syndrome.

Nursing considerations

• Tell the patient that he'll be conscious during catheterization and that he may feel temporary local discomfort from the administration of the local anesthetic. Catheter insertion takes about 30 minutes.
• After catheter insertion, you may inflate the balloon with a syringe to take PAWP readings. Don't inflate the balloon with more than 1.5 cc of air because overinflation could distend the pulmonary artery, causing vessel rupture. Never leave the balloon wedged for a prolonged period; doing so may lead to a pulmonary infarction.
• After each PAWP reading, flush the line; if you encounter difficulty, notify the doctor.
• Maintain 300 mm Hg pressure in the pressure bag to permit a flush flow of 3 to 6 ml/hour.
• If fever develops when the catheter is in place, inform the doctor; he may remove the catheter and send its tip to the laboratory for culture.

Tight is right

• Make sure stopcocks are properly positioned and connections are secure. Loose connections may introduce air into the system or cause blood backup, leakage of deoxygenated blood, or inaccurate pressure readings. Also make sure the lumen hubs are properly identified to serve the appropriate catheter ports. (See *Identifying hemodynamic pressure monitoring problems*, pages 76 and 77.)
• Because the catheter can slip back into the right ventricle and irritate it, check the monitor for a right ventricular waveform to detect this problem promptly.
• To minimize valvular trauma, make sure the balloon is deflated whenever the catheter is withdrawn from the pulmonary artery to the right ventricle or from the right ventricle to the right atrium.
• Adhere to your facility's policy for dressing, tubing, catheter, and flush changes.
• Document the date, time, and site of catheter insertion; the doctor who performed the procedure; pressure waveforms and values for the various heart chambers; balloon inflation volume required

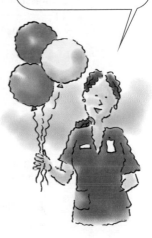

When taking PAWP readings, don't inflate the balloon with more than 1.5 cc of air. Overinflation could cause the vessel to rupture.

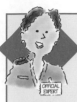

Advice from the experts

Identifying hemodynamic pressure monitoring problems

This chart reviews common hemodynamic pressure monitoring problems, their possible causes, and appropriate interventions.

Problem	Possible causes	Interventions
Line fails to flush	• Stopcocks positioned incorrectly	• Make sure the stopcocks are positioned correctly.
	• Inadequate pressure from pressure bag	• Make sure the pressure bag gauge reads 300 mm Hg.
	• Kink in pressure tubing	• Check the pressure tubing for kinks.
	• Blood clot in catheter	• Try to aspirate the clot with a syringe. If the line still won't flush, notify the doctor and prepare to replace the line, if necessary. Important: Never use a syringe to flush a hemodynamic line.
Damped waveform	• Air bubbles	• Secure all connections. • Remove air from the lines and the transducer. • Check for and replace cracked equipment.
	• Blood clot in catheter	• Refer to "Line fails to flush" (above).
	• Blood flashback in line	• Make sure stopcock positions are correct; tighten loose connections and replace cracked equipment; flush the line with the fast-flush valve; replace the transducer dome if blood backs up into it.
	• Incorrect transducer position	• Make sure the transducer is kept at the level of the right atrium at all times. Improper levels give false-high or false-low pressure readings.
	• Arterial catheter out of blood vessel or pressed against vessel wall	• Reposition the catheter if it's against the vessel wall. • Try to aspirate blood to confirm proper placement in the vessel. If you can't aspirate blood, notify the doctor and prepare to replace the line. *Note:* Bloody drainage at the insertion site may indicate catheter displacement. Notify the doctor immediately.
	• Inadequate pressure from pressure bag	• Make sure the pressure bag gauge reads 300 mm Hg.

Identifying hemodynamic pressure monitoring problems *(continued)*

Problem	Possible causes	Interventions
Pulmonary artery wedge pressure tracing unobtainable	• Ruptured balloon	• If you feel no resistance when injecting air or if you see blood leaking from the balloon inflation lumen, stop injecting air and notify the doctor. If the catheter is left in, label the inflation lumen with a warning not to inflate.
	• Incorrect amount of air in balloon	• Deflate the balloon. Check the label on the catheter for correct volume. Reinflate slowly with the correct amount. To avoid rupturing the balloon, never use more than the stated volume.
	• Catheter malpositioned	• Notify the doctor. Obtain a chest X-ray.

to obtain a wedge tracing; arrhythmias that occurred during or after the procedure; type of flush solution used and its heparin concentration (if any); type of dressing applied; and the patient's tolerance of the procedure.

Cardiac output monitoring

Cardiac output—the amount of blood ejected by the heart in 1 minute—is monitored to evaluate cardiac function. The normal range for cardiac output is 4 to 8 L/minute.

The most widely used method for monitoring cardiac output is the bolus thermodilution technique. Other methods include the Fick method (see *Calculating cardiac output*, page 78) and the dye dilution test.

On the rocks or room temperature

To measure cardiac output using the bolus thermodilution technique, a solution is injected into the right atrium through the proximal port on a PA catheter. Iced or room-temperature injectant may be used depending on your facility's policy and on the patient's status.

This indicator solution mixes with the blood as it travels through the right ventricle into the pulmonary artery, and a thermistor on the catheter registers the change in temperature of the flowing blood. A computer then plots the temperature change over time as a curve and calculates flow based on the area under the curve. (See *Doppler-based hemodynamic monitoring*, page 79.)

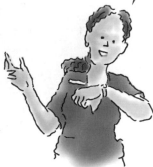

Cardiac output is a measure of the blood ejected from the heart in 1 minute.

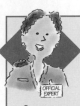

Advice from the experts

Calculating cardiac output

One way to calculate cardiac output (CO) is by using the Fick method. In this method, the blood's oxygen content is measured before and after it passes through the lungs. First, a blood sample is obtained from the pulmonary and brachial arteries and analyzed for oxygen content. Next, a spirometer is used to measure oxygen consumption (the amount of air entering the lungs each minute).

Use this formula to calculate CO:

$$CO \text{ (L/minute)} = \frac{\text{oxygen consumption (ml/minute)}}{\text{arterial oxygen content} - \text{venous oxygen content (ml/minute)}}$$

Cardiac index: The better assessor

Cardiac output is better assessed by calculating the cardiac index, which takes body size into account. To calculate the patient's cardiac index, divide his cardiac output by his body surface area, a function of height and weight. The normal cardiac index for adults ranges from 2.5 to 4.2 L/minute/m^2; for pregnant women, 3.5 to 6.5 L/minute/m^2.

Nursing considerations

• Make sure the patient doesn't move during the procedure because movement can cause an error in measurement.
• Perform cardiac output measurements at least every 2 to 4 hours, especially if the patient is receiving vasoactive or inotropic agents or if fluids are being added or restricted. Monitor for changes.
• Discontinue cardiac output measurements when the patient is hemodynamically stable and weaned from his vasoactive and inotropic medications.
• Monitor the patient for signs and symptoms of inadequate perfusion, including restlessness, fatigue, changes in level of consciousness, decreased capillary refill time, diminished peripheral pulses, oliguria, and pale, cool skin.
• Add the fluid volume injected for cardiac output determinations to the patient's total intake.
• Record the patient's cardiac output, cardiac index, and other hemodynamic values and vital signs at the time of measurement. Also, note the patient's position during measurement.

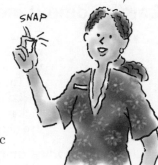

Calculating the patient's cardiac index is a snap. Divide his cardiac output by his body surface area.

SNAP

Doppler-based hemodynamic monitoring

Esophageal Doppler echocardiography is a noninvasive method of measuring cardiac output that's currently being studied. It calculates cardiac output by measuring blood flow through the heart valves or ventricular outflow tracts.

Pros

This type of monitoring has several advantages. First, it's noninvasive. Second, it allows for immediate evaluation of hemodynamic status in the doctor's office, emergency department, or operating room. Finally, it allows for periods of activity or exercise without the risk of dislodging invasive lines.

Cons

With this method of hemodynamic monitoring, it's difficult to align the ultrasound beam with the flow of blood. If the beam isn't properly angled, the results are affected. The quality of the imaging is another limitation.

Cardiac catheterization

Cardiac catheterization involves passing a catheter into the right, left, or both sides of the heart.

A multipurpose procedure

This procedure permits measurement of blood pressure and blood flow in the chambers of the heart. It's used to determine valve competence and cardiac wall contractility and to detect intracardiac shunts. The procedure is also used for blood sample collection and can be used to obtain diagnostic images of the ventricles (contrast ventriculography) and arteries (coronary arteriography or angiography).

Cardiac calculations

Use of thermodilution catheters allows calculation of cardiac output. Such calculations are used to evaluate valvular insufficiency or stenosis, septal defects, congenital anomalies, myocardial function and blood supply, and heart wall motion.

Confirming common problems

Common abnormalities and defects that can be confirmed by cardiac catheterization include CAD, myocardial incompetence, valvular heart disease, and septal defects.

Nursing considerations

When caring for a patient undergoing a cardiac catheterization, describe the procedure and events after it and take steps to prevent postoperative complications.

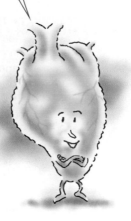

Cardiac catheterization can confirm the presence of CAD, myocardial incompetence, valvular heart disease, and septal defects. Pretty thorough!

Before the procedure

• Explain that this test is used to evaluate the function of the heart and its vessels. Instruct the patient to restrict food and fluids for at least 6 hours before the test. Tell him that the procedure takes 1 to 2 hours and that he may receive a mild sedative during the procedure.

• Tell the patient that the catheter is inserted into an artery or vein in the arm or leg. Tell him that he'll experience a transient stinging sensation when a local anesthetic is injected to numb the catheter insertion site.

• Inform the patient that injection of the contrast medium through the catheter may produce a hot, flushing sensation or nausea that quickly passes; instruct him to follow directions to cough or breathe deeply. Explain that he'll be given medication if he experiences chest pain during the procedure. Explain that he may also be given nitroglycerin periodically to dilate coronary vessels and aid visualization. Reassure him that complications, such as MI and thromboembolism, are rare.

• Make sure that the patient or a responsible family member has signed an informed consent form.

• Check for and tell the doctor about hypersensitivity to shellfish, iodine, or contrast media used in other diagnostic tests.

• Discontinue anticoagulant therapy, as ordered, to reduce the risk of complications from bleeding.

• Review activity restrictions and position requirements that may be necessary for the patient after the procedure, such as lying flat with the limb extended for 4 to 6 hours and using sandbags to apply pressure to the insertion site if a femoral sheath is used.

• Document the presence of peripheral pulses, noting their intensity. Mark the pulses so they may be easily located after the procedure.

Be sure to discuss postprocedure instructions with your patient.

After the procedure

• Determine if a hemostatic device, such as a collagen plug or suture closure system, was used to close the vessel puncture site. If either method was used, inspect the site for bleeding or oozing, redness, swelling, or hematoma formation. Maintain the patient on bed rest for 1 to 2 hours.

• Enforce bed rest for 8 hours if no hemostatic device was used. If the femoral route was used for catheter insertion, keep the patient's leg extended for 6 to 8 hours; if the antecubital fossa route was used, keep the arm extended for at least 3 hours.

• Monitor vital signs every 15 minutes for 2 hours, then every 30 minutes for the next 2 hours, and then every hour for 2 hours. If

no hematoma or other problems arise, check every 4 hours. If signs are unstable, check every 5 minutes and notify the doctor.
• Continually assess the insertion site for a hematoma or blood loss, and reinforce the pressure dressing as needed.
• Check the patient's color, skin temperature, and peripheral pulse below the puncture site.
• Administer I.V. fluids as ordered (usually 100 ml/hour) to promote excretion of the contrast medium. Monitor for signs of fluid overload.
• Watch for signs of chest pain, shortness of breath, abnormal heart rate, dizziness, diaphoresis, nausea or vomiting, or extreme fatigue. Notify the doctor immediately if these complications occur.

Imaging and radiographic tests

Imaging and radiographic testing produces detailed images of the heart and its ability to function. These tests include echocardiography, cardiac magnetic resonance imaging (MRI), cardiac positron-emission tomography (PET) scanning, cardiac blood pool imaging, technetium-99m (^{99m}Tc) pyrophosphate scanning, thallium scanning, duplex ultrasonography, and venography.

Imaging and radiographic tests can produce detailed images of the heart.

Are you getting my good side?

Echocardiography

Echocardiography is used to examine the size, shape, and motion of cardiac structures. In this procedure, a transducer is placed at an acoustic window (an area where bone and lung tissue are absent) on the patient's chest. The transducer directs sound waves toward cardiac structures, which reflect these waves.

Echo, echo

The transducer picks up the echoes, converts them to electrical impulses, and relays them to an echocardiography machine for display on a screen and for recording on a strip chart or videotape. The most commonly used echocardiographic techniques are M-mode (motion mode) and two-dimensional.

How picky

In M-mode echocardiography, a single, pencil-like ultrasound beam strikes the heart, producing an "ice pick," or vertical, view of cardiac structures. This mode is especially useful for precisely viewing cardiac structures.

A big fan of two-dimensional echocardiography

In two-dimensional echocardiography, the ultrasound beam rapidly sweeps through an arc, producing a cross-sectional, or fan-shaped, view of cardiac structures; this technique is useful for recording lateral motion and providing the correct spatial relationship between cardiac structures. In many cases, both techniques are performed to complement each other.

TEE combination

In transesophageal echocardiography (TEE), ultrasonography is combined with endoscopy to provide a better view of the heart's structures. (See *A closer look at TEE.*)

In exercise echocardiography and dobutamine stress echocardiography, a two-dimensional echocardiogram records cardiac wall motion during exercise or while dobutamine is being infused. (See *Teaching about cardiac stress testing.*)

Echo abnormalities

The echocardiogram may detect mitral stenosis, mitral valve prolapse, aortic insufficiency, wall motion abnormalities, and pericardial effusion (excess pericardial fluid).

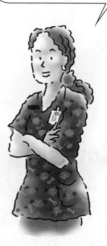

Echocardiography can give you an "ice pick" vertical view of heart structures or a fan-shaped cross section of the heart.

A closer look at TEE

In transesophageal echocardiography (TEE), ultrasonography is combined with endoscopy to provide a better view of the heart's structures.

How it's done

A small transducer is attached to the end of a gastroscope and inserted into the esophagus so that images of the heart's structure can be taken from the posterior of the heart. This test causes less tissue penetration and interference from chest wall structures and produces high-quality images of the thoracic aorta (except for the superior ascending aorta, which is shadowed by the trachea).

And why

TEE is used to evaluate valvular disease or repairs. It's also used to diagnose:

• thoracic and aortic disorders
• endocarditis
• congenital heart disease
• intracardiac thrombi
• tumors.

Teaching about cardiac stress testing

Exercise echocardiography and dobutamine stress echocardiography are types of cardiac stress testing that detect changes in heart wall motion through the use of two-dimensional echocardiography during exercise or a dobutamine infusion. Imaging is done before and after either exercise or dobutamine administration. Usually, these tests are performed to:

* identify the cause of chest pain
* detect heart abnormalities, obstructions, or damage
* determine the heart's functional capacity after myocardial infarction or cardiac surgery
* evaluate myocardial perfusion
* measure the heart chambers
* set limits for an exercise program.

Preparing your patient

When preparing your patient for these tests, cover the following points:

* Explain that this test will evaluate how his heart performs under stress and how specific heart structures work under stress.
* Instruct the patient not to eat, smoke, or drink alcohol or caffeinated beverages for at least 4 hours before the test.
* Advise him to ask his doctor whether he should withhold current medications before the test.
* Tell him to wear a two-piece outfit because he'll be removing all clothing above the waist and will wear a hospital gown.
* Explain that electrodes will be placed on his chest and arms to obtain an initial electrocardiogram (ECG). Mention that the areas where electrodes are placed will be cleaned with alcohol and that the skin will be abraded for optimal electrode contact.
* Tell him that an initial echocardiogram will be performed while he's lying down. Conductive gel, which feels warm, will be placed on his chest. Then a special transducer will be placed at various angles on his chest to visualize different parts of his heart. Emphasize that he must remain still to prevent distorting the images.
* Inform the patient that the entire procedure should take 60 to 90 minutes. Explain that the doctor will compare these echocardiograms to diagnose his heart condition.

Explaining exercise echocardiography

If the patient will have an exercise stress test after the initial echocardiogram, cover these teaching points:

* Tell him he'll walk on the treadmill at a prescribed rate for a predetermined time to raise his heart rate. After he reaches the prescribed heart rate, he'll lie down and a second echocardiogram will be done.
* Explain that he may feel tired, sweaty, and slightly short of breath during the test. If his symptoms are severe or chest pain develops, the test will be stopped.
* Reassure him that his blood pressure will be monitored during the test. After the test is complete, his ECG and blood pressure will be monitored for 10 minutes.

Describing the dobutamine stress test

If the patient will undergo a dobutamine stress test after the initial echocardiogram, cover these teaching points:

* Explain that an I.V. line will be inserted into his vein for the dobutamine infusion. Tell him that this drug will increase his heart rate without exercise. Tell him to expect initial discomfort when the I.V. line is inserted. Mention that, during the infusion, he may feel palpitations, shortness of breath, and fatigue.
* Inform the patient that a second echocardiogram will be done during the dobutamine infusion. After the drug is infused and his heart rate reaches the desired level, a third echocardiogram will be obtained.
* Reassure the patient that his blood pressure will be monitored during the test.

Nursing considerations

* Explain the procedure to the patient, and advise him to remain still during the test because movement can distort results. Tell him that conductive gel is applied to the chest and a quarter-sized transducer is placed directly over the gel. Because pressure is exerted to keep the transducer in contact with the skin, warn the patient that he may feel minor discomfort.
* After the procedure, remove the conductive gel from the skin.

Cardiac magnetic resonance imaging

Also known as *nuclear magnetic resonance*, MRI yields high-resolution, tomographic, three-dimensional images of body structures. It takes advantage of certain magnetically aligned body nuclei that fall out of alignment after radio frequency transmission. The MRI scanner records the signals the nuclei emit as they realign in a process called *precession* and then translates the signals into detailed pictures of body structures. The resulting images show tissue characteristics without lung or bone interference.

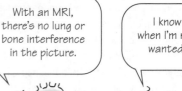

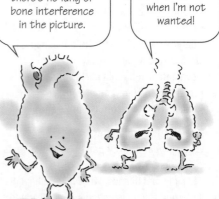

With an MRI, there's no lung or bone interference in the picture.

I know when I'm not wanted!

Look at leaflets

A cardiac MRI permits visualization of valve leaflets and structures, pericardial abnormalities and processes, ventricular hypertrophy, cardiac neoplasm, infarcted tissue, anatomic malformations, and structural deformities. It can be used to monitor the progression of ischemic heart disease and the effectiveness of treatment.

Nursing considerations

- Instruct the patient that he'll need to lie still during the test.
- Warn him that he'll hear a thumping noise.

Lose the jewels

- Have the patient remove all jewelry and other metallic objects before testing. A patient with an internal surgical clip, scalp vein needle, pacemaker, gold fillings, heart valve prosthesis, or other metal object in his body can't undergo an MRI.
- Permit the patient to resume activities as ordered.

Cardiac positron-emission tomography

Cardiac PET scanning combines elements of computed tomography scanning and conventional radionuclide imaging. Here's how it works: Radioisotopes are administered to the patient. These isotopes emit particles called *positrons*, which the PET scanner detects and reconstructs to form an image. One distinct advantage of PET scans is that positron emitters can be chemically "tagged" to biologically active molecules, such as glucose, enabling study of their uptake and distribution in tissue.

Cardiac PET scanning is used to detect CAD, evaluate myocardial metabolism and contractility, and distinguish viable cardiac tissue from infarcted tissue, especially during the early stages of MI. Reduced blood flow with increased glucose use indicates ischemia. Reduced blood flow with decreased glucose use indicates necrotic, scarred tissue. Normally, no areas of ischemic tissue are present on the scan.

Nursing considerations

• Warn the patient that cigarette smoking is restricted and medication use may be restricted before the test.
• Make sure the patient has signed an informed consent form.
• Document and report all allergies.
• Advise the patient that he may be connected to a cardiac monitor.
• Instruct the patient that he'll need to lie still during the test.
• Explain to the patient that he'll be given a radioactive substance, either by injection, inhalation, or I.V. infusion.
• Tell the patient that the test is usually painless. If an I.V. infusion is planned, the patient may experience slight discomfort from the needle puncture and tourniquet. If the radioisotope will be inhaled, explain to the patient that this procedure is painless.

Cardiac blood pool imaging

Cardiac blood pool imaging (multiple-gated acquisition [MUGA] scan) is used to evaluate regional and global ventricular performance. During a MUGA scan, the camera records 14 to 64 points of a single cardiac cycle, yielding sequential images that can be studied like a motion picture film to evaluate regional wall motion and determine the ejection fraction and other indices of cardiac function.

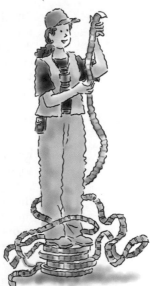

A MUGA scan of the heart can be studied just like a moving picture.

Various variations

There are many variations of the MUGA scan. In the stress MUGA test, the same test is performed at rest and after exercise to detect changes in ejection fraction and cardiac output. In the nitroglycerin MUGA test, the scintillation camera records points in the cardiac cycle after the sublingual administration of nitroglycerin to assess the drug's effect on ventricular function.

Nursing considerations

• An ECG is required to signal the computer and the camera to take images for each cardiac cycle.
• If arrhythmias interfere with a reliable ECG, the test may need to be postponed.

^{99m}Tc pyrophosphate scanning

^{99m}Tc pyrophosphate scanning, also known as *hot spot imaging* or PYP scanning, helps diagnose acute myocardial injury by showing the location and size of newly damaged myocardial tissue. Especially useful for diagnosing transmural infarction, this test works best when performed 12 hours to 6 days after symptom onset. It also helps diagnose right ventricular infarctions; locate true posterior infarctions; assess trauma, ventricular aneurysm, and heart tumors; and detect myocardial damage from a recent electric shock such as defibrillation.

Scanning the hot spots

In this test, the patient receives an injection of ^{99m}Tc pyrophosphate, a radioactive material absorbed by injured cells. A scintillation camera scans the heart and displays damaged areas as "hot spots," or bright areas. A spot's size usually corresponds to the injury size.

Nursing considerations

• Tell the patient that the doctor will inject ^{99m}Tc pyrophosphate into an arm vein about 3 hours before the start of this 45-minute test. Reassure him that the injection causes only transient discomfort and that it involves only negligible radiation exposure.
• Instruct the patient to remain still during the test.
• Permit the patient to resume activities, as ordered.

Thallium scanning

Also known as *cold spot imaging*, thallium scanning evaluates myocardial blood flow and myocardial cell status. This test helps determine areas of ischemic myocardium and infarcted tissue. It can also help evaluate coronary artery and ventricular function as well as pericardial effusion. Thallium imaging can also detect an MI in its first few hours. (See *Understanding thallium scanning*.)

Cold-hearted

The test uses thallium-201, a radioactive isotope that emits gamma rays and closely resembles potassium. When injected I.V., the isotope enters healthy myocardial tissue rapidly but enters areas with poor blood flow and damaged cells slowly. A camera counts the gamma rays and displays an image. Areas with heavy isotope uptake appear light, while areas with poor uptake, known as "cold spots," look dark. Cold spots represent areas of reduced myocardial perfusion.

Now I get it!

Understanding thallium scanning

In thallium scanning, areas with poor blood flow and ischemic cells fail to take up the isotope (thallium-201 or Cardiolite) and thus appear as cold spots on a scan. Thallium imaging should show normal distribution of the isotope throughout the left ventricle with no defects (cold spots).

What resting reveals

To distinguish normal from infarcted myocardial tissue, the doctor may order an exercise thallium scan followed by a resting perfusion scan. A resting perfusion scan helps differentiate between an ischemic area and an infarcted or scarred area of the myocardium. Ischemic myocardium appears as a reversible defect (the cold spot disappears). Infarcted myocardium shows up as a nonreversible defect (the cold spot remains).

Nursing considerations

- Tell the patient to avoid heavy meals, cigarette smoking, and strenuous activity for 24 hours before the test.
- If the patient is scheduled for an exercise thallium scan, advise him to wear comfortable clothes or pajamas and appropriate exercise shoes.
- After the procedure, permit the patient to resume activities, as ordered.

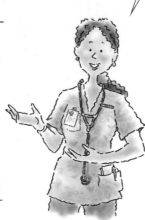

With duplex ultrasonography, a handheld transducer directs high-frequency sound waves that help to evaluate blood flow.

Duplex ultrasonography

Duplex ultrasonography is a noninvasive method used to evaluate blood flow in the major arteries and veins of the arms, legs, abdomen, and extracranial cerebrovascular system. The procedure involves using a handheld transducer to direct high-frequency sound waves into an artery or vein and its surrounding tissues.

Two-step process

In the first part of the test, the sound waves reflect off the blood vessel and surrounding tissues, creating images that are displayed on a monitor. Then additional sound waves are directed specifically into the vessel to be studied. These sound waves strike moving red blood cells within the vessel at one frequency and are reflected back to the transducer at another frequency. This change in frequency produces an audible Doppler signal that corresponds to blood flow velocity within the vessel. The speed, direction, and pattern of the blood flow are displayed on the monitor as a spectral waveform. The size and shape of the imaged blood vessel can also be measured.

Diagnosing duplex

Duplex ultrasonography can be used to diagnose diseases of the arteries and the veins, such as atherosclerotic blockages, arterial thrombosis or emboli, aneurysms, pseudoaneuryms, arterial dissections, congenital abnormalities, arteriovenous fistulae, thrombophlebitis, and venous insufficiency. It can also be used to create maps of a patient's arteries and veins prior to transplant or bypass surgery.

Additional arterial analysis

Pulse volume recorder testing may be performed along with arterial duplex ultrasonography. This test yields quantitative recordings of the differences in arterial blood flow between various segments of the arms or legs. Several blood pressure cuffs are placed on the extremity and a handheld Doppler is used to record segmental systolic pressures and spectral waveforms from each cuff. By comparing the difference between each segment, the presence, location, and extent of arterial blockage can be determined.

Nursing considerations

• Explain the test to the patient. Emphasize that the test is noninvasive and that he won't feel the sound waves.
• Inform the patient that water-soluble conductive gel will be applied to his skin to conduct the sound waves into his tissues.
• Check with the vascular laboratory to determine whether special instructions or preparation is necessary. Note that some tests may require the patient to fast.

Venography of the lower limb

Also known as *ascending contrast phlebography*, a venography is a radiographic examination of veins in the lower extremity that may be used to assess the condition of the deep leg veins after injection of a contrast medium.

Not for everyone

This procedure isn't used for routine screening because it exposes the patient to relatively high doses of radiation and can cause such complications as phlebitis, local tissue damage and, occasionally, deep vein thrombosis (DVT). It's used in patients whose duplex ultrasound findings are unclear.

Nursing considerations

- Make sure the patient has signed an informed consent form.
- Document and report all allergies.
- Check the patient's history for and report hypersensitivity to iodine, iodine-containing foods, or contrast media.
- Reassure the patient that contrast media complications are rare, but tell him to immediately report nausea, severe burning or itching, constriction in the throat or chest, or dyspnea.
- Discontinue anticoagulant therapy as ordered.
- Administer sedation as ordered.
- Instruct the patient to restrict food and to drink only clear liquids for 4 hours before the test.
- Warn the patient that he might experience a burning sensation in the leg when the contrast medium is injected as well as some discomfort during the procedure.
- If DVT is documented, initiate therapy (anticoagulant therapy, bed rest, leg elevation or support) as ordered.

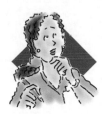

Quick quiz

1. Which test provides the best means of standardizing measurement of PT to monitor oral anticoagulant therapy?
  A. Plasma thrombin time
  B. INR
  C. Partial thromboplastin time
  D. Activated bleeding time

Answer: B. The INR is the best means of standardizing measurement of PT to monitor anticoagulant therapy.

2. The test that's most specific for myocardial damage is:
  A. CK.
  B. CK-MB.
  C. troponin I.
  D. myoglobin.

Answer: C. Troponin I is found only in the myocardium; it's more specific to myocardial damage than the other choices.

3.   Cardiac enzyme levels are monitored in the patient with chest pain for which reason?

A.   Serial measurement of enzyme levels reveals the extent of cardiac damage and helps monitor healing progress.

B.   Cardiac enzymes help identify the area of myocardial damage.

C.   Decreasing enzyme levels help to estimate the recovery time for the patient with myocardial damage.

D.   Cardiac enzyme results will reveal if the patient is truly having chest pain.

Answer: A. Serial enzymes indicate whether cardiac damage is occurring.

4.   TEE combines ultrasonography with which other procedure?

A.   Electrocardiography

B.   Endoscopic retrograde cholangiopancreatography

C.   Endoscopy

D.   Sigmoidoscopy

Answer: C. In TEE, ultrasonography is combined with endoscopy to provide a better view of the heart's structures.

5.   A noninvasive method of evaluating blood flow is:

A.   Duplex ultrasonography.

B.   venography.

C.   angiography.

D.   cardiac catheterization.

Answer: A. Duplex ultrasonography evaluates blood flow in the major blood vessels of the arms, legs, abdomen, and extracranial cerebrovascular system through use of high-frequency sound waves and a handheld transducer.

Scoring

☆☆☆   If you answered all five questions correctly, terrific! You test about tests with the best.

☆☆   If you answered four questions correctly, fab! You have the drop on diagnosing.

☆   If you answered fewer than four questions correctly, no need for a stress test. Another look at the chapter will get you the right results.

Treatments

Just the facts

In this chapter, you'll learn:

♦ treatments for cardiovascular disorders

♦ patient preparation for specific types of cardiovascular treatments

♦ monitoring and home care techniques for the patient after discharge.

A look at treatments for cardiovascular disorders

Many treatments are available for patients with cardiovascular disorders; the dramatic ones, such as heart transplantation and artificial heart insertion, have received a lot of publicity. However, some more commonly used treatment measures include drug therapy, surgery, balloon catheter treatments, defibrillation, synchronized cardioversion, and pacemaker insertion.

Drug therapy

Several types of drugs are critical to the treatment of cardiovascular disorders. These drugs include:
- adrenergics
- antianginals
- antiarrhythmics
- anticoagulants
- antihypertensives
- antilipemics
- diuretics
- thrombolytics.

Looks like we're on!

Many drug types play critical roles in the treatment of cardiovascular disorders.

Detailed information about cardiovascular drugs can be found in the appendix, Guide to cardiovascular drugs.

Surgery

Despite successful advances, such single- and multiple-organ transplants, improved immunosuppressants, and improved ventricular assist devices (VADs), far more patients undergo conventional surgeries. Surgeries for the treatment of disorders of the cardiovascular system include coronary artery bypass graft (CABG), minimally invasive direct coronary artery bypass (MIDCAB), heart transplantation, vascular repair, valve surgery, and VAD insertion.

Coronary artery bypass graft

A CABG circumvents an occluded coronary artery with an autogenous graft (usually a segment of the saphenous vein or internal mammary artery), thereby restoring blood flow to the myocardium. CABG techniques vary according to the patient's condition and the number of arteries needing bypass.

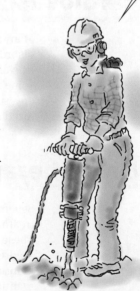

The most common bypass builds a new road from the aorta to a coronary artery.

Construction ahead

The most common procedure, aortocoronary bypass, involves suturing one end of the autogenous graft to the ascending aorta and the other end to a coronary artery distal to the occlusion. (See *Bypassing coronary occlusions*.)

CABG candidates

More than 200,000 Americans (most of them male) undergo CABG each year, making it one of the most common cardiac surgeries. Prime candidates include patients with severe angina from atherosclerosis and others with coronary artery disease who have a high risk of myocardial infarction (MI). Successful CABG can relieve anginal pain, improve cardiac function and, possibly, enhance the patient's quality of life.

CABG caveat

Although the surgery relieves pain in about 90% of patients, its long-term effectiveness is unclear. (See *Relieving anginal pain with EECP*, page 94.) In addition, such problems as graft closure and development of atherosclerosis in other coronary arteries may make repeat surgery necessary. In addition, because CABG doesn't resolve the underlying disease associated with arterial blockage, CABG may not reduce the risk of MI recurrence.

Bypassing coronary occlusions

After the patient receives general anesthesia, autocoronary by-pass surgery begins with graft harvesting. The surgeon makes a series of incisions in the patient's thigh or calf and removes a saphenous vein segment for grafting. Most surgeons prefer to use a segment of the internal mammary artery.

Exposing the heart
Once the autografts are obtained, the surgeon performs a me-dial sternotomy to expose the heart and then initiates car-diopulmonary bypass.

To reduce myocardial oxygen demands during surgery and to protect the heart, the surgeon induces cardiac hypothermia and standstill by injecting a cold, cardioplegic solution (potassi-um-enriched saline solution) into the aortic root.

One fine sewing lesson
After the patient is prepared, the surgeon sutures one end of the venous graft to the ascending aorta and the other end to a patent coronary artery that's distal to the occlusion. The graft is sutured in a reversed position to promote proper blood flow. The surgeon repeats this procedure for each occlusion to be bypassed.

In the example depicted below, saphenous vein segments bypass occlusions in three sections of the coronary artery.

Finishing up
When the grafts are in place, the surgeon flushes the cardio-plegic solution from the heart and discontinues cardiopul-monary bypass. He then implants epicardial pacing electrodes, inserts a chest tube, closes the incision, and applies a sterile dressing.

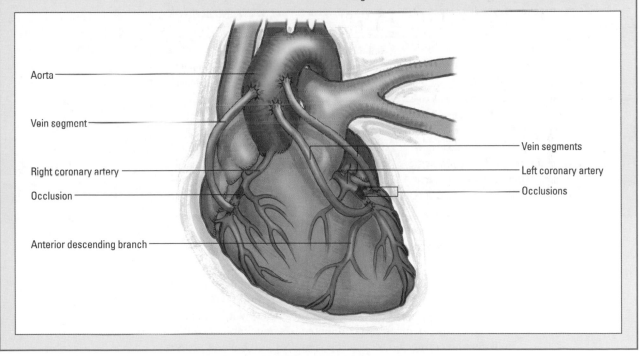

Relieving anginal pain with EECP

Enhanced external counterpulsation (EECP) can be used to provide pain relief to people with recurrent stable angina when standard treatments fail. It can reduce coronary ischemia, improve exercise tolerance, and stimulate the development of collateral circulation.

Candidates for EECP

A patient may be considered for EECP if he:
• isn't a candidate for revascularization or if the risk of these procedures is too high
• has recurrent angina even with drug therapy and revascularization
• declines invasive procedures.

Patients with diabetes may benefit from EECP because of their increased risk of cardiovascular disease and unfavorable outcomes to revascularization procedures.

Understanding EECP

In EECP, pneumatic cuffs are wrapped around the patient's calves, thighs, and lower buttocks. During diastole, the cuffs are sequentially inflated, starting with the calves and moving up the legs. The compression of arteries in the legs promotes retrograde arterial blood flow and coronary perfusion, similar to intra-aortic counterpulsation. At the end of diastole, cuff pressure is instantly released, reducing vascular resistance and decreasing the heart's workload. EECP may also stimulate collateral circulation around stenosed or occluded coronary arteries.

In contrast to intra-aortic counterpulsation, EECP enhances venous return, increasing the filling pressures of the heart and, consequently, cardiac output.

Adverse effects of EECP

Although rare, the patient may experience leg discomfort, bruising, blisters, or skin abrasions from frequent cuff inflation. Because EECP increases venous return, patients with decreased left ventricular ejection fraction or heart failure should be monitored closely for pulmonary congestion or edema during and after the procedure.

Other uses of EECP

Therapeutic uses of EECP may be expanded to the treatment of other cardiovascular diseases. Studies are currently looking at using EECP to treat moderate and severe left ventricular dysfunction and cardiomyopathy. Research is also being conducted on the use of EECP as an interim treatment in acute coronary syndromes and acute myocardial infarction until revascularization can be performed.

Patient preparation

• Reinforce the doctor's explanation of the surgery.
• Explain the complex equipment and procedures used in the intensive care unit (ICU) or postanesthesia care unit (PACU).
• Explain that the patient awakens from surgery with an endotracheal (ET) tube in place and connected to a mechanical ventilator. He'll also be connected to a cardiac monitor and have in place a nasogastric (NG) tube, a chest tube, an indwelling urinary catheter, arterial lines, epicardial pacing wires and, possibly, a pulmonary artery (PA) catheter. Tell him that discomfort is minimal and that the equipment is removed as soon as possible.

• Review incentive spirometry techniques and range-of-motion (ROM) exercises with the patient. Also teach him to splint his incision.
• Make sure that the patient or a responsible family member has signed a consent form.
• Before surgery, prepare the patient's skin as ordered.
• Immediately before surgery, begin cardiac monitoring and then assist with PA catheterization and insertion of arterial lines. Some facilities insert PA catheters and arterial lines in the operating room, before surgery.

Monitoring and aftercare

• After a CABG, look for signs of hemodynamic compromise, such as severe hypotension, decreased cardiac output, and shock.
• Begin warming procedures according to your facility's policy.
• Check and record vital signs and hemodynamic parameters every 5 to 15 minutes until the patient's condition stabilizes. Administer medications as ordered and titrate according to the patient's response.
• Monitor electrocardiograms (ECGs) continuously for disturbances in heart rate and rhythm. If you detect serious abnormalities, notify the doctor and be prepared to assist with epicardial pacing or, if necessary, cardioversion or defibrillation.

Reading the map

• To ensure adequate myocardial perfusion, keep arterial pressure within the limits set by the doctor. Usually, mean arterial pressure (MAP) less than 70 mm Hg results in inadequate tissue perfusion; pressure greater than 110 mm Hg can cause hemorrhage and graft rupture. Monitor pulmonary artery pressure (PAP), central venous pressure (CVP), left atrial pressure, and cardiac output as ordered.
• Frequently evaluate the patient's peripheral pulses, capillary refill time, and skin temperature and color and auscultate for heart sounds; report abnormalities.
• Evaluate tissue oxygenation by assessing breath sounds, chest excursion, and symmetry of chest expansion. Check arterial blood gas (ABG) results every 2 to 4 hours, and adjust ventilator settings to keep arterial blood gas values within ordered limits.
• Maintain chest tube drainage at the ordered negative pressure (usually –10 to –40 cm H_2O), and assess regularly for hemorrhage, excessive drainage (greater than 200 ml/hour), and sudden decrease or cessation of drainage.

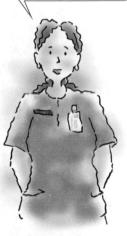

After a CABG, be on the lookout for severe hypotension, decreased cardiac output, and shock. These signs indicate hemodynamic compromise.

In and out

- Monitor the patient's intake and output, and assess for electrolyte imbalance, especially hypokalemia and hypomagnesemia. Assess urine output at least hourly during the immediate postoperative period and then less frequently as the patient's condition stabilizes.
- As the patient's incisional pain increases, give an analgesic or other drugs, as ordered.
- Throughout the recovery period, assess for signs and symptoms of stroke, pulmonary embolism, and impaired renal perfusion.
- After weaning the patient from the ventilator and removing the ET tube, provide chest physiotherapy. Start with incentive spirometry, and encourage the patient to splint his incision, cough, turn frequently, and deep-breathe. Assist with ROM exercises, as ordered, to enhance peripheral circulation and prevent thrombus formation.

Postperi problems

- Explain that postpericardiotomy syndrome commonly develops after open-heart surgery. Instruct the patient about signs and symptoms, such as fever, muscle and joint pain, weakness, and chest discomfort.
- Prepare the patient for the possibility of postoperative depression, which may not develop until weeks after discharge. Reassure him that this depression is normal and should pass quickly.
- Maintain nothing-by-mouth status until bowel sounds return. Then begin the patient on clear liquids and advance his diet as tolerated and as ordered. Tell the patient to expect sodium and cholesterol restrictions and explain that this diet can help reduce the risk of recurrent arterial occlusion.
- Monitor for postoperative complications, such as stroke, pulmonary embolism, pneumonia, and impaired renal perfusion.
- Gradually allow the patient to increase activities as ordered. (See *Using cardiac rehab*.)

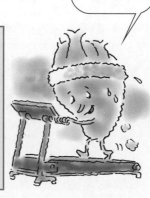

> Cardiac rehab can help me get back in shape.

Using cardiac rehab

Cardiac rehab is an exercise program to monitor and improve cardiovascular status and help the patient learn how to manage heart disease.

Elements of cardiac rehab include:
- individualized exercise program
- diet, nutrition, and weight control
- stress management
- reduction of risk factors
- lipid and cholesterol control.

Sessions are held weekly, based on patient need and tolerance. Heart rate, blood pressure, and symptoms are continuously monitored during the session. Education is provided based on the patient's individual needs.

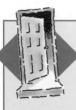

No place like home

Teaching the patient after CABG

Before discharge from the hospital, instruct the patient to:
• watch for and immediately notify the doctor of any signs of infection (redness, swelling, or drainage from the leg or chest incisions; fever; or sore throat) or possible arterial reocclusion (angina, dizziness, dyspnea, rapid or irregular pulse, or prolonged recovery time from exercise)
• call the doctor in the case of weight gain greater than 3 lb (1.4 kg) in 1 week
• follow his prescribed diet, especially sodium and cholesterol restrictions
• maintain a balance between activity and rest by trying to sleep at least 8 hours each night,

scheduling a short rest period each afternoon, and resting frequently when engaging in tiring physical activity
• participate in an exercise program or cardiac rehabilitation, if prescribed
• follow lifestyle modifications (no smoking, improved diet, and regular exercise) to reduce atherosclerotic progression
• contact a local chapter of the Mended Hearts Club and the American Heart Association for information and support
• make sure he understands the dose, frequency of administration, and possible adverse effects of prescribed medications.

• Monitor the incision site for signs of infection or drainage.
• Provide support to the patient and his family to help them cope with recovery and lifestyle changes. (See *Teaching the patient after CABG*.)

Minimally invasive direct coronary artery bypass

Until recently, cardiac surgery required stopping the heart and using cardiopulmonary bypass to oxygenate and circulate blood. Now, MIDCAB can be performed on a pumping heart through a small thoracotomy incision. The patient may receive only right lung ventilation along with drugs, such as beta-adrenergic blockers, to slow the heart rate and reduce heart movement during surgery.

It's a good thing

Advantages of MIDCAB include shorter hospital stays, use of shorter-acting anesthetic agents, fewer postoperative complications (such as infection), earlier extubation, reduced cost, smaller incisions, and earlier return to work. Patients eligible for MIDCAB include those with proximal left anterior descending lesions and some lesions of the right coronary and circumflex arteries.

Wow! MIDCAB can be performed while I pump!

Patient preparation

• Review the procedure with the patient and answer his questions. Tell the patient that he'll be extubated in the operating room or within 2 to 4 hours after surgery.
• Teach the patient to splint his incision, cough and breathe deeply, and use an incentive spirometer.
• Explain the use of pain medications after surgery as well as nonpharmacologic methods to control pain.
• Let the patient know that he should be able to walk with assistance the first postoperative day and be discharged within 48 hours.

Monitoring and aftercare

• After a MIDCAB, look for signs of hemodynamic compromise, such as severe hypotension, decreased cardiac output, and shock.
• Check and record vital signs and hemodynamic parameters every 5 to 15 minutes until the patient's condition stabilizes. Administer medications as ordered and titrate according to the patient's response.
• Monitor ECGs continuously for disturbances in heart rate and rhythm. If you detect serious abnormalities, notify the doctor and be prepared to assist with epicardial pacing or, if necessary, cardioversion or defibrillation.
• To ensure adequate myocardial perfusion, keep arterial pressure within the limits set by the doctor. Usually, MAP less than 70 mm Hg results in inadequate tissue perfusion; pressure greater than 110 mm Hg can cause hemorrhage and graft rupture. Monitor PAP, CVP, left atrial pressure, and cardiac output if a PA catheter was inserted.
• Frequently evaluate the patient's peripheral pulses, capillary refill time, and skin temperature and color and auscultate for heart sounds; report abnormalities.
• Evaluate tissue oxygenation by assessing breath sounds, chest excursion, and symmetry of chest expansion.
• Monitor the patient's intake and output, and assess for electrolyte imbalance, especially hypokalemia and hypomagnesemia. Assess urine output at least hourly during the immediate postoperative period and then less frequently as the patient's condition stabilizes.
• Provide analgesia or encourage the use of patient-controlled analgesia, if appropriate.

> After a MIDCAB, check and record vital signs and hemodynamic parameters every 5 to 15 minutes until the patient's condition stabilizes.

• Throughout the recovery period, assess for symptoms of stroke, pulmonary embolism, and impaired renal perfusion.
• Provide chest physiotherapy and incentive spirometry, and encourage the patient to splint his incision, cough, turn frequently, and deep-breathe. Assist with ROM exercises, as ordered, to enhance peripheral circulation and prevent thrombus formation.
• Explain that postpericardiotomy syndrome commonly develops after open-heart surgery. Instruct the patient about signs and symptoms, such as fever, muscle and joint pain, weakness, and chest discomfort.
• Prepare the patient for the possibility of postoperative depression, which may not develop until weeks after discharge. Reassure him that this depression is normal and should pass quickly.
• Maintain nothing-by-mouth status until bowel sounds return. Then begin the patient on clear liquids and advance his diet as tolerated and as ordered. Tell the patient to expect sodium and cholesterol restrictions and explain that this diet can help reduce the risk of recurrent arterial occlusion.
• Gradually allow the patient to increase activities as ordered.
• Monitor the incision site for signs of infection or drainage.
• Provide support to the patient and his family to help them cope with recovery and lifestyle changes. (See *Teaching the patient after MIDCAB*.)

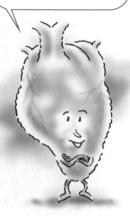

Coughing is encouraged following cardiac procedures such as MIDCAB.

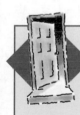

No place like home

Teaching the patient after MIDCAB

Before discharge from the facility following minimally invasive direct coronary artery bypass (MIDCAB), instruct the patient to:
• continue with the progressive exercise started in the facility
• perform coughing and deep-breathing exercises (while splinting the incision with a pillow to reduce pain) and use the incentive spirometer to reduce pulmonary complications
• avoid lifting objects that weigh more than 10 lb (4.5 kg) for the next 4 to 6 weeks
• wait 2 to 4 weeks before resuming sexual activity

• check the incision site daily and immediately notify the doctor of signs of infection (redness, foul-smelling drainage, or swelling) or possible graft occlusion (slow, rapid, or irregular pulse; angina; dizziness; or dyspnea)
• perform necessary incisional care
• follow lifestyle modifications
• take medications as prescribed and report adverse effects to the doctor
• consider participation in a cardiac rehabilitation program.

Heart transplantation

Heart transplantation involves the replacement of a person's heart with a donor heart. It's the treatment of choice for patients with end-stage cardiac disease who have a poor prognosis, estimated survival of 6 to 12 months, and poor quality of life. A heart transplant candidate typically has uncontrolled symptoms and no other surgical options.

No guarantee

Transplantation doesn't guarantee a cure. Serious postoperative complications include infection and tissue rejection. Most patients experience one or both of these complications post-operatively.

Rejection and infection

Rejection typically occurs in the first 6 weeks after surgery, but it may still occur after this time. The patient is treated with mono-clonal antibodies and potent immunosuppressants. The resulting immunosuppression places the patient at risk for life-threatening infection.

Patient preparation

• Reinforce the doctor's explanation of the surgery.
• Explain the complex equipment and procedures used in the ICU and PACU.
• Explain that the patient awakens from surgery with an ET tube in place and connected to a mechanical ventilator. He'll also be connected to a cardiac monitor and have in place an NG tube, a chest tube, an indwelling urinary catheter, arterial lines, epicardial pacing wires and, possibly, a PA catheter. Tell him that discomfort is minimal and that the equipment is removed as soon as possible.
• Review incentive spirometry techniques and ROM exercises with the patient.
• Make sure that the patient or a responsible family member has signed an informed consent form.
• Before surgery, prepare the patient's skin as ordered.
• Immediately before surgery, begin cardiac monitoring and then assist with PA catheterization and insertion of arterial lines. Some facilities insert PA catheters and arterial lines in the operating room, before surgery.

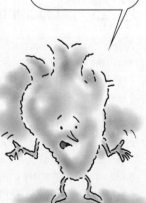

Most patients experience infection, tissue rejection, or both after heart transplantation.

Monitoring and aftercare

• Provide emotional support to the patient and his family. Begin to address their fears by discussing the procedure, possible complications, and the impact of transplantation and a prolonged recovery period on the patient's life.

• After surgery, maintain reverse isolation.

• Administer immunosuppressants, and monitor the patient closely for signs of infection. Transplant recipients may exhibit only subtle signs because immunosuppressants mask obvious signs.

• Monitor vital signs every 15 minutes until stabilized, and assess the patient for signs of hemodynamic compromise, such as hypotension, decreased cardiac output, and shock.

• If necessary, administer nitroprusside (Nipride) during the first 24 to 48 hours to control blood pressure. An infusion of dopamine can improve contractility and renal perfusion.

• Volume replacement with normal saline, plasma expanders, or blood products may be necessary to maintain CVP. Monitor the patient for signs and symptoms of fluid overload, such as edema, jugular vein distention, and increased PAPs.

• Patients with elevated PAP may receive prostaglandin E to produce pulmonary vasodilation and reduced right ventricular afterload.

• Monitor ECGs for rhythm disturbances.

• Maintain the chest tube drainage system at the prescribed negative pressure. Regularly assess for hemorrhage or sudden cessation of drainage.

When the body says no

• Continually assess the patient for signs of tissue rejection (decreased electrical activity on the ECG, right-axis shift, atrial arrhythmias, conduction defects, weight gain, lethargy, ventricular failure, jugular vein distention, and increased T-cell count).

• Keep in mind that the effects of denervated heart muscle or denervation (in which the vagus nerve is cut during heart transplant surgery) makes such drugs as edrophonium (Tensilon) and anticholinergics (such as atropine) ineffective. (See *Teaching the patient after heart transplantation*, page 102.)

> Since my surgery, I've experienced such problems as atrial arrhythmias, conduction defects, and jugular vein distention. I feel so rejected!

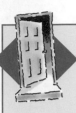

No place like home

Teaching the patient after heart transplantation

Before discharge from the facility, instruct the patient to:
• continue with the progressive exercise started in the facility
• perform coughing and deep-breathing exercises (while splinting the incision with a pillow to reduce pain) and use the incentive spirometer to reduce pulmonary complications
• avoid lifting objects that weigh more than 10 lb (4.5 kg) for the next 4 to 6 weeks
• wait 2 to 4 weeks before resuming sexual activity
• check the incision site daily and immediately notify the doctor of any signs of infection (such as redness, foul-smelling drainage, or swelling)
• perform necessary incisional care
• follow lifestyle modifications
• take medications (which will be lifelong), as prescribed, and report adverse effects to the doctor
• consider participation in a cardiac rehabilitation program, as advised
• immediately report any episodes of chest pain or shortness of breath
• avoid crowds and anyone with an infectious illness
• comply with follow-up visits as instructed.

Vascular repair

Vascular repair includes aneurysm resection, aneurysm exclusion, grafting, embolectomy, vena caval filtering, endarterectomy, vein stripping, and vein ablation. The specific surgery used depends on the type, location, and extent of vascular occlusion or damage. (See *Types of vascular repair.*)

Life and limb

Vascular repair can be used to treat:
• vessels damaged by arteriosclerotic or thromboembolic disorders (such as aortic aneurysm or arterial occlusive disease), trauma, infections, or congenital defects
• vascular obstructions that severely compromise blood flow
• vascular disease that doesn't respond to drug therapy or nonsurgical treatments such as balloon catheterization
• life-threatening dissecting or ruptured aortic aneurysms
• limb-threatening acute arterial occlusion.

Repair despairs

All vascular surgeries have the potential for vessel trauma, emboli, hemorrhage, infection, and other complications. Grafting carries added risks because the graft may occlude, narrow, dilate, or rupture.

Types of vascular repair

Several procedures exist to repair damaged or diseased vessels. These options include aortic aneurysm repair, vena caval filter insertion, embolectomy, and bypass grafting.

Aortic aneurysm repair

Aortic aneurysm repair involves removing or excluding an aneurysmal segment of the aorta. The surgeon first makes an incision to expose the aneurysm site. If necessary, the patient is placed on a cardiopulmonary bypass machine. Next, the surgeon clamps the aorta, resects the aneurysm, and repairs the damaged portion of the aorta. A synthetic bypass graft may be used.

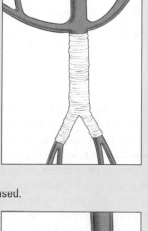

Vena caval filter insertion

A vena caval filter traps emboli in the vena cava, preventing them from reaching the pulmonary vessels. Inserted percutaneously by catheter, the vena caval filter, or *umbrella*, traps emboli but allows venous blood flow.

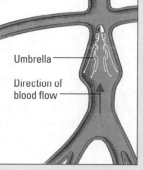

Umbrella

Direction of blood flow

Embolectomy

To remove an embolism from an artery, a surgeon may perform an embolectomy. In this procedure, he inserts a balloon-tipped indwelling catheter in the artery and passes it through the thrombus (as shown below left). He then inflates the balloon and withdraws the catheter to remove the thrombus (as shown below right).

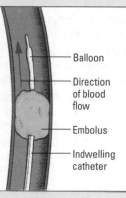

Balloon

Direction of blood flow

Embolus

Indwelling catheter

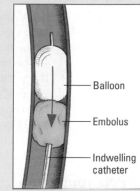

Balloon

Embolus

Indwelling catheter

Bypass grafting

Bypass grafting serves to bypass an arterial obstruction resulting from arteriosclerosis. After exposing the affected artery, the surgeon anastomoses a synthetic or autogenous graft to divert blood flow around the occluded arterial segment. The autogenous graft may be a vein or artery harvested from elsewhere in the patient's body. This illustration shows a femoropopliteal bypass.

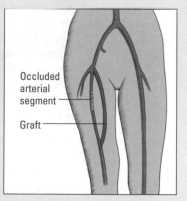

Occluded arterial segment

Graft

Patient preparation

• Make sure the patient and his family understand the doctor's explanation of the surgery and its possible complications.
• Tell the patient that he'll receive a general anesthetic and will awaken from the anesthetic in the ICU or PACU. Explain that he'll have an I.V. line in place, ECG electrodes for continuous cardiac monitoring and, possibly, an arterial line or a PA catheter to provide continuous pressure monitoring. He may also have a urinary catheter in place to allow accurate output measurement. If appropriate, explain that he'll be intubated and placed on mechanical ventilation.

Flow check

• Before surgery, perform a complete vascular assessment. Take vital signs to provide a baseline. Evaluate the strength and sound of the blood flow and the symmetry of the pulses, and note bruits. Record the temperature of the extremities, their sensitivity to motor and sensory stimuli, and pallor, cyanosis, or redness. Rate peripheral pulse volume and strength on a scale of 0 (pulse absent) to 4 (bounding pulse), and check capillary refill time by blanching the fingernail or toenail; normal refill time is less than 3 seconds.
• As ordered, instruct the patient to restrict food and fluids for at least 12 hours before surgery.

Keep your guard

• If the patient is awaiting surgery for aortic aneurysm repair, be on guard for signs and symptoms of acute dissection or rupture. Especially note sudden, severe, tearing pain in the chest, abdomen, or lower back; severe weakness; diaphoresis; tachycardia; or a precipitous drop in blood pressure. If any of these signs or symptoms occurs, notify the doctor immediately.

Monitoring and aftercare

• Check and record the patient's vital signs every 15 minutes until his condition stabilizes, then every 30 minutes for 1 hour, and hourly thereafter for 2 to 4 hours. Report hypotension and hypertension immediately.
• Auscultate heart, breath, and bowel sounds, and report abnormal findings. Monitor the ECG for abnormalities in heart rate or rhythm. Also monitor other pressure readings, and carefully record intake and output.
• Check the patient's dressing regularly for excessive bleeding.
• Assess the patient's neurologic and renal function, and report abnormalities.
• Provide analgesics, as ordered, for incisional pain.
• Frequently assess peripheral pulses, using a handheld Doppler if palpation is difficult. Mark on the skin the location of the Doppler

signals. Check all extremities bilaterally for muscle strength and movement, color, temperature, and capillary refill time.

• Change dressings and provide incision care, as ordered. Position the patient to avoid pressure on grafts and to reduce edema. Administer antithrombotics, as ordered, and monitor appropriate laboratory values to evaluate effectiveness.

• Assess for complications, and immediately report relevant signs and symptoms. (See *Vascular repair complications*.)

• As the patient's condition improves, take steps to wean him from the ventilator, if appropriate. To promote good pulmonary

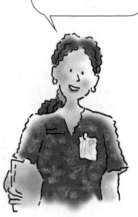

After vascular repair, position the patient to avoid pressure on grafts and to reduce edema.

Vascular repair complications

After a patient has undergone vascular repair surgery, monitor for these potential complications.

Complication	Signs and symptoms
Pulmonary infection	• Fever • Cough • Congestion • Dyspnea • Abnormal lung sounds
Infection	• Redness • Warmth • Drainage • Pain • Fever • Increased heart rate • Hypertension or hypotension
Renal dysfunction	• Low urine output • Elevated blood urea nitrogen and serum creatinine levels
Occlusion	• Reduced or absent peripheral pulses • Paresthesia • Severe pain • Cyanosis • Loss of Doppler signal in bypass graft
Hemorrhage	• Hypotension • Tachycardia • Restlessness and confusion • Shallow respirations • Abdominal pain • Increased abdominal girth

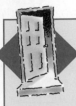

hygiene, encourage the patient to cough, turn, and deep-breathe frequently.
• Assist the patient with ROM exercises, as ordered, to prevent thrombus formation. Assist with early ambulation to prevent complications of immobility.
• Provide support to the patient and his family to help them cope with recovery and lifestyle changes. (See *Teaching the patient after vascular repair.*)

Valve surgery

Types of valve surgery include valvuloplasty (valvular repair), commissurotomy (separation of the adherent, thickened leaflets of the mitral valve), and valve replacement (with a mechanical or prosthetic valve).

Attention to prevention

Valve surgery is typically used to prevent heart failure in a patient with valvular stenosis or insufficiency accompanied by severe, unmanageable symptoms.

Pressure points

Because of the high pressure generated by the left ventricle during contraction, stenosis and insufficiency most commonly affect the mitral and aortic

Because they're under the most pressure, the mitral and aortic valves are the most likely to need repair.

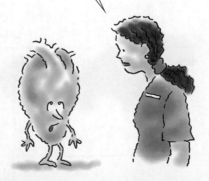

valves. Other indications for valve surgery depend on the patient's symptoms and on the affected valve:

• *aortic insufficiency*—valve replacement indicated after symptoms (palpitations, dizziness, dyspnea on exertion, angina, and murmurs) have developed or chest X-ray and ECG reveal left ventricular hypertrophy

• *aortic stenosis*—possibly produces no symptoms; valve replacement (or balloon valvuloplasty) recommended if cardiac catheterization reveals significant stenosis

• *mitral stenosis*—valvuloplasty or commissurotomy indicated if the patient develops fatigue, dyspnea, hemoptysis, arrhythmias, pulmonary hypertension, or right ventricular hypertrophy

• *mitral insufficiency*—valvuloplasty or valve replacement indicated when symptoms (dyspnea, fatigue, and palpitations) interfere with patient activities or in acute insufficiency (as in papillary muscle rupture).

It gets complicated

Although valve surgery carries a low risk of mortality, it can cause serious complications. Hemorrhage, for instance, may result from unligated vessels, anticoagulant therapy, or coagulopathy resulting from cardiopulmonary bypass during surgery. Stroke may result from thrombus formation caused by turbulent blood flow through the prosthetic valve or from poor cerebral perfusion during cardiopulmonary bypass. In valve replacement, bacterial endocarditis can develop within days of implantation or months later. Valve dysfunction or failure may occur as the prosthetic device wears out.

Patient preparation

• As necessary, reinforce and supplement the doctor's explanation of the procedure.
• Tell the patient that he'll awaken from surgery in an ICU or a PACU. Mention that he'll be connected to a cardiac monitor and have I.V. lines, an arterial line and, possibly, a PA or left atrial catheter in place.
• Explain that he'll breathe through an ET tube connected to a mechanical ventilator and that he'll have a chest tube in place.

Monitoring and aftercare

• Closely monitor the patient's hemodynamic status for signs of compromise. Watch especially for severe hypotension, decreased cardiac output, and shock. Check and record vital signs every 15 minutes until his condition stabilizes. Frequently assess heart

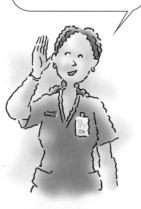

Distant heart sounds or new murmurs may indicate prosthetic valve failure.

sounds; report distant heart sounds or new murmurs, which may indicate prosthetic valve failure.

• Monitor the ECG continuously for disturbances in heart rate and rhythm, such as bradycardia, ventricular tachycardia, and heart block. Such disturbances may signal injury of the conduction system, which may occur during valve replacement from proximity of the atrial and mitral valves to the atrioventricular node. Arrhythmias may also result from myocardial irritability or ischemia, fluid and electrolyte imbalance, hypoxemia, or hypothermia. If you detect serious abnormalities, notify the doctor and be prepared to assist with temporary epicardial pacing.

Blood check

• Take steps to maintain the patient's MAP between 70 and 100 mm Hg. Also, monitor PAP and left atrial pressure as ordered.
• Frequently assess the patient's peripheral pulses, capillary refill time, and skin temperature and color and auscultate for heart sounds. Evaluate tissue oxygenation by assessing breath sounds, chest excursion, and symmetry of chest expansion. Report abnormalities.

Breathing check

• Check ABG values every 2 to 4 hours, and have the ventilator settings adjusted as needed.
• Maintain chest tube drainage at the prescribed negative pressure (usually –10 to –40 cm H_2O for adults). Assess chest tubes frequently for signs of hemorrhage, excessive drainage (greater than 200 ml/hour), and a sudden decrease or cessation of drainage.

Med check

• As ordered, administer analgesic, anticoagulant, antibiotic, antiarrhythmic, inotropic, and pressor medications as well as I.V. fluids and blood products. Monitor intake and output, and assess for electrolyte imbalances, especially hypokalemia. When anticoagulant therapy begins, evaluate its effectiveness by monitoring prothrombin time (PT) and International Normalized Ratio (INR) daily.
• After weaning from the ventilator and removing the ET tube, promote chest physiotherapy. Start the patient on incentive spirometry, and encourage him to splint the incision, cough, turn frequently, and deep-breathe.
• Throughout the patient's recovery period, observe him carefully for complications. (See *Teaching the patient after valve surgery*.)

> The effectiveness of anticoagulant therapy can be evaluated by monitoring PT and INR daily.

Teaching the patient after valve surgery

Before discharge from the facility, instruct the patient to:
• immediately report chest pain, fever, or redness, swelling, or drainage at the incision site
• immediately notify the doctor if signs or symptoms of heart failure (weight gain, dyspnea, or edema) develop
• notify the doctor if signs or symptoms of postpericardiotomy syndrome (fever, muscle and joint pain, weakness, or chest discomfort) develop

• follow the prescribed medication regimen and report adverse effects
• follow his prescribed diet, especially sodium and fat restrictions
• maintain a balance between activity and rest
• follow his exercise or rehabilitation program, if prescribed
• inform his dentist and other doctors of his prosthetic valve before undergoing surgery or dental work and to take prophylactic antibiotics before such procedures.

Ventricular assist device insertion

A VAD is a device that's implanted to support a failing heart. A VAD consists of a blood pump, cannulas, and a pneumatic or electrical drive console.

More output, less work

VADs are designed to decrease the heart's workload and increase cardiac output in patients with ventricular failure.

A temporary diversion

A VAD is commonly used while a patient waits for a heart transplant. In a surgical procedure, blood is diverted from a ventricle to an artificial pump. This pump, which is synchronized to the patient's ECG, then functions as the ventricle. (See *VAD: Help for a failing heart*, page 110.)

Right or left or both?

A VAD is used to provide systemic or pulmonary support, or both:
• A right VAD (RVAD) provides pulmonary support by diverting blood from the failing right ventricle to the VAD, which then pumps the blood to the pulmonary circulation by way of the VAD connection to the pulmonary artery.
• With a left VAD (LVAD), blood flows from the left ventricle to the VAD, which then pumps blood back to the body by way of the VAD connection to the aorta.
• When biventricular support is needed, both may be used.

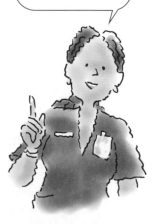

A VAD can help when the patient is waiting for a heart transplant.

VAD: Help for a failing heart

A ventricular assist device (VAD), which is commonly called a "bridge to transplant," is a mechanical pump that relieves the workload of the ventricle as the heart heals or until a donor heart is located.

Implantable

The typical VAD is implanted in the upper abdominal wall. An inflow cannula drains blood from the left ventricle into a pump, which then pushes the blood into the aorta through the outflow cannula.

Pump options

VADs are available as continuous flow or pulsatile pumps. A continuous flow pump fills continuously and returns blood to the aorta at a constant rate. A pulsatile pump may work in one of two ways: It may fill during systole and pump blood into the aorta during diastole, or it may pump irrespective of the patient's cardiac cycle.

Many types of VAD systems are available. This illustration shows a VAD implanted in the left abdominal wall and

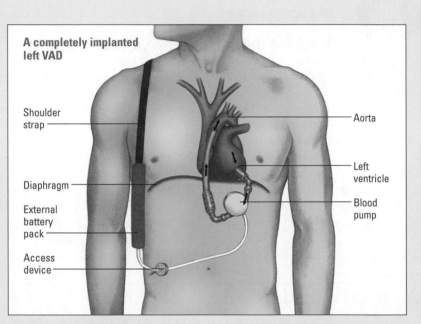

A completely implanted left VAD

- Shoulder strap
- Diaphragm
- External battery pack
- Access device
- Aorta
- Left ventricle
- Blood pump

connected to an external battery pack by a percutaneous lead.

Potential complications

Despite the use of anticoagulants, the VAD may cause thrombi formation, leading to pulmonary embolism or stroke. Other complications may include heart failure, bleeding, cardiac tamponade, or infection.

Patient preparation

- Prepare the patient and his family for VAD insertion; be sure to explain how the device works, what its purpose is, and what to expect after insertion.
- Make sure that informed consent is obtained.
- Continue close patient monitoring, including continuous ECG monitoring, pulmonary artery and hemodynamic status monitoring, and intake and output monitoring.

Monitoring and aftercare

- Assess the patient's cardiovascular status at least every 15 minutes until stable, and then hourly. Monitor blood pressure and hemodynamic parameters, including cardiac output and cardiac index, ECG, and peripheral pulses.

• Inspect the incision and dressing at least every hour initially, and then every 2 to 4 hours as indicated by the patient's condition.
• Monitor urine output hourly, and maintain I.V. fluid therapy, as ordered. Watch for signs of fluid overload or decreasing urine output.
• Assess chest tube drainage and function frequently. Notify the doctor if drainage is greater than 150 ml over 2 hours. Auscultate lungs for evidence of abnormal breath sounds. Evaluate oxygen saturation or mixed venous oxygen saturation levels, and administer oxygen as needed and as ordered.
• Obtain hemoglobin levels, hematocrit, and coagulation studies as ordered. Administer blood component therapy as indicated and as ordered.
• Assess for signs and symptoms of bleeding.
• Turn the patient every 2 hours and begin ROM exercises when he's stable.
• Administer antibiotics prophylactically, if ordered. (See *Teaching the patient after VAD insertion*.)

> Notify the doctor if chest tube drainage is greater than 150 ml over 2 hours.

Caution!

No place like home

Teaching the patient after VAD insertion

Before discharge following the insertion of a ventricular assist device (VAD), instruct the patient to:
• immediately report redness, swelling, or drainage at the incision site; chest pain; or fever
• immediately notify the doctor if signs or symptoms of heart failure (weight gain, dyspnea, or edema) develop
• follow the prescribed medication regimen and report adverse effects
• follow his prescribed diet, especially sodium and fat restrictions
• maintain a balance between activity and rest
• follow his exercise or rehabilitation program (if prescribed)
• comply with the laboratory schedule for monitoring International Normalized Ratio if the patient is receiving warfarin (Coumadin).

Balloon catheter treatments

Balloon catheter treatments for cardiovascular disorders include percutaneous balloon valvuloplasty, percutaneous transluminal coronary angioplasty (PTCA) and intra-aortic balloon pump (IABP) counterpulsation.

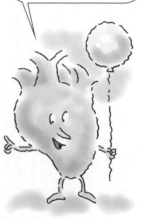

Percutaneous balloon valvuloplasty enlarges the orifice of a stenotic heart valve. That's my kind of inflation!

Percutaneous balloon valvuloplasty

Percutaneous balloon valvuloplasty may be performed in the cardiac catheterization laboratory. It's intended to improve valvular function by enlarging the orifice of a stenotic heart valve caused by congenital defect, calcification, rheumatic fever, or aging. A small balloon valvuloplasty catheter is introduced through the skin at the femoral vein.

Although valve surgery remains the treatment of choice for valvular heart disease, percutaneous balloon valvuloplasty offers an alternative for individuals who are considered poor candidates for surgery.

Balloon bungles

Unfortunately, elderly patients with aortic disease commonly experience restenosis 1 to 2 years after undergoing balloon valvuloplasty. In addition, despite decreasing the risks associated with more invasive procedures, balloon valvuloplasty can lead to complications, including:
• worsening valvular insufficiency by misshaping the valve so that it doesn't close completely
• pieces breaking off of the calcified valve, which may travel to the brain or lungs and cause embolism (rare)
• severely damaging delicate valve leaflets, requiring immediate surgery to replace the valve (rare)
• bleeding and hematoma at the arterial puncture site
• MI (rare), arrhythmias, myocardial ischemia, and circulatory defects distal to the catheter entry site.

Patient preparation

• Describe the procedure to the patient and his family, and tell them that it takes 1 to 4 hours to complete.
• Explain that a catheter will be inserted into an artery or a vein in the patient's groin and that he may feel pressure as the catheter moves along the vessel.
• Reassure the patient that although he'll be awake during the procedure, he'll be given a sedative. Instruct him to report any angina during the procedure.

• Check the patient's history for allergies; if he has had allergic reactions to shellfish, iodine, or contrast media, notify the doctor.
• Make sure the patient signs an informed consent form.
• Restrict food and fluids for at least 6 hours before the procedure.
• Make sure that the results of coagulation studies, complete blood count (CBC), serum electrolyte studies, blood typing and crossmatching, blood urea nitrogen (BUN), and serum creatinine are available.
• Obtain baseline vital signs and assess peripheral pulses.
• Apply ECG electrodes and insert an I.V. line if not already in place.
• Administer oxygen through a nasal cannula.
• Perform skin preparation according to your facility's policy.
• Give the patient a sedative, as ordered.

Monitoring and aftercare

• Assess the patient's vital signs and oxygen saturation every 15 minutes for the first hour and then every 30 minutes for 4 hours, unless his condition warrants more frequent checking. Monitor I.V. infusions, such as heparin or nitroglycerin, as indicated.
• Assess peripheral pulses distal to the catheter insertion site as well as the color, sensation, temperature, movement, and capillary refill time of the affected extremity.
• Monitor cardiac rhythm continuously, and assess hemodynamic parameters closely for changes.
• Instruct the patient to remain in bed for 8 hours and to keep the affected extremity straight. Maintain sandbags in position, if used to apply pressure to the catheter site. Elevate the head of the bed 15 to 30 degrees. If a hemostatic device was used to close the catheter insertion site, anticipate that the patient may be allowed out of bed in only a few hours.
• Assess the catheter site for hematoma, ecchymosis, and hemorrhage. If bleeding occurs, locate the artery and apply manual pressure; then notify the doctor.
• Administer I.V. fluids as ordered (usually 100 ml/hour) to promote excretion of the contrast medium. Be sure to assess for signs of fluid overload.
• Document the patient's tolerance of the procedure and status after it, including vital signs, hemodynamic parameters, appearance of the catheter site, ECG findings, condition of the extremity distal to the insertion site, complications, and necessary interventions.
(See *Teaching the patient after percutaneous balloon valvuloplasty.*)

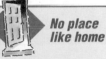

No place like home

Teaching the patient after percutaneous balloon valvuloplasty

Before discharge from the facility, instruct the patient to:
• resume normal activity
• notify the doctor if he experiences bleeding or increased bruising at the puncture site or recurrence of symptoms of valvular insufficiency, such as breathlessness or decreased exercise tolerance
• comply with regular follow-up visits.

Percutaneous transluminal coronary angioplasty

PTCA offers a nonsurgical alternative to coronary artery bypass surgery. The doctor uses a balloon-tipped catheter to dilate a coronary artery that has become narrowed because of atherosclerotic plaque. (See *Looking at PTCA.*)

Looking at PTCA

Percutaneous transluminal coronary angioplasty (PTCA) can open an occluded coronary artery without opening the chest. This procedure is outlined in the steps below.

First, the doctor must thread the catheter into the artery. The illustration below shows the entrance of a guide catheter into the coronary artery.

When angiography shows the guide catheter positioned at the occlusion site, the doctor carefully inserts a smaller double-lumen balloon catheter through the guide catheter and directs the balloon through the occlusion.

The doctor then inflates the balloon, causing arterial stretching and plaque fracture, as shown below. The balloon may need to be inflated or deflated several times until successful arterial dilation occurs.

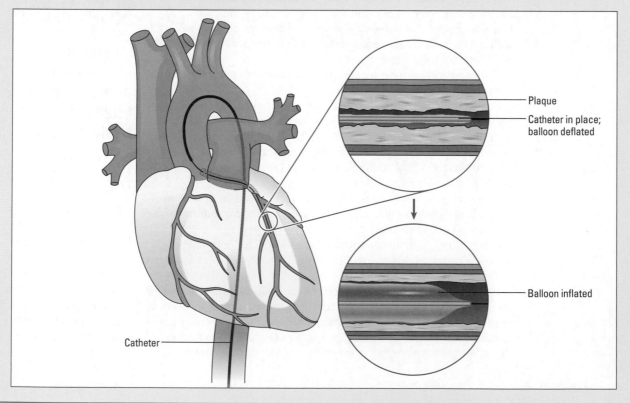

Plaque

Catheter in place; balloon deflated

Balloon inflated

Catheter

Shorter stay, fewer bucks

Performed in the cardiac catheterization laboratory under local anesthesia, PTCA doesn't involve a thoracotomy, so it's less costly and requires shorter hospitalization. Patients can usually walk the next day and return to work in 2 weeks.

Best working conditions

PTCA works best when lesions are readily accessible, non-calcified, less than 10 mm, concentric, discrete, and smoothly tapered. Patients with a history of less than 1 year of disabling angina make good candidates because their lesions tend to be softer and more compressible.

Harrowing narrowing

Complications of PTCA are acute vessel closure and late restenosis. To prevent restenosis, such procedures as stenting, atherectomy, and laser angioplasty may be performed. Also, vascular brachytherapy and new drug-eluting stents may decrease the incidence of restenosis. (See *Preventing restenosis*.)

> Although they may not be ready for the treadmill, patients can usually walk the day after PTCA.

Now I get it!

Preventing restenosis

Standard angioplasty is performed to remove the plaque blockage in the coronary artery. However, restenosis of the vessel is a frequent complication that occurs from scar tissue formation rather than plaque buildup.

Vascular brachytherapy

Vascular brachytherapy is the use of radiation in the coronary vessels to inhibit the development of this scar tissue, thus preventing restenosis of the vessel. The procedure involves a specialized radiation catheter that's inserted after angioplasty to direct beta radiation to the treated area for a few minutes. The radiation and catheter are then removed, with no radiation source being left in the body.

Coronary drug-eluting stents

Stents are used to open arteries that feed the heart, thereby improving circulation to myocardial tissue. One complication of stents is restenosis of the vessel. Drug-eluting stents open the artery and also release a drug to the implantation site that helps reduce restenosis. The drug works by blocking proliferation of smooth muscle cells.

Placement of drug-eluting stents during a cardiac catheterization or angioplasty procedure is the same as for regular stents. Post-procedural care is also the same.

Patient preparation

- Describe the procedure to the patient and his family, and tell them that it takes 1 to 4 hours to complete.
- Explain that a catheter will be inserted into an artery or a vein in the patient's groin and that he may feel pressure as the catheter moves along the vessel.
- Reassure the patient that although he'll be awake during the procedure, he'll be given a sedative. Instruct him to report any angina during the procedure.
- Explain that the doctor injects a contrast medium to outline the lesion's location. Warn the patient that he may feel a hot, flushing sensation or transient nausea during the injection.
- Check the patient's history for allergies; if he has had allergic reactions to shellfish, iodine, or contrast media, notify the doctor.
- Give 650 mg of aspirin the evening before the procedure, if ordered, to prevent platelet aggregation.
- Make sure that the patient has signed an informed consent form.
- Restrict food and fluids for at least 6 hours before the procedure.
- Make sure that the results of coagulation studies, CBC, serum electrolyte studies, blood typing and crossmatching, BUN, and serum creatinine are available.
- Obtain baseline vital signs and assess peripheral pulses.
- Apply ECG electrodes and insert an I.V. line if not already in place.
- Administer oxygen through a nasal cannula.
- Perform skin preparation according to your facility's policy.
- Give the patient a sedative as ordered.

Monitoring and aftercare

- Assess the patient's vital signs and oxygen saturation every 15 minutes for the first hour and then every 30 minutes for 4 hours, unless his condition warrants more frequent checking. Monitor I.V. infusions, such as heparin or nitroglycerin, as indicated.
- Assess peripheral pulses distal to the catheter insertion site as well as the color, sensation, temperature, movement, and capillary refill time of the affected extremity.
- Monitor cardiac rhythm continuously, and assess hemodynamic parameters closely for changes.
- Instruct the patient to remain in bed for 8 hours and to keep the affected extremity straight. Maintain sandbags in position, if used to apply pressure to the catheter site. Elevate the head of the bed 15 to 30 degrees. If a hemostatic device was used to close the catheter insertion site, anticipate that the patient may be allowed out of bed in only a few hours.

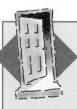

No place like home

Teaching the patient after PTCA

If the patient doesn't experience complications from percutaneous transluminal coronary angioplasty (PTCA), he may go home in 6 to 12 hours. Before discharge, instruct the patient to:

• call his doctor if he experiences any bleeding or bruising at the arterial puncture site

• return for a stress thallium imaging test and follow-up angiography, as recommended by his doctor

• report chest pain to the doctor because restenosis can occur after PTCA.

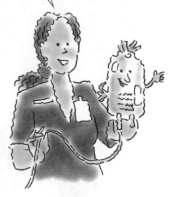

Administer I.V. fluids to promote excretion of the contrast medium.

• Administer I.V. fluids as ordered (usually 100 ml/hour) to promote excretion of the contrast medium. Be sure to assess for signs of fluid overload.

• Assess the catheter site for hematoma, ecchymosis, and hemorrhage. If bleeding occurs, locate the artery and apply manual pressure; then notify the doctor.

• After the doctor removes the catheter, apply direct pressure for at least 10 minutes and assess the site often.

• Document the patient's tolerance of the procedure and status afterward, including vital signs, hemodynamic parameters, appearance of the catheter site, ECG findings, condition of the extremity distal to the insertion site, complications, and necessary interventions. (See *Teaching the patient after PTCA*.)

Intra-aortic balloon pump counterpulsation

IABP counterpulsation temporarily reduces left ventricular workload and improves coronary perfusion. (See *Understanding a balloon pump*, page 118.)

What for?

IABP counterpulsation may benefit patients with:
• cardiogenic shock due to acute MI
• septic shock
• intractable angina before surgery
• intractable ventricular arrhythmias
• ventricular septal or papillary muscle ruptures.

It's also used for patients who suffer pump failure before or after cardiac surgery.

Now I get it!

Understanding a balloon pump

An intra-aortic balloon pump consists of a polyurethane balloon attached to an external pump console by means of a large-lumen catheter. It's inserted percutaneously through the femoral artery and positioned in the descending aorta just distal to the left subclavian artery and above the renal arteries.

Push...

This external pump works in precise counterpoint to the left ventricle, inflating the balloon with helium early in diastole and deflating it just before systole. As the balloon inflates, it forces blood toward the aortic valve, thereby raising pressure in the aortic root and augmenting diastolic pressure to improve coronary perfusion. It also improves peripheral circulation by forcing blood through the brachiocephalic, common carotid, and subclavian arteries arising from the aortic trunk.

...And pull

The balloon deflates rapidly at the end of diastole, creating a vacuum in the aorta. This vacuum action reduces aortic volume and pressure, thereby decreasing the resistance to left ventricular ejection (afterload). This decreased workload, in turn, reduces the heart's oxygen requirements and, combined with the improved myocardial perfusion, helps prevent or diminish myocardial ischemia.

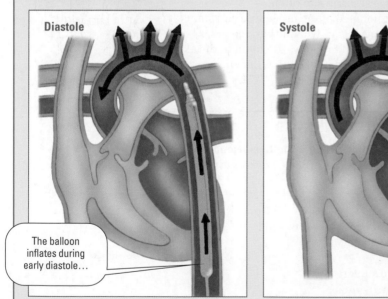

Diastole

Systole

The balloon inflates during early diastole...

...and deflates just before systole.

How so?

The doctor may perform balloon catheter insertion at the patient's bedside as an emergency procedure or in the operating room.

An IABP can be inserted right in the patient's room.

Patient preparation

• Explain to the patient that the doctor is going to place a catheter in the aorta to help his heart pump more easily. Tell him that, while the catheter is in place, he can't sit up, bend his knee, or flex his hip more than 30 degrees.
• Attach the patient to a continuous ECG monitor, and make sure he has an arterial line, a PA catheter, and a peripheral I.V. line in place.
• Gather a surgical tray for percutaneous catheter insertion, heparin, normal saline solution, the IABP catheter, and the pump console. Connect the ECG monitor to the pump console. Then prepare the femoral site.

Monitoring and aftercare

• After the IABP catheter is inserted, select either the ECG or the arterial waveform to regulate inflation and deflation of the balloon. With the ECG waveform, the pump inflates the balloon in the middle of the T wave (diastole) and deflates with the R wave (before systole). With the arterial waveform, the upstroke of the arterial wave triggers balloon inflation. (See *Timing IABP counterpulsation,* page 120.)
• Frequently assess the insertion site. Don't elevate the head of the bed more than 30 degrees, to prevent upward migration of the catheter and occlusion of the left subclavian artery. If the balloon occludes the artery, you may see a diminished left radial pulse, and the patient may report dizziness. Incorrect balloon placement may also cause flank pain or a sudden decrease in urine output.
• Assess distal pulses, color, temperature, and capillary refill of the patient's extremities every 15 minutes for the first 4 hours after insertion. After 4 hours, assess hourly for the duration of IABP therapy.
• Watch for signs of thrombus formation, such as a sudden weakening of pedal pulses, pain, and motor or sensory loss.
• Apply antiembolism stockings or antithrombic pumps as ordered.
• Encourage active ROM exercises every 2 hours for the arms, the unaffected leg, and the affected ankle.
• Maintain adequate hydration to help prevent thrombus formation.
• If bleeding occurs at the catheter insertion site, apply direct pressure and notify the doctor.

IABP counterpulsation patients should be watched for signs of thrombus formation, such as sudden weakening of pedal pulses, pain, and motor or sensory loss.

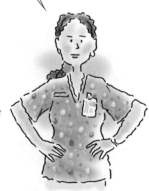

Now I get it!

Timing IABP counterpulsation

Intra-aortic balloon pump (IABP) counter-pulsation is synchronized with either the electrocardiogram or the arterial wave-form. Ideally, balloon inflation should begin when the aortic valve closes—at the dicrotic notch on the arterial waveform. Deflation should occur just before systole.

Proper timing is crucial

Early inflation can damage the aortic valve by forcing it closed, whereas late inflation permits most of the blood emerging from the ventricle to flow past the balloon, reducing pump effectiveness.

Late deflation increases the resistance against which the left ventricle must pump, possibly causing cardiac arrest.

At the peak

The illustration below depicts how IABP counterpulsation boosts peak diastolic pressure and lowers peak systolic and end-diastolic pressures.

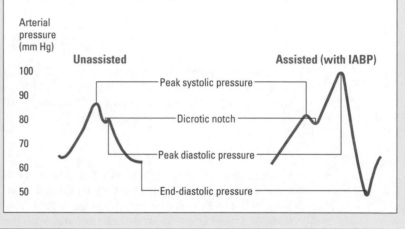

How timing affects waveforms

The arterial waveforms below show correctly and incorrectly timed balloon inflation and deflation.

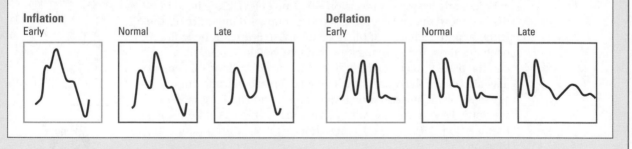

Quick response required

• An alarm on the console may indicate a gas leak from a damaged catheter or ruptured balloon. If the alarm sounds or you see blood in the catheter, shut down the pump console and immediately place the patient in Trendelenburg's position to prevent an embolus from reaching the brain. Then notify the doctor.

> **No place like home**
>
> ## Teaching the patient after IABP treatment
>
> Before discharge from the facility, instruct the patient to:
> - call his doctor if he experiences bleeding, bruising, or a pulsatile mass at the insertion site
> - return for follow-up testing as recommended by his doctor
> - report chest pain to the doctor.

Weaning ways

- After the patient's signs and symptoms of left-sided heart failure diminish, only minimal drug support is required, and the doctor begins weaning the patient from IABP counterpulsation by reducing the frequency of pumping or decreasing the balloon volume. A minimum volume or pumping ratio must be maintained to prevent thrombus formation. Most consoles have a flutter function that moves the balloon to prevent clot formation. Use the flutter function when the patient has been weaned from counterpulsation but the catheter hasn't yet been removed.
- To discontinue the IABP, the doctor deflates the balloon, clips the sutures, removes the catheter, and allows the site to bleed for 5 seconds to expel clots.
- After the doctor discontinues the IABP, apply direct pressure for 30 minutes and then apply a pressure dressing. Evaluate the site for bleeding and hematoma formation hourly for the next 4 hours. (See *Teaching the patient after IABP treatment.*)

Cardiovascular resynchronization techniques

When the electrical conduction of the heart is disrupted, cardiac output is diminished and perfusion of blood and oxygen to all body tissues is affected. Treatment to restore the heart's conduction needs to begin quickly. Such treatments include defibrillation, an implantable cardioverter-defibrillator (ICD), synchronized cardioversion, and pacemaker insertion.

Defibrillation

In defibrillation, electrode paddles are used to direct an electric current through the patient's heart. The current causes the myo-

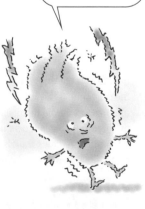

Shock it to me! In defibrillation, an electric current is directed through the heart.

cardium to depolarize, which in turn encourages the SA node to resume control of the heart's electrical activity.

The electrode paddles delivering the current may be placed on the patient's chest or, during cardiac surgery, directly on the myocardium. (See *Biphasic defibrillators*.)

Act early and quickly

Because some arrhythmias, such as ventricular fibrillation, can cause death if not corrected, the success of defibrillation depends on early recognition and quick treatment.

In addition to treating ventricular fibrillation, defibrillation may also be used to treat ventricular tachycardia that doesn't produce a pulse.

Automated external defibrillators

An automated external defibrillator (AED) has a cardiac rhythm analysis system. The AED interprets the patient's cardiac rhythm and gives the operator step-by-step directions on how to proceed if defibrillation is indicated. Most AEDs have a "quick-look" feature that allows visualization of the rhythm with the paddles before electrodes are connected.

Biphasic defibrillators

Most hospital defibrillators are monophasic, delivering a single current of electricity that travels in one direction between the two pads or paddles on the patient's chest. A large amount of electrical current is required for effective monophasic defibrillation.

Current flows to and fro
Biphasic defibrillators have recently been introduced into hospitals. Pad or paddle placement is the same as with the monophasic defibrillator. The difference is that during biphasic defibrillation, the electrical current discharged from the pads or paddles travels in a positive direction for a specified duration and then reverses and flows in a negative direction for the remaining time of the electrical discharge.

Energy efficient…
The biphasic defibrillator delivers two currents of electricity and lowers the defibrillation threshold of the heart muscle, making it possible to successfully defibrillate ventricular fibrillation with smaller amounts of energy. Instead of using 200 joules, an initial shock of 150 joules is usually effective.

… And adjustable…
The biphasic defibrillator is able to adjust for differences in impedance (the resistance of the current through the chest). This functionality reduces the number of shocks needed to terminate ventricular fibrillation.

…With less myocardial damage
Because the biphasic defibrillator requires lower energy levels and fewer shocks, damage to the myocardial muscle is reduced. Biphasic defibrillators used at the clinically appropriate energy level may be used for defibrillation and, in the synchronized mode, for synchronized cardioversion.

Who's in charge here?

The AED is equipped with a microcomputer that analyzes a patient's heart rhythm at the push of a button. It then audibly or visually prompts you to deliver a shock.

Patient preparation

• Assess the patient to determine if he lacks a pulse. Call for help, and perform cardiopulmonary resuscitation (CPR) until the defibrillator and other emergency equipment arrive.

• Connect the monitoring leads of the defibrillator to the patient, and assess his cardiac rhythm in two leads.

• Expose the patient's chest, and apply conductive pads at the paddle placement positions. (See *Defibrillator paddle placement.*)

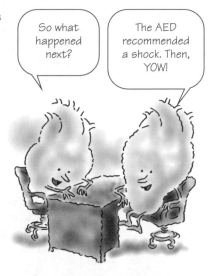

Peak technique

Defibrillator paddle placement

Here's a guide to correct paddle placement for defibrillation.

Anterolateral placement

For anterolateral placement, place one paddle to the right of the upper sternum, just below the right clavicle, and the other over the fifth or sixth intercostal space at the left anterior axillary line.

Anteroposterior placement

For anteroposterior placement, place the anterior paddle directly over the heart at the precordium, to the left of the lower sternal border. Place the flat posterior paddle under the patient's body beneath the heart and immediately below the scapulae.

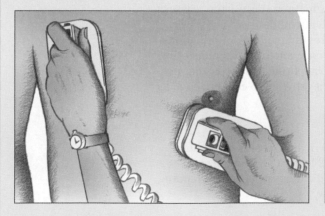

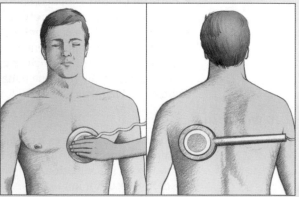

Monitoring and aftercare

• Turn on the defibrillator. If performing manual external defibrillation, set the energy level at 200 joules (for a manual biphasic defibrillator) or 360 joules (for a monophasic defibrillator).
• Charge the paddles by pressing the CHARGE buttons, which are located on either the machine or the paddles.

Ready...

• Place the paddles over the conductive pads and press firmly against the patient's chest, using 25 lb (11.3 kg) of pressure.
• Reassess the patient's cardiac rhythm in two leads.

...Set...

• If the patient remains in ventricular fibrillation or pulseless ventricular tachycardia, instruct all personnel to stand clear of the patient and the bed. Also, make a visual check to make sure everyone is clear of the patient and the bed.

...Go!

• Discharge the current by pressing both paddle DISCHARGE buttons simultaneously.
• Leave the paddles in position on the patient's chest while you reassess his cardiac rhythm; have someone else assess his pulse.
• If necessary, continue CPR and prepare to defibrillate a second time. Instruct someone to reset the energy level on the defibrillator to 200 or more joules (for a biphasic defibrillator) or 360 joules (for a monophasic defibrillator). Announce that you're preparing to defibrillate, and follow the procedure described above.

One more time

• Reassess the patient. If defibrillation is again necessary, follow the same procedure as before.
• Perform the three counter-shocks in rapid succession, reassessing the patient's rhythm before each attempt.
• If the patient still has no pulse after three initial defibrillations, resume CPR, give supplemental oxygen, and begin administering appropriate medications such as epinephrine. Also, consider possible causes for failure of the patient's rhythm to convert, such as acidosis and hypoxia.

It worked!

• If defibrillation restores a normal rhythm, assess the patient. Obtain baseline ABG levels and a 12-lead ECG. Provide supplemental oxygen, ventilation, and medications as needed. Prepare the defibrillator for immediate reuse.

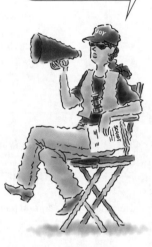

I want everyone to step back from the patient and the bed! And defibrillate!

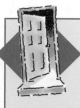

No place like home

Teaching the patient after defibrillation

Before discharge from the facility, instruct the patient to:
• report episodes of chest pain to the doctor
• encourage the family to learn cardiopulmonary resuscitation as well as how to use an automated external defibrillator
• consider an implantable cardioverter-defibrillator, if recommended by his doctor.

• Document the procedure, including the patient's ECG rhythms before and after defibrillation; the number of times defibrillation was performed; the voltage used during each attempt; whether a pulse returned; the dosage, route, and time of any drugs administered; whether CPR was used; how the airway was maintained; and the patient's outcome. (See *Teaching the patient after defibrillation.*)

Implantable cardioverter-defibrillator

An ICD has a programmable pulse generator and lead system that monitors the heart's activity, detects ventricular bradyarrhythmias and tachyarrhythmias, and responds with appropriate therapies. It's used for antitachycardia and bradycardia pacing, cardioversion, and defibrillation. Some ICDs also have the ability to pace the atrium and the ventricle.

Power station nearby

To implant an ICD, the cardiologist positions the lead (or leads) transvenously in the endocardium of the right ventricle (and the right atrium, if both chambers require pacing). The lead connects to a generator box, which is implanted in the right or left upper chest near the clavicle. (See *Location of an ICD*, page 126.)

Patient preparation

• Reinforce the cardiologist's instructions to the patient and his family, answering any questions they may have.
• Be sure to emphasize the need for the device, the potential complications, and ICD terminology.
• Restrict food and fluid for 12 hours before the procedure.
• Provide a sedative on the morning of the procedure, as ordered, to help the patient relax.

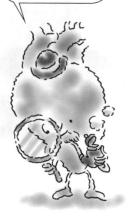

An ICD detects problems with the heart's activity and responds with appropriate therapies.

Location of an ICD

To insert an implantable cardioverter-defibrillator (ICD), the cardiologist makes a small incision near the collarbone and accesses the subclavian vein. The leadwires are inserted through the subclavian vein, threaded into the heart, and placed in contact with the endocardium.

Pocket placement

The leads are connected to the pulse generator, which is placed under the skin in a specially prepared pocket in the right or left upper chest. (Placement is similar to that used for a pacemaker.) The cardiologist then closes the incision and programs the device.

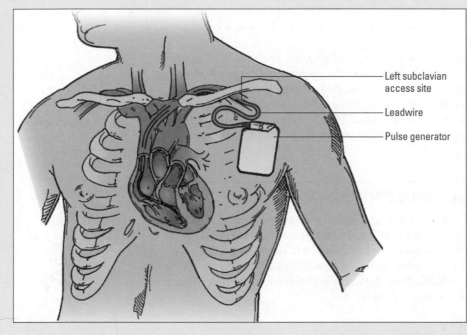

Left subclavian access site

Leadwire

Pulse generator

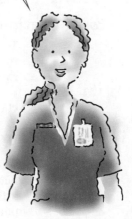

Family members of patients who have undergone ICD implantation should be encouraged to learn CPR.

Monitoring and aftercare

- The patient will be monitored on a telemetry unit.
- Monitor for arrhythmias and proper device functioning.
- Gradually allow the patient to increase activities, as ordered.
- Monitor the incision site for signs of infection or drainage.
- Provide support to the patient and his family to help them cope with recovery and lifestyle changes.
- Encourage family members to learn CPR. (See *Teaching the patient after ICD implantation.*)

No place like home

Teaching the patient after ICD implantation

Before discharge from the facility, instruct the patient to:
• avoid placing excessive pressure over the insertion site or moving or jerking the area until the postoperative visit
• check the incision site daily and immediately notify the doctor of signs and symptoms of infection

• wear medical alert identification and carry information regarding his implantable cardioverter-defibrillator (ICD) at all times
• increase exercise and sexual activity as allowed by the doctor
• take medications as prescribed and report adverse effects to the doctor.

Synchronized cardioversion

Cardioversion (synchronized countershock) is an elective or emergency procedure used to correct tachyarrhythmias (such as atrial tachycardia, atrial flutter, atrial fibrillation, and symptomatic ventricular tachycardia). It's also the treatment of choice for patients with arrhythmias that don't respond to drug therapy.

Small shock

In synchronized cardioversion, an electric current is delivered to the heart to correct an arrhythmia. Compared with defibrillation, it uses much lower energy levels and is synchronized to deliver an electric charge to the myocardium at the peak R wave.

Back in control

The procedure causes immediate depolarization, interrupting reentry circuits (abnormal impulse conduction that occurs when cardiac tissue is activated two or more times, causing reentry arrhythmias) and allowing the sinoatrial node to resume control.

Synchronizing the electrical charge with the R wave ensures that the current won't be delivered on the vulnerable T wave and disrupt repolarization. Thus, it reduces the risk that the current will strike during the relative refractory period of a cardiac cycle and induce ventricular fibrillation.

Patient preparation

• Describe this elective procedure to the patient, and make sure informed consent is obtained.

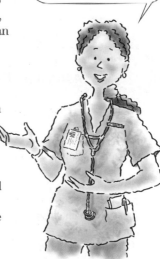

Cardioversion interrupts reentry circuits, allowing normal heart rhythms to regain control.

• Withhold all food and fluids for 6 to 12 hours before the procedure. If cardioversion is urgent, withhold food beginning as soon
as possible.
• Obtain a baseline 12-lead ECG.
• Connect the patient to a pulse oximeter and blood pressure
cuff.
• If the patient is awake, administer a sedative as ordered.
• Place the leads on the patient's chest and assess his cardiac
rhythm.
• Apply conductive gel to the paddles or attach defibrillation pads
to the chest wall; position the pads so that one pad is to the right
of the sternum, just below the clavicle, and the other is at the fifth
or sixth intercostal space in the left anterior axillary line.

Monitoring and aftercare

• Turn on the defibrillator and select the ordered energy level,
usually between 50 and 100 joules. (See *Choosing the correct car-
dioversion energy level*.)
• Activate the synchronized mode by depressing the synchronizer
switch.
• Check that the machine is sensing the R wave correctly.
• Place the paddles on the chest and apply firm pressure.
• Charge the paddles.
• Instruct other personnel to stand clear of the patient and the
bed to avoid the risk of an electric shock.

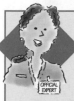

Advice from the experts

Choosing the correct cardioversion energy level

When choosing an energy level for cardioversion, try the lowest energy level first. If the arrhythmia isn't corrected, repeat the procedure using the next energy level.

Try, try again
Repeat this procedure until the arrhythmia is corrected or until the highest energy level is
reached. The monophasic energy doses (or clinically equivalent biphasic energy dose) used for
cardioversion are:
• 100, 200, 300, 360 joules for unstable ventricular tachycardia with a pulse
• 50, 100, 200, 300, 360 joules for unstable paroxysmal supraventricular tachycardia
• 100, 200, 300, 360 joules for unstable atrial fibrillation with a rapid ventricular response
• 50, 100, 200, 300, 360 joules for unstable atrial flutter with a rapid ventricular response.

• Discharge the current by pushing both paddles' DISCHARGE buttons simultaneously.
• If cardioversion is unsuccessful, repeat the procedure two or three times, as ordered, gradually increasing the energy with each additional counter-shock.
• If normal rhythm is restored, continue to monitor the patient and provide supplemental ventilation as long as needed.
• If the patient's cardiac rhythm changes to ventricular fibrillation, switch the mode from SYNCHRONIZED to DEFIBRILLATE and defibrillate the patient immediately after charging the machine.

Use your hands

• When using handheld paddles, continue to hold the paddles on the patient's chest until the energy is delivered.
• Remember to reset the SYNC MODE on the defibrillator after each synchronized cardioversion. Resetting this switch is necessary because most defibrillators automatically reset to an unsynchronized mode.

Write it down

• Document the use of synchronized cardioversion, the rhythm before and after cardioversion, the amperage used, and how the patient tolerated the procedure. (See *Teaching the patient after synchronized cardioversion.*)

> What rhythm! Always document the rhythm before and after cardioversion.

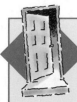

No place like home

Teaching the patient after synchronized cardioversion

Before discharge from the facility, instruct the patient to:
• report chest pain or palpitations to his doctor
• encourage family members to learn cardiopulmonary resuscitation and use of an automated external defibrillator
• take medication and attend follow-up visits with the doctor, as recommended.

Permanent pacemaker insertion

A permanent pacemaker is a self-contained device that's surgically implanted in a pocket under the patient's skin. This implantation is usually performed in an operating room or a cardiac catheterization laboratory.

Permanent pacemakers function in the DEMAND mode, allowing the patient's heart to beat on its own but preventing it from falling below a preset rate.

> Complete heart block is just one reason I might need a pacemaker.

And the nominees for insertion are...

Permanent pacemakers are indicated for patients with:
• persistent bradyrhythmia
• complete heart block
• congenital or degenerative heart disease
• Stokes-Adams syndrome
• Wolff-Parkinson-White syndrome
• sick sinus syndrome.

Setting the pace

Pacing electrodes can be placed in the atria, the ventricles, or both chambers (atrioventricular sequential or dual chamber). Biventricular pacemakers are also available for cardiac resynchronization therapy in some patients with heart failure. (See *Understanding pacemaker codes.*)

The most common pacing codes are VVI for single-chamber pacing and DDD for dual-chamber pacing. To keep the patient healthy and active, newer pacemakers are designed to increase the heart rate with exercise. (See *Biventricular pacemaker*, page 132.)

Patient preparation

• Explain the procedure to the patient.
• Before pacemaker insertion, shave the patient's chest from the axilla to the midline and from the clavicle to the nipple line on the side selected by the doctor.
• Establish an I.V. line.
• Obtain baseline vital signs and a baseline ECG.
• Provide sedation as ordered.

Monitoring and aftercare

• Monitor the patient's ECG to check for arrhythmias and to ensure correct pacemaker functioning.
• Check the dressing for signs of bleeding and infection.

Now I get it!

Understanding pacemaker codes

The capabilities of pacemakers are described by a five-letter coding system, although typically only the first three letters are used.

First letter

The first letter identifies which heart chambers are paced. Here are the letters used to signify these options:
- V = Ventricle
- A = Atrium
- D = Dual (ventricle and atrium)
- O = None.

Second letter

The second letter signifies the heart chamber where the pacemaker senses the intrinsic activity:
- V = Ventricle
- A = Atrium
- D = Dual
- O = None.

Third letter

The third letter shows the pacemaker's response to the intrinsic electrical activity it senses in the atrium or ventricle:
- T = Triggers pacing
- I = Inhibits pacing
- D = Dual; can be triggered or inhibited depending on the mode and where intrinsic activity occurs
- O = None; the pacemaker doesn't change its mode in response to sensed activity.

Fourth letter

The fourth letter denotes the pacemaker's programmability; it tells whether the pacemaker can be modified by an external programming device:
- P = Basic functions programmable
- M = Multiprogrammable parameters
- C = Communicating functions such as telemetry
- R = Rate responsiveness (rate adjusts to fit the patient's metabolic needs and achieve normal hemodynamic status)
- O = None.

Fifth letter

The fifth letter denotes the pacemaker's response to a tachyarrhythmia:
- P = Pacing ability—pacemaker's rapid burst paces the heart at a rate above its intrinsic rate to override the tachycardia source
- S – Shock—an implantable cardioverter-defibrillator identifies ventricular tachycardia and delivers a shock to stop the arrhythmia
- D = Dual ability to shock and pace
- O = None.

- Change the dressing according to your facility's policy.
- Check vital signs and level of consciousness (LOC) every 15 minutes for the first hour, every hour for the next 4 hours, and then every 4 hours.
- Provide the patient with an identification card that lists the pacemaker type and manufacturer, serial number, pacemaker rate setting, date implanted, and the doctor's name. (See *Teaching the patient after permanent pacemaker insertion*, page 133.)

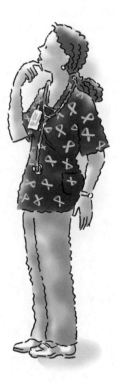

Now I get it!

Biventricular pacemaker

A biventricular pace-maker is a type of pacemaker that's currently being used to treat heart failure.

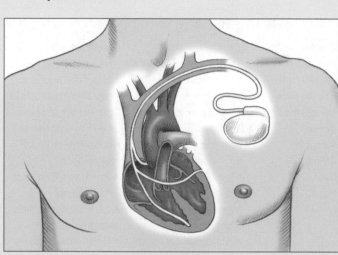

All together now
It works by sending tiny electrical signals to the left and right ventricles at the same time, ultimately causing the walls of the left ventricle to pump together. The result is more efficient pumping of the heart, improved circulation, and decreased fluid backup in the heart muscle and lungs.

Another lead
Insertion is similar to a regular pacemaker. However, in addition to the two leads that are used in most pacemakers, a third lead is placed into a cardiac vein and paces the left ventricle.

Temporary pacemaker insertion

A temporary pacemaker is typically used in an emergency. The device consists of an external, battery-powered pulse generator and a lead or electrode system.

Temporary pacemakers usually come in three types:
- transcutaneous
- transvenous
- epicardial.

Dire straits

In a life-threatening situation, a transcutaneous pacemaker is the best choice. This device works by sending an electrical impulse from the pulse generator to the patient's heart by way of two electrodes, which are placed on the front and back of the patient's chest.

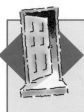

No place like home

Teaching the patient after permanent pacemaker insertion

Before discharge from the facility, instruct the patient to:
• report chest pain or palpitations to his doctor
• carry information regarding his pacemaker with him at all times
• wear medical alert identification regarding his pacemaker
• follow instructions from his doctor regarding check-ups on pacemaker function.

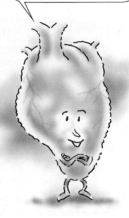

When you have enough time, a transvenous pacemaker is the more comfortable—and more reliable—choice.

Transcutaneous pacing is quick and effective, but it's used only until the doctor can institute transvenous or permanent pacing.

When you have more time

In addition to being more comfortable for the patient, a transvenous pacemaker is more reliable than a transcutaneous pacemaker.

Transvenous pacing involves threading an electrode catheter through a vein into the patient's right atrium or right ventricle. The electrode is attached to an external pulse generator that can provide an electrical stimulus directly to the endocardium.

When to use...

Indications for a temporary transvenous pacemaker include:
• management of bradycardia
• presence of tachyarrhythmias
• other conduction system disturbances.

The purposes of temporary transvenous pacemaker insertion are:
• to maintain circulatory integrity by providing for standby pacing in case of sudden complete heart block
• to increase heart rate during periods of symptomatic bradycardia
• occasionally, to control sustained supraventricular or ventricular tachycardia.

...And when not to

Among the contraindications to pacemaker therapy are electromechanical dissociation and ventricular fibrillation.

Suited for surgery

Epicardial pacing is used during cardiac surgery, when the surgeon may insert electrodes through the epicardium of the right ventricle and, if he wants to institute atrioventricular sequential pacing, the right atrium. From there, the electrodes pass through the chest wall, where they remain available if temporary pacing becomes necessary.

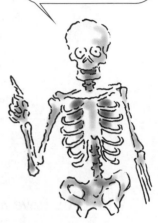

Transcutaneous pacemaker electrodes shouldn't be placed over bony areas because bone is a poor conductor of current.

Patient preparation

• Teach measures to prevent microshock; warn the patient not to use any electrical equipment that isn't grounded.
• When using a transcutaneous pacemaker, don't place the electrodes over a bony area because bone conducts current poorly. With a female patient, place the anterior electrode under the patient's breast but not over her diaphragm.
• If the doctor inserts the transvenous pacer wire through the brachial or femoral vein, immobilize the patient's arm or leg to avoid putting stress on the pacing wires.

Monitoring and aftercare

• After instituting use of any temporary pacemaker, assess the patient's vital signs, skin color, LOC, and peripheral pulses to determine the effectiveness of the paced rhythm. Perform a 12-lead ECG to serve as a baseline, and then perform additional ECGs daily or with clinical changes. Also, if possible, obtain a rhythm strip before, during, and after pacemaker placement; anytime the pacemaker settings are changed; and whenever the patient receives treatment because of a complication due to the pacemaker.
• Continuously monitor the ECG reading, noting capture, sensing, rate, intrinsic beats, and competition of paced and intrinsic rhythms. If the pacemaker is sensing correctly, the sense indicator on the pulse generator should flash with each beat.
• Record the date and time of pacemaker insertion, the type of pacemaker, the reason for insertion, and the patient's response. Record the pacemaker settings. Document any complications and the measures taken to resolve them.
• If the patient has epicardial pacing wires in place, clean the insertion site and change the dressing daily. At the same time, monitor the site for signs of infection. Always keep the pulse generator nearby in case pacing becomes necessary.
• Prepare the patient for permanent pacemaker surgery as appropriate.

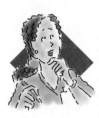

Quick quiz

1. Which measures should be performed immediately following a CABG?

    A.   Ambulation, 12-lead ECG, and clear liquid diet
    B.   Vital signs, cardiac rhythm, and pulse oximetry
    C.   Vital signs, cardiac rhythm, and clear liquid diet
    D.   12-lead ECG, vital signs, and ambulation

Answer: B. Immediately following a CABG, the patient's vital signs should be obtained, his cardiac rhythm evaluated, and a pulse oximetry reading obtained to assess oxygenation.

2. What are the signs of hemodynamic compromise?

    A.   Hypotension, decreased cardiac output, and shock
    B.   Tachycardia, hypertension, and increased urine output
    C.   Shock, diaphoresis, and increased cardiac output
    D.   Bradycardia, hypertension, and decreased urine output

Answer: A. Signs of hemodynamic compromise include hypotension, decreased cardiac output, and signs of shock (cool, clammy skin; decreased urine output; initially tachycardia, then bradycardia).

3. What's an important teaching point for the patient receiving a heart transplant?

    A.   He'll need to stay indoors during the winter months.
    B.   He'll need to take immunosuppressants for at least 6 months following surgery.
    C.   He'll be at risk for life-threatening infections because of the medications he'll be taking.
    D.   After 6 weeks, he'll no longer be at risk for rejection.

Answer: C. After a heart transplant, the patient is treated with monoclonal antibodies and potent immunosuppressants. The resulting immunosuppression places the patient at risk for life-threatening infection.

4. In a life-threatening situation, which pacemaker is the best choice?

    A.   Permanent pacemaker
    B.   Transcutaneous pacemaker
    C.   Transvenous pacemaker
    D.   Epicardial pacemaker

Answer: B. A transcutaneous pacemaker provides quick and effective pacing, but it's used only until a doctor can institute transvenous or permanent pacing.

5. What's a nonsurgical alternative to coronary artery bypass surgery?

    A.   PTCA

    B.   VAD

    C.   ICD

    D.   MIDCAB

Answer: A. PTCA offers a nonsurgical alternative to coronary artery bypass surgery. Performed in the cardiac catheterization laboratory under local anesthesia, PTCA doesn't involve a thoracotomy, so it's less costly and requires shorter hospitalization. Patients can usually walk the next day and return to work in 2 weeks.

Scoring

☆☆☆ If you answered all five questions correctly, perfect! You're a pro at cardiac procedures.

☆☆ If you answered four questions correctly, terrific! From transplants to PTCA, you have this information down.

☆ If you answered fewer than four questions correctly, stay mellow. The best treatment is to reread the chapter.

Arrhythmias

Just the facts

In this chapter, you'll learn:

♦ ways to identify various arrhythmias

♦ causes of each type of arrhythmia

♦ significance of, treatment for, and nursing implications of each type of arrhythmia

♦ assessment findings for each type of arrhythmia.

A look at arrhythmias

Cardiac arrhythmias are variations in the normal pattern of electrical stimulation of the heart. Arrhythmias vary in severity—from those that are mild, cause no symptoms, and require no treatment (such as sinus arrhythmia) to those that require emergency intervention (such as catastrophic ventricular fibrillation). Arrhythmias are generally classified according to their origin (ventricular or supraventricular). Their effects on cardiac output and blood pressure determine their clinical significance. Lethal arrhythmias, such as pulseless ventricular tachycardia and ventricular fibrillation, are a major cause of cardiac death.

The most common types of arrhythmias include sinus node arrhythmias, atrial arrhythmias, junctional arrhythmias, ventricular arrhythmias, and atrioventricular (AV) blocks.

> Arrhythmias are variations in my normal pattern of electrical stimulation. Bummer!

Sinus node arrhythmias

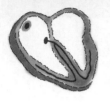

When a heart is functioning normally, the sinoatrial (SA) node, also called the *sinus node*, acts as the primary pacemaker. The sinus node assumes this role because its automatic firing rate exceeds that of the heart's other pacemakers. In an adult at rest, the sinus node has an inherent firing rate of 60 to 100 times per minute.

What nerve!

The SA node's blood supply comes from the right coronary artery and left circumflex artery. The autonomic nervous system richly innervates the sinus node through the vagal nerve, a parasympathetic nerve, and several sympathetic nerves. Stimulation of the vagus nerve decreases the node's firing rate, and stimulation of the sympathetic system increases it.

Types of sinus node arrhythmias include sinus arrhythmia, sinus bradycardia, sinus tachycardia, sinus arrest, and sick sinus syndrome.

Sinus arrhythmia

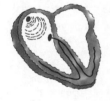

In sinus arrhythmia, the pacemaker cells of the SA node fire irregularly. The cardiac rate stays within normal limits, but the rhythm is irregular and corresponds to the respiratory cycle. Sinus arrhythmias commonly occur in athletes, children, and elderly people but rarely occur in infants. Conditions unrelated to respiration may also produce sinus arrhythmia, including inferior-wall myocardial infarction (MI), advanced age, use of digoxin (Lanoxin) or morphine, and increased intracranial pressure.

How it happens

During inspiration, blood flow to the heart increases. This increase reduces vagal tone, which in turn increases heart rate. During expiration, venous return decreases. This increases vagal tone, slowing the heart rate. (See *Breathing and sinus arrhythmia.*)

What to look for

To identify sinus arrhythmia, observe the patient's heart rhythm during respiration. The atrial and ventricular rates should be within normal limits (60 to 100 beats/minute) but increase during inspiration and slow with expiration. Electrocardiogram (ECG) complexes fall closer together during inspiration, shortening the P-P interval (the time elapsed between two consecutive P waves).

Breathing and sinus arrhythmia

When sinus arrhythmia is related to respirations, you'll see an increase in heart rate with inspiration and a decrease with expiration, as shown here.

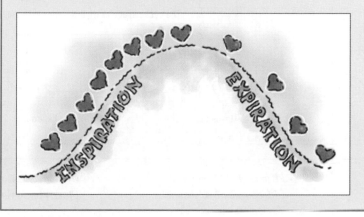

During expiration, the P-P interval lengthens. The difference between the shortest and longest P-P intervals exceeds 0.12 second. (See *Recognizing sinus arrhythmia*, page 140.)

Breathing easy

Check the patient's peripheral pulse rate. It, too, should increase during inspiration and decrease during expiration. If the arrhythmia is caused by an underlying condition, you may note signs and symptoms of that condition as well.

When evaluating sinus arrhythmia, be sure to check the monitor carefully. A marked variation in P-P intervals in an elderly patient may indicate sick sinus syndrome, a related but more serious phenomenon. (See *A longer look at sinus arrhythmia*, page 140.)

How you intervene

Unless the patient is symptomatic, treatment usually isn't necessary. If sinus arrhythmia is unrelated to respiration, the underlying cause may require treatment.

On the alert

If sinus arrhythmia is caused by drugs, such as morphine or other sedatives, the doctor may decide to continue those medications. If a patient taking digoxin suddenly develops sinus arrhythmia, notify the doctor immediately. The patient may be experiencing digoxin toxicity.

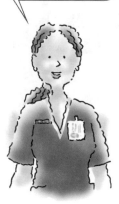

Sinus arrhythmia is easier to detect when the patient's heart rate is slow; it may disappear when the heart rate increases, such as with exercise or after atropine administration.

Recognizing sinus arrhythmia

Take a look at this example of how sinus arrhythmia appears on a rhythm strip. Notice its distinguishing characteristics.

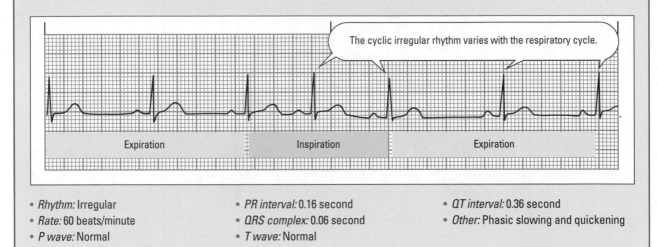

The cyclic irregular rhythm varies with the respiratory cycle.

Expiration | Inspiration | Expiration

- *Rhythm:* Irregular
- *Rate:* 60 beats/minute
- *P wave:* Normal

- *PR interval:* 0.16 second
- *QRS complex:* 0.06 second
- *T wave:* Normal

- *QT interval:* 0.36 second
- *Other:* Phasic slowing and quickening

Sinus bradycardia

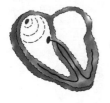

In sinus bradycardia, the sinus rate falls below 60 beats/minute while the rhythm remains regular. It may occur normally during sleep or in a person with a well-conditioned heart—an athlete, for instance. That's because a well-conditioned heart can pump more blood with each contraction, maintaining a normal cardiac output with fewer beats.

How it happens

Sinus bradycardia usually occurs as a normal response to a reduced demand for blood flow. In this case, vagal stimulation increases and sympathetic stimulation decreases. As a result, automaticity (the tendency of cells to initiate their own impulses) in the SA node diminishes.

Sinus bradycardia commonly occurs after an inferior-wall MI involving the right coronary artery, which supplies blood to the SA node. Numerous other conditions and the use of certain drugs may also cause sinus bradycardia. (See *Causes of sinus bradycardia.*)

Advice from the experts

A longer look at sinus arrhythmia

Don't mistake sinus arrhythmia for other rhythms. At first glance, it may look like atrial fibrillation, normal sinus rhythm with premature atrial contractions, sinoatrial block, or sinus pauses. Observe the monitor and the patient's respiratory pattern for several minutes to determine the rate and rhythm. As always, check the patient's pulse.

Causes of sinus bradycardia

Sinus bradycardia may be caused by:
• noncardiac disorders, such as hyperkalemia, increased intracranial pressure, hypothyroidism, hypothermia, sleep, and glaucoma
• conditions producing excess vagal stimulation or decreased sympathetic stimulation, such as sleep, deep relaxation, Valsalva's maneuver, carotid sinus massage, and vomiting
• cardiac diseases, such as sinoatrial node disease, cardiomyopathy, myocarditis, myocardial ischemia, and heart block; sinus bradycardia can also occur immediately following an inferior-wall myocardial infarction
• certain drugs, especially beta-adrenergic blockers, digoxin (Lanoxin), calcium channel blockers, lithium (Eskalith), and antiarrhythmics, such as sotalol (Betapace), amiodarone (Cordarone), propafenone (Rhythmol), and quinidine.

What to look for

In sinus bradycardia, the heartbeat is regular with a rate less than 60 beats/minute. All other ECG findings are normal: a P wave precedes each QRS complex and the PR interval, QRS complex, T wave, and QT interval are all normal. (See *Recognizing sinus bradycardia*, page 142.)

No symptoms? No problem.

The clinical significance of sinus bradycardia depends on the rate and whether the patient is symptomatic. Most adults can tolerate a sinus bradycardia of 45 to 59 beats/minute.

Symptoms? Problem!

However, if the rate falls below 45 beats/minute, patients usually have signs and symptoms of decreased cardiac output, such as hypotension, dizziness, confusion, or syncope (Stokes-Adams attack). Keep in mind, too, that patients with underlying cardiac disease may be less tolerant of a drop in heart rate.

Bradycardia may also trigger more serious arrhythmias, such as ventricular tachycardia and ventricular fibrillation. Ectopic beats, such as premature atrial, junctional, or ventricular contractions, may also occur, causing palpitations and an irregular pulse.

In a patient with acute inferior-wall MI, sinus bradycardia is considered a favorable prognostic sign, unless it's accompanied by hypotension. That's because, with a slower heart rate, the heart uses less oxygen and avoids ischemia.

Sinus bradycardia rarely affects children. When it occurs in an ill child, it's considered an ominous sign.

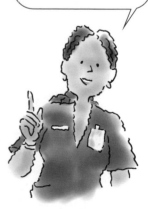

If it occurs without hypotension, sinus bradycardia is a favorable prognostic sign in acute inferior-wall MI.

Recognizing sinus bradycardia

Take a look at this example of how sinus bradycardia appears on a rhythm strip. Notice its distinguishing characteristics.

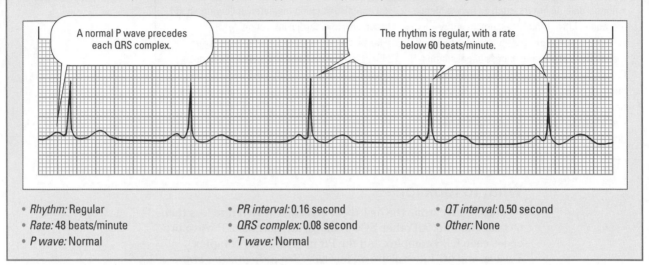

A normal P wave precedes each QRS complex.

The rhythm is regular, with a rate below 60 beats/minute.

- *Rhythm:* Regular
- *Rate:* 48 beats/minute
- *P wave:* Normal
- *PR interval:* 0.16 second
- *QRS complex:* 0.08 second
- *T wave:* Normal
- *QT interval:* 0.50 second
- *Other:* None

How you intervene

If the patient is asymptomatic and his vital signs are stable, treatment isn't necessary. Continue to observe his heart rhythm, monitoring the progression and duration of bradycardia. Evaluate his tolerance of the rhythm at rest and with activity. Also, review the drugs he's taking. Check with the doctor about stopping medications that may be depressing the SA node, such as digoxin, beta-adrenergic blockers, and calcium channel blockers. Before giving those drugs, make sure the heart rate is within a safe range.

If the patient is symptomatic, treatment aims to identify and correct the underlying cause. Meanwhile, drugs such as atropine, epinephrine, and dopamine, or a temporary pacemaker, help to maintain an adequate heart rate. Patients with chronic, symptom-producing sinus bradycardia may require insertion of a permanent pacemaker. (See *Treating symptom-producing bradycardia.*)

Check the ABCs

If the patient abruptly develops a significant sinus bradycardia, assess his airway, breathing, and circulation (ABCs). If these are adequate, determine whether the patient has an effective cardiac output. If not, he may develop these signs and symptoms:
- hypotension
- cool, clammy skin

Sinus badycardia in a child is an ominous sign.

Peak technique

Treating symptom-producing bradycardia

This algorithm shows the steps for treating bradycardia in a patient not in cardiac arrest.

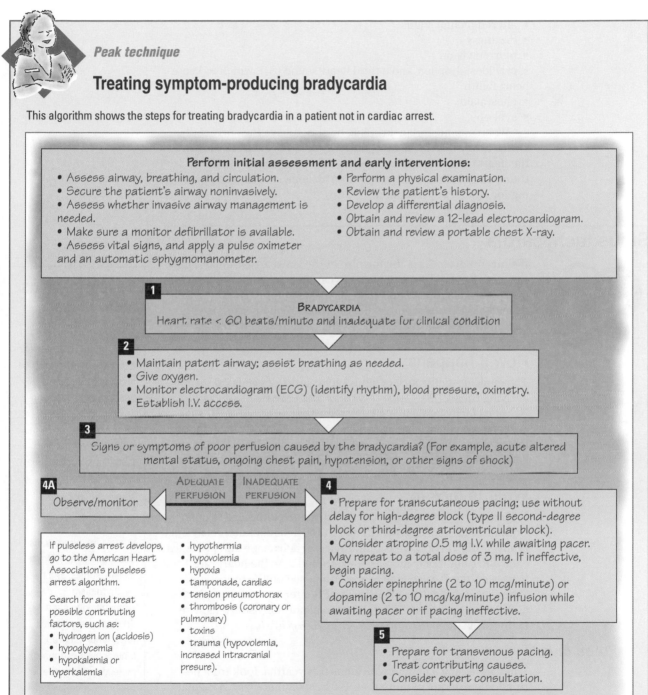

Perform initial assessment and early interventions:

- Assess airway, breathing, and circulation.
- Secure the patient's airway noninvasively.
- Assess whether invasive airway management is needed.
- Make sure a monitor defibrillator is available.
- Assess vital signs, and apply a pulse oximeter and an automatic sphygmomanometer.

- Perform a physical examination.
- Review the patient's history.
- Develop a differential diagnosis.
- Obtain and review a 12-lead electrocardiogram.
- Obtain and review a portable chest X-ray.

1

BRADYCARDIA
Heart rate < 60 beats/minute and inadequate for clinical condition

2

- Maintain patent airway; assist breathing as needed.
- Give oxygen.
- Monitor electrocardiogram (ECG) (identify rhythm), blood pressure, oximetry.
- Establish I.V. access.

3

Signs or symptoms of poor perfusion caused by the bradycardia? (For example, acute altered mental status, ongoing chest pain, hypotension, or other signs of shock)

ADEQUATE PERFUSION   INADEQUATE PERFUSION

4A

Observe/monitor

If pulseless arrest develops, go to the American Heart Association's pulseless arrest algorithm.

Search for and treat possible contributing factors, such as:
- hydrogen ion (acidosis)
- hypoglycemia
- hypokalemia or hyperkalemia

- hypothermia
- hypovolemia
- hypoxia
- tamponade, cardiac
- tension pneumothorax
- thrombosis (coronary or pulmonary)
- toxins
- trauma (hypovolemia, increased intracranial presure).

4

- Prepare for transcutaneous pacing; use without delay for high-degree block (type II second-degree block or third-degree atrioventricular block).
- Consider atropine 0.5 mg I.V. while awaiting pacer. May repeat to a total dose of 3 mg. If ineffective, begin pacing.
- Consider epinephrine (2 to 10 mcg/minute) or dopamine (2 to 10 mcg/kg/minute) infusion while awaiting pacer or if pacing ineffective.

5

- Prepare for transvenous pacing.
- Treat contributing causes.
- Consider expert consultation.

Reproduced with permission. *2005 American Heart Association Guidelines for Cardiopulmonary Resuscitation and Emergency Cardiovascular Care.* © 2005, American Heart Association.

- altered mental status
- dizziness
- blurred vision
- crackles, dyspnea, and a third heart sound (S_3), which indicate heart failure
- chest pain
- syncope.

When administering atropine, be sure to give the correct dose: Doses lower than 0.5 mg may have a paradoxical effect, slowing the heart rate even further. Keep in mind that a patient with a transplanted heart won't respond to atropine and may require pacing for emergency treatment.

Sinus tachycardia

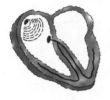

If sinus bradycardia is the tortoise of the sinus arrhythmias, sinus tachycardia is the hare. Sinus tachycardia in an adult is characterized by a sinus rate greater than 100 beats/minute. The rate rarely exceeds 180 beats/minute except during strenuous exercise; the maximum rate achievable with exercise decreases with age.

How it happens

The clinical significance of sinus tachycardia depends on the underlying cause. (See *Causes of sinus tachycardia*.)

Sinus tachycardia in a patient who has had an acute MI suggests massive heart damage and is a poor prognostic sign. Persistent tachycardia may also signal impending heart failure or cardiogenic shock.

What to look for

In sinus tachycardia, atrial and ventricular rhythms are regular. Both rates are equal, generally 100 to 160 beats/minute. As in sinus bradycardia, the P wave is of normal size and shape and precedes each QRS, but it may increase in amplitude. As the heart rate increases, the P wave may be superimposed on the preceding T wave and difficult to identify. The PR interval, QRS complex, and T wave are normal. The QT interval normally shortens with tachycardia. (See *Recognizing sinus tachycardia*.)

Pulse check!

When assessing a patient with sinus tachycardia, look for a peripheral pulse rate of more than 100 beats/minute with a regular rhythm. Usually, the patient will be asymptomatic.

Causes of sinus tachycardia

Sinus tachycardia may be a normal response to exercise, pain, stress, fever, or strong emotions, such as fear and anxiety. It can also occur:
- with certain cardiac conditions, such as heart failure, cardiogenic shock, and pericarditis
- as a compensatory mechanism in shock, anemia, respiratory distress, pulmonary embolism, sepsis, and hyperthyroidism
- when taking such drugs as atropine, isoproterenol (Isuprel), aminophylline, dopamine, dobutamine, epinephrine, alcohol, caffeine, nicotine, and amphetamines.

Recognizing sinus tachycardia

Take a look at this example of how sinus tachycardia appears on a rhythm strip. Notice its distinguishing characteristics.

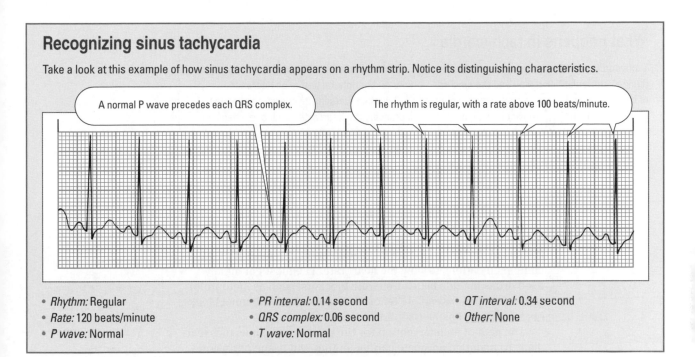

A normal P wave precedes each QRS complex.

The rhythm is regular, with a rate above 100 beats/minute.

- *Rhythm:* Regular
- *Rate:* 120 beats/minute
- *P wave:* Normal
- *PR interval:* 0.14 second
- *QRS complex:* 0.06 second
- *T wave:* Normal
- *QT interval:* 0.34 second
- *Other:* None

If cardiac output falls and compensatory mechanisms fail, the patient may experience hypotension, syncope, and blurred vision. He may report chest pain and palpitations, commonly described as a pounding chest or a sensation of skipped heartbeats. He may also report a sense of nervousness or anxiety. If heart failure develops, he may exhibit lung crackles, an extra heart sound (S_3), and jugular vein distention. (See *What happens in tachycardia,* page 146.)

Hard on the heart

Because the heart demands more oxygen at higher rates, tachycardia can trigger chest pain in patients with coronary artery disease (CAD). An increase in heart rate can also be detrimental for patients with obstructive types of heart conditions, such as aortic stenosis and hypertrophic cardiomyopathy.

How you intervene

No treatment for sinus tachycardia is necessary if the patient is asymptomatic or if the rhythm is the result of physical exertion. In other cases, the underlying cause may be treated, which usually resolves the arrhythmia. For example, if sinus tachycardia is caused by hemorrhage, treatment includes stopping the bleeding and replacing blood and fluid.

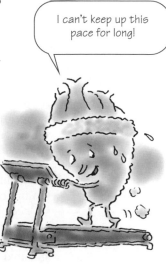

I can't keep up this pace for long!

What happens in tachycardia

Tachycardia can lower cardiac output by reducing ventricular filling time and the amount of blood pumped by the ventricles during each contraction. Normally, ventricular volume reaches 120 to 130 ml during diastole. In tachycardia, decreased ventricular volume leads to hypotension and decreased peripheral perfusion.

As cardiac output plummets, arterial pressure and peripheral perfusion decrease. Tachycardia worsens myocardial ischemia by increasing the heart's demand for oxygen and reducing the duration of diastole—the period of greatest coronary flow.

Slow it down

If sinus tachycardia leads to cardiac ischemia, treatment may include medications to slow the heart rate. The most commonly used drugs include beta-adrenergic blockers, such as metoprolol (Lopressor) and atenolol (Tenormin), and calcium channel blockers such as verapamil (Isoptin).

The goal of an intervention for the patient with sinus tachycardia is to maintain adequate cardiac output and tissue perfusion and to identify and correct the underlying cause.

Getting at the history

Check the patient's medication history. Over-the-counter sympathomimetic agents, which mimic the effects of the sympathetic nervous system, may contribute to sinus tachycardia. These agents may be contained in nose drops and cold formulas.

You should also ask about the patient's use of caffeine, nicotine, herbal supplements, alcohol, and such illicit drugs as cocaine and amphetamines—any of which can trigger tachycardia. Advise him to avoid these substances.

Achoo! Over-the-counter cold medicines may contribute to sinus tachycardia.

Part of the plan

Here are other steps you should take for the patient with sinus tachycardia:
• Because sinus tachycardia can lead to injury of the heart muscle, check for chest pain or angina. Also assess for signs and symptoms of heart failure, including crackles, an S_3 heart sound, and jugular vein distention.
• Monitor intake and output as well as daily weight.
• Check the patient's level of consciousness (LOC) to assess cerebral perfusion.
• Provide the patient with a calm environment. Help reduce fear and anxiety, which can fuel the arrhythmia.

- Teach about procedures and treatments. Include relaxation techniques in the information you provide.
- Be aware that a sudden onset of sinus tachycardia after an MI may signal extension of the infarction. Prompt recognition is vital so treatment can be started.

Sinus arrest

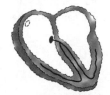

A disorder of impulse formation, sinus arrest results from a lack of electrical activity in the atrium (atrial standstill). During atrial standstill, the atria aren't stimulated and an entire PQRST complex is missing from the ECG strip.

Except for this missing complex, or pause, the ECG usually remains normal. Atrial standstill is called *sinus pause* when one or two beats aren't formed and *sinus arrest* when three or more beats aren't formed.

Sinus arrest closely resembles third-degree SA block, also called *exit block*, on the ECG strip. (See *Understanding sinoatrial blocks*, pages 148 and 149.)

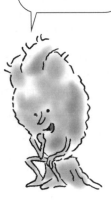

Sometimes I just like to pause and reflect.

How it happens

Sinus arrest occurs when the SA node fails to generate an impulse. Such failure may result from several conditions, including acute infection, heart disease, and vagal stimulation. Pauses of 2 to 3 seconds normally occur in healthy adults during sleep and occasionally in patients with increased vagal tone or hypersensitive carotid sinus disease. Sinus arrest may be associated with sick sinus syndrome. (See *Causes of sinus arrest*, page 150.)

What to look for

When assessing for sinus pause, you'll find on the ECG that atrial and ventricular rhythms are regular except for a missing complex at the onset of atrial standstill. Atrial and ventricular rates are equal and are usually within normal limits. The rate may vary, however, as a result of the pauses. (See *Recognizing sinus arrest*, page 151.)

Failing to make an appearance

A P wave that's of normal size and shape precedes each QRS complex but is absent during a pause. The PR interval is normal and constant when the P wave is present and not measurable when it's absent. The QRS complex, the T wave, and the QT interval are normal when present and are absent during a pause.

(Text continues on page 150.)

Now I get it!

Understanding sinoatrial blocks

In sinoatrial (SA) block, the SA node discharges impulses at regular intervals. Some of those impulses, though, are delayed on their way to the atria. Based on the length of the delay, SA blocks are divided into three categories: first-, second-, and third-degree. Second-degree block is further divided into type I (Wenckebach block) and type II.

First-degree SA block consists of a delay between the firing of the sinus node and depolarization of the atria. Because the electrocardiogram (ECG) doesn't show sinus node activity, you can't detect first-degree SA block. However, you can detect the other three types of SA block.

Second-degree type I block

In second-degree type I block, conduction time between the sinus node and the surrounding atrial tissue becomes progressively longer until an entire cycle is dropped. The pause is less than twice the shortest P-P interval.

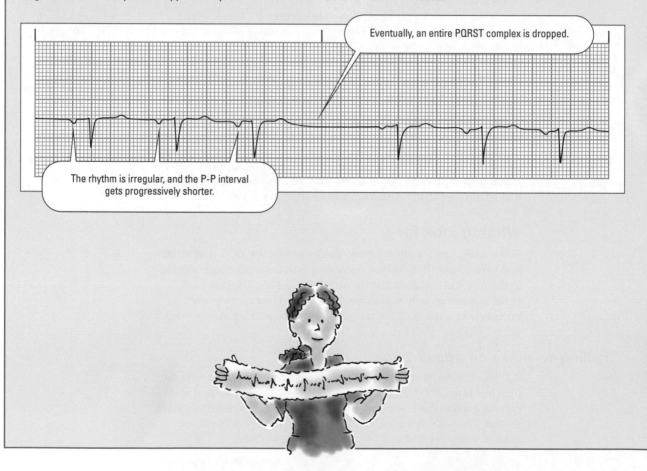

Eventually, an entire PQRST complex is dropped.

The rhythm is irregular, and the P-P interval gets progressively shorter.

Second-degree type II block

In second-degree type II block, conduction time between the sinus node and atrial tissue is normal until an impulse is blocked. The duration of the pause is a multiple of the P-P interval.

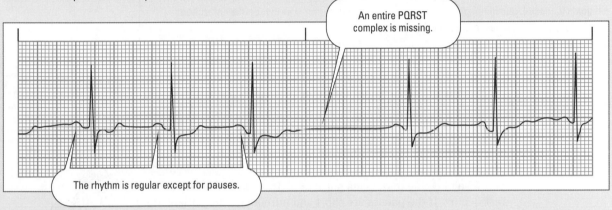

An entire PQRST complex is missing.

The rhythm is regular except for pauses.

Third-degree block

In third-degree block, some impulses are blocked, causing long sinus pauses. The pause isn't a multiple of the sinus rhythm. On an ECG, third-degree SA block looks similar to sinus arrest but results from a different cause.

Third-degree SA block is caused by a failure to conduct impulses; sinus arrest results from failure to form impulses. Failure in each case causes atrial activity to stop.

In sinus arrest, the pause commonly ends with a junctional escape beat. In third-degree block, the pause lasts for an indefinite period and ends with a sinus beat.

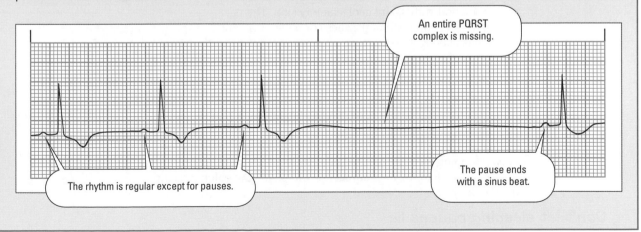

An entire PQRST complex is missing.

The rhythm is regular except for pauses.

The pause ends with a sinus beat.

Causes of sinus arrest

Sinus arrest can be caused by:
• sinus node disease, such as fibrosis and idiopathic degeneration
• increased vagal tone, as occurs with Valsalva's maneuver, carotid sinus massage, and vomiting
• digoxin (Lanoxin), quinidine, procainamide (Pronestyl), and salicylates, especially if given at toxic levels

• excessive doses of beta-adrenergic blockers, such as metoprolol (Lopressor) and propranolol (Inderal)
• cardiac disorders, such as chronic coronary artery disease, acute myocarditis, cardiomyopathy, and hypertensive heart disease
• acute inferior-wall myocardial infarction.

Junctional escape beats, including premature atrial, junctional, or ventricular contractions, may also be present. With sinus arrest, the length of the pause isn't a multiple of the previous R-R intervals.

Taking a break

You won't be able to detect a pulse or heart sounds when sinus arrest occurs. If the pauses are short and infrequent, the patient will most likely be asymptomatic and won't require treatment. He may have a normal sinus rhythm for days or weeks between episodes of sinus arrest, and he may not be able to feel the arrhythmias at all.

Too many for too long

Recurrent and prolonged pauses may cause signs of decreased cardiac output, such as low blood pressure, altered mental status, and cool, clammy skin. The patient may also complain of dizziness or blurred vision. The arrhythmias can produce syncope or near-syncopal episodes within 7 seconds of asystole.

How you intervene

An asymptomatic patient needs no treatment. For a patient displaying mild symptoms, treatment focuses on maintaining cardiac output and identifying the cause of the sinus arrest. That may involve stopping medications that contribute to SA node suppression, such as digoxin, beta-adrenergic blockers, and calcium channel blockers.

Don't let sleeping pauses lie

Examine the circumstances under which sinus pauses occur. A sinus pause may be insignificant if detected while the patient is

> This silence is certainly a cause for concern.

Recognizing sinus arrest

Take a look at this example of how sinus arrest. appears on a rhythm strip. Notice its distinguishing characteristics.

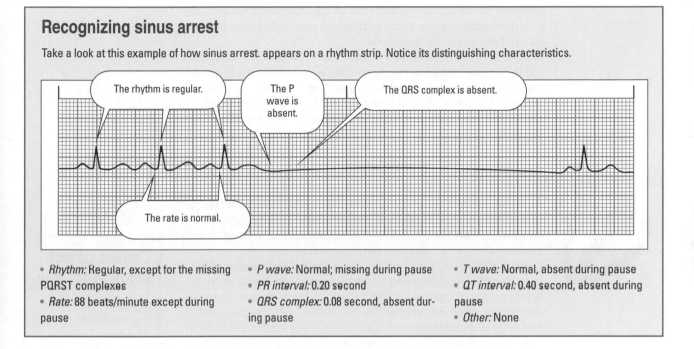

The rhythm is regular.

The P wave is absent.

The QRS complex is absent.

The rate is normal.

- *Rhythm:* Regular, except for the missing PQRST complexes
- *Rate:* 88 beats/minute except during pause
- *P wave:* Normal; missing during pause
- *PR interval:* 0.20 second
- *QRS complex:* 0.08 second, absent during pause
- *T wave:* Normal, absent during pause
- *QT interval:* 0.40 second, absent during pause
- *Other:* None

sleeping. If the pauses are recurrent, assess the patient for evidence of decreased cardiac output, such as altered mental status, low blood pressure, and cool, clammy skin.

Ask him whether he's dizzy or light-headed or has blurred vision. Does he feel as if he has passed out? If so, he may be experiencing syncope from a prolonged sinus arrest.

Document the patient's vital signs and how he feels during pauses as well as what activities he was involved in when they occurred. Activities that increase vagal stimulation, such as Valsalva's maneuver or vomiting, increase the likelihood of sinus pauses.

When matters get even worse

Assess for a progression of the arrhythmia. Notify the doctor immediately if the patient becomes unstable. Withhold medications that may contribute to sinus pauses and check with the doctor about whether those drugs should be continued.

If appropriate, be alert for signs of digoxin (Lanoxin), quinidine, or procainamide (Pronestyl) toxicity. Obtain a serum digoxin level and a serum electrolyte level.

Arresting the arrest

A patient who develops signs of circulatory collapse needs immediate treatment. As with sinus bradycardia, emergency treatment includes administration of atropine or epinephrine and insertion of a temporary pacemaker. A permanent pacemaker may be implanted for long-term management.

The goal for the patient with sinus arrest is to maintain adequate cardiac output and perfusion. Be sure to record and document the frequency and duration of pauses. Determine whether a pause is the result of sinus arrest or SA block. If a pacemaker is implanted, give the patient discharge instructions about pacemaker care.

Sick sinus syndrome

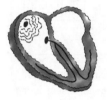

Also called *sinus nodal dysfunction*, sick sinus syndrome refers to a wide spectrum of SA node abnormalities. The syndrome is caused by disturbances in the way impulses are generated or the inability to conduct impulses to the atrium.

Sick sinus syndrome usually shows up as bradycardia, with episodes of sinus arrest and SA block interspersed with sudden, brief periods of rapid atrial fibrillation. Patients are also prone to paroxysms of other atrial tachyarrhythmias, such as atrial flutter and ectopic atrial tachycardia, a condition sometimes referred to as *bradycardia-tachycardia (or brady-tachy) syndrome*.

Most patients with sick sinus syndrome are older than age 60, but anyone can develop the arrhythmia. It's rare in children except after open-heart surgery that results in SA node damage. The arrhythmia affects men and women equally. The onset is progressive, insidious, and chronic.

How it happens

Sick sinus syndrome results either from a dysfunction of the sinus node's automaticity or from abnormal conduction or blockages of impulses coming out of the nodal region. These conditions, in turn, stem from a degeneration of the area's autonomic nervous system and partial destruction of the sinus node, as may occur with an interrupted blood supply after an inferior-wall MI. (See *Causes of sick sinus syndrome*.)

Blocked exits

In addition, certain conditions can affect the atrial wall surrounding the SA node and cause exit blocks. Conditions that cause inflammation or degeneration of atrial tissue can also lead to sick sinus syndrome. In many patients, though, the exact cause of sick sinus syndrome is never identified.

Causes of sick sinus syndrome

Sick sinus syndrome may result from:
• conditions leading to fibrosis of the sinoatrial (SA) node, such as increased age, atherosclerotic heart disease, hypertension, and cardiomyopathy
• trauma to the SA node caused by open-heart surgery (especially valvular surgery), pericarditis, or rheumatic heart disease
• autonomic disturbances affecting autonomic innervation, such as hypervagatonia and degeneration of the autonomic system
• cardioactive medications, such as digoxin (Lanoxin), beta-adrenergic blockers, and calcium channel blockers.

What to look for

Sick sinus syndrome encompasses several potential rhythm disturbances that may be intermittent or chronic. (See *Recognizing sick sinus syndrome.*) Those rhythm disturbances include one or a combination of the following conditions:

- sinus bradycardia
- SA block
- sinus arrest
- sinus bradycardia alternating with sinus tachycardia
- episodes of atrial tachyarrhythmias, such as atrial fibrillation and atrial flutter
- failure of the sinus node to increase heart rate with exercise.

Check for speed bumps

Look for an irregular rhythm with sinus pauses and abrupt rate changes. Atrial and ventricular rates may be fast, slow, or alternating periods of fast rates and slow rates interrupted by pauses.

The P wave varies with the rhythm and usually precedes each QRS complex. The PR interval is usually within normal limits but varies with changes in the rhythm. The QRS complex and T wave are usually normal, as is the QT interval, which may vary with rhythm changes.

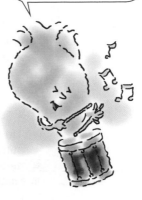

I know I'm supposed to be a regular guy, but sometimes I just get a crazy beat.

Recognizing sick sinus syndrome

Take a look at this example of how sick sinus syndrome appears on a rhythm strip. Notice its distinguishing characteristics.

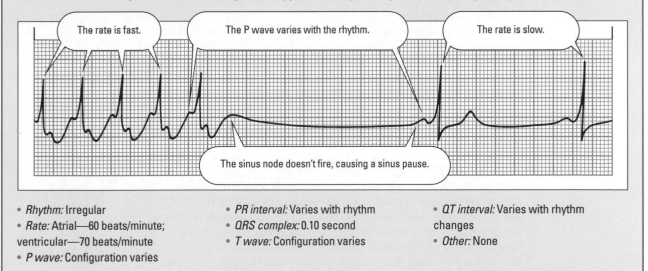

- *Rhythm:* Irregular
- *Rate:* Atrial—60 beats/minute; ventricular—70 beats/minute
- *P wave:* Configuration varies
- *PR interval:* Varies with rhythm
- *QRS complex:* 0.10 second
- *T wave:* Configuration varies
- *QT interval:* Varies with rhythm changes
- *Other:* None

Make up your mind!

The patient's pulse rate may be fast, slow, or normal, and the rhythm may be regular or irregular. You can usually detect an irregularity on the monitor or when palpating the pulse, which may feel inappropriately slow and then become rapid.

If you monitor the patient's heart rate during exercise or exertion, you may observe an inappropriate response to exercise such as a failure of the heart rate to increase. You may also detect episodes of brady-tachy syndrome, atrial flutter, atrial fibrillation, SA block, or sinus arrest on the monitor.

That sinking feeling

The patient may show signs and symptoms of decreased cardiac output, such as hypotension, blurred vision, and syncope, a common experience with this arrhythmia. The length of a pause significant enough to cause syncope varies with the patient's age, posture at the time, and cerebrovascular status. Consider any pause that lasts 2 to 3 seconds significant.

Other assessment findings depend on the patient's condition. For instance, he may have crackles in the lungs, an S_3 heart sound, or a dilated and displaced left ventricular apical impulse if he has underlying cardiomyopathy.

How you intervene

The significance of sick sinus syndrome depends on the patient's age, the presence of other diseases, and the type and duration of the specific arrhythmias that occur. If atrial fibrillation is involved, the prognosis is worse, most likely because of the risk of thromboembolic complications.

As with other sinus node arrhythmias, no treatment is necessary if the patient is asymptomatic. If the patient is symptomatic, however, treatment aims to alleviate signs and symptoms and correct the underlying cause of the arrhythmia.

Atropine or epinephrine may be given initially for an acute attack. A pacemaker may be used until the underlying disorder resolves. Tachyarrhythmias may be treated with antiarrhythmic medications, such as metoprolol and digoxin.

When the solution is part of the problem

Unfortunately, medications used to suppress tachyarrhythmias may worsen underlying SA node disease and bradyarrhythmias. The patient may need anticoagulants if he develops sudden bursts, or paroxysms, of atrial fibrillation. The anticoagulants help prevent thromboembolism and stroke, a complication of the condition. Because the syndrome is progressive and chronic, a symptomatic patient needs lifelong treatment.

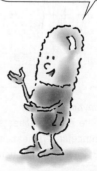

Drugs that suppress tachyarrhythmias may worsen underlying SA node disease.

Keep a running total

When caring for a patient with sick sinus syndrome, monitor and document all arrhythmias he experiences and signs or symptoms he develops. Assess how his rhythm responds to activity and pain and look for changes in the rhythm.

Watch the patient carefully after starting calcium channel blockers, beta-adrenergic blockers, or other antiarrhythmic medications. If treatment includes anticoagulant therapy and the insertion of a pacemaker, make sure the patient and his family receive appropriate instruction.

Atrial arrhythmias

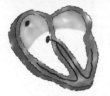

Atrial arrhythmias, the most common cardiac rhythm disturbances, result from impulses originating in areas outside the SA node. These arrhythmias can affect ventricular filling time and diminish the strength of the atrial kick, a contraction that normally provides the ventricles with up to 30% of their blood.

Triple play

Atrial arrhythmias are thought to result from three mechanisms—altered automaticity, circuit reentry, and afterdepolarization. Let's take a look at each cause and review specific atrial arrhythmias:
• Altered automaticity—An increase in the automaticity (the ability of cardiac cells to initiate impulses on their own) of the atrial fibers can trigger abnormal impulses. Causes of increased automaticity include extracellular factors, such as hypoxia, hypocalcemia, and digoxin toxicity, and conditions in which the function of the heart's normal pacemaker, the SA node, is diminished. For example, increased vagal tone or hypokalemia can increase the refractory period of the SA node and allow atrial fibers to fire impulses.
• Circuit reentry—In circuit reentry, an impulse is delayed along a slow conduction pathway. Despite the delay, the impulse remains active enough to produce another impulse during myocardial repolarization. Circuit reentry may occur with CAD, cardiomyopathy, or an MI.
• Afterdepolarization—Afterdepolarization can occur with cell injury, digoxin toxicity, and other conditions. An injured cell sometimes only partly repolarizes. Partial repolarization can lead to a repetitive ectopic firing called *triggered activity*. The depolarization produced by triggered activity is known as *afterdepolarization* and can lead to atrial or ventricular tachycardia.

> Those atrial arrhythmias think they're so popular just because they're the most common rhythm disturbances.

Atrial arrhythmias include premature atrial contractions (PACs), atrial flutter, atrial fibrillation, and atrial tachycardia. Let's examine each atrial arrhythmia in detail.

Premature atrial contractions

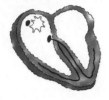

PACs originate outside the SA node and usually result from an irritable spot, or focus, in the atria that takes over as pacemaker for one or more beats. The SA node fires an impulse, but then an irritable focus jumps in, firing its own impulse before the SA node can fire again.

PACs may not be conducted through the AV node and the rest of the heart, depending on their prematurity and the status of the AV and intraventricular conduction system. Nonconducted or blocked PACs don't trigger a QRS complex.

How it happens

PACs commonly occur in a normal heart and are rarely dangerous in a patient who doesn't have heart disease. In fact, they usually cause no symptoms and can go unrecognized for years. (See *Causes of PACs*.)

A sign of things to come

However, in patients with heart disease, PACs may lead to more serious arrhythmias, such as atrial fibrillation and atrial flutter. In a patient who has had an acute MI, PACs can serve as an early sign of heart failure or an electrolyte imbalance. PACs can also result from the release of the neurohormone catecholamine during episodes of pain or anxiety.

What to look for

With PACs, atrial and ventricular rates are irregular, but the underlying rhythm may be regular. When the PAC is conducted through the ventricles, the QRS complex appears normal on the patient's ECG.

Because the PAC depolarizes the SA node early, the SA node must reset itself. This action causes a pause after the PAC, disrupting the normal cycle. The next sinus beat then occurs sooner than it normally would, causing the P-P interval between two normal beats that have been interrupted by a PAC to be shorter than three consecutive sinus beats. This occurrence is referred to as *noncompensatory pause*. (See *Recognizing PACs*.)

Causes of PACs

Premature atrial contractions (PACs) may be triggered by:
• alcohol and cigarette use
• anxiety
• fatigue
• fever
• infection
• coronary or valvular heart disease
• acute respiratory failure or hypoxia
• pulmonary disease
• digoxin toxicity
• electrolyte imbalances.

Recognizing PACs

Take a look at this example of how premature atrial contractions (PACs) appear on a rhythm strip. Notice the distinguishing characteristics.

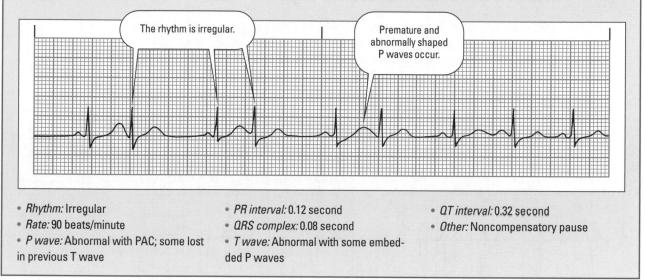

- *Rhythm:* Irregular
- *Rate:* 90 beats/minute
- *P wave:* Abnormal with PAC; some lost in previous T wave

- *PR interval:* 0.12 second
- *QRS complex:* 0.08 second
- *T wave:* Abnormal with some embedded P waves

- *QT interval:* 0.32 second
- *Other:* Noncompensatory pause

A hallmark moment

The hallmark ECG characteristic of a PAC is a premature P wave with an abnormal configuration (when compared with a sinus P wave). It may be lost in the previous T wave, distorting that wave's configuration. (The T wave might be bigger or have an extra bump.) Varying configurations of the P wave indicate more than one ectopic site. (See *Nonconducted PACs and second-degree AV block*, page 158.)

The PR interval is usually normal but may be shortened or slightly prolonged, depending on the origin of the ectopic focus. If no QRS complex follows the premature P wave, a nonconducted PAC has occurred.

PACs may occur in bigeminy (every other beat is a PAC), trigeminy (every third beat is a PAC), or couplets (two PACs at a time). The patient may have an irregular peripheral or apical pulse rhythm when the PACs occur. He may complain of palpitations, skipped beats, or a fluttering sensation. In a patient with heart disease, signs and symptoms of decreased cardiac output—such as hypotension and syncope—may occur.

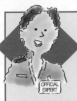

Advice from the experts

Nonconducted PACs and second-degree AV block

Don't confuse nonconducted premature atrial contractions (PACs) with type II second-degree atrioventricular (AV) block. In type II second-degree AV block, the P-P interval is regular. A nonconducted PAC, however, is an atrial impulse that arrives early to the AV node, when the node isn't yet repolarized.

As a result, the premature P wave fails to be conducted to the ventricle. The rhythm strip below shows a P wave embedded in the preceding T wave.

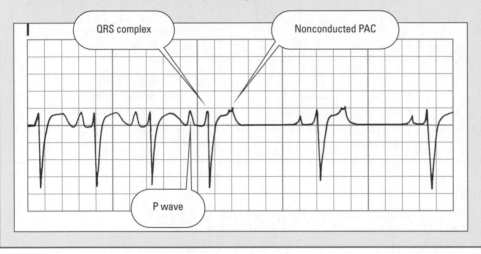

How you intervene

Most patients who are asymptomatic don't need treatment. If the patient is symptomatic, however, treatment may focus on eliminating the cause, such as caffeine and alcohol. People who have frequent PACs may be treated with drugs that prolong the refractory period of the atria. Those drugs include digoxin, procainamide, and quinidine.

The patient's part

When caring for a patient with PACs, assess him to help determine what's triggering the ectopic beats. Tailor your patient teaching to help the patient correct or avoid the underlying cause. For example, the patient might need to avoid caffeine or smoking or learn stress reduction techniques to lessen his anxiety.

If the patient has ischemic or valvular heart disease, monitor him for signs and symptoms of heart failure, electrolyte imbalances, and the development of more severe atrial arrhythmias.

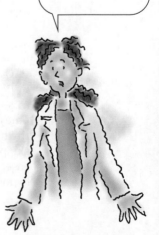

Too much caffeine and stress can cause PACs.

Atrial flutter

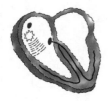

Atrial flutter, a supraventricular tachycardia, is characterized by an atrial rate of 250 to 400 beats/minute, although it's generally around 300 beats/minute. Originating in a single atrial focus, this rhythm results from circuit reentry and possibly increased automaticity.

How it happens

Atrial flutter is commonly associated with second-degree block. In that instance, the AV node fails to allow conduction of all the impulses to the ventricles. As a result, the ventricular rate is slower. Atrial flutter rarely occurs in a healthy person. When it does, it may indicate intrinsic cardiac disease. (See *Causes of atrial flutter.*)

What to look for

Atrial flutter is characterized by abnormal P waves that lose their distinction because of the rapid atrial rate. The waves blend together, creating a saw-toothed appearance and are called *flutter waves*, or *F waves*. Varying degrees of AV block produce ventricular rates one-half to one-fourth of the atrial rate. The QRS complex is usually normal but may be widened if flutter waves are buried in the complex. You won't be able to identify a T wave, nor will you be able to measure the QT interval. (See *Recognizing atrial flutter*, page 160.)

A flitter, a flutter

The atrial rhythm may vary between fibrillatory waves and flutter waves, an arrhythmia commonly referred to as *atrial fibrillation and flutter*. Fibrillatory waves are uneven baseline fibrillation waves caused by the initiation of chaotic impulses from multiple ectopic sites in the atria. Depolarization can't spread in an organized manner because the atria quiver instead of contract.

Rating the ratio

The clinical significance of atrial flutter is determined by the number of impulses conducted through the node—expressed as a conduction ratio, for example, 2:1 or 4:1—and the resulting ventricular rate. If the ventricular rate is too slow (less than 40 beats/minute) or too fast (more than 150 beats/minute), cardiac output may be seriously compromised.

Usually the faster the ventricular rate, the more dangerous the arrhythmia. The rapid rate reduces ventricular filling time and

Causes of atrial flutter

Atrial flutter may be caused by:
• conditions that enlarge atrial tissue and elevate atrial pressures, such as severe mitral valve disease, hyperthyroidism, pericardial disease, and primary myocardial disease
• cardiac surgery
• acute myocardial infarction
• chronic obstructive pulmonary disease
• systemic arterial hypoxia.

Recognizing atrial flutter

Take a look at this example of how atrial flutter appears on a rhythm strip. Notice its distinguishing characteristics.

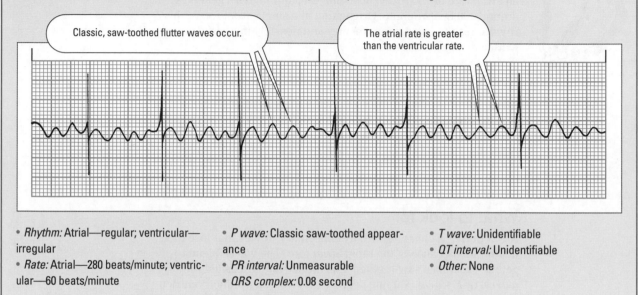

Classic, saw-toothed flutter waves occur.

The atrial rate is greater than the ventricular rate.

- *Rhythm:* Atrial—regular; ventricular—irregular
- *Rate:* Atrial—280 beats/minute; ventricular—60 beats/minute

- *P wave:* Classic saw-toothed appearance
- *PR interval:* Unmeasurable
- *QRS complex:* 0.08 second

- *T wave:* Unidentifiable
- *QT interval:* Unidentifiable
- *Other:* None

coronary perfusion, which can cause angina, heart failure, pulmonary edema, hypotension, and syncope.

One of the most common rates is 150 beats/minute. With an atrial rate of 300, that rhythm is referred to as a 2:1 block. (See *Atrial flutter and sinus tachycardia.*)

Misleading pulses

When caring for a patient with atrial flutter, you may note that his peripheral or apical pulse is normal in rate and rhythm. That's because the pulse reflects the number of ventricular contractions, not the number of atrial impulses.

If the ventricular rate is normal, the patient may be asymptomatic. However, if the ventricular rate is rapid, the patient may exhibit signs and symptoms of reduced cardiac output and cardiac decompensation.

How you intervene

Atrial flutter with a rapid ventricular response and reduced cardiac output requires immediate intervention. Therapy aims to control the ventricular rate and convert the atrial ectopic rhythm to a

Advice from the experts

Atrial flutter and sinus tachycardia

Whenever you see sinus tachycardia with a rate of 150 beats/minute, take another look. That rate is a common one for atrial flutter with 2:1 conduction. Look closely for flutter waves, which may be difficult to see if they're hidden in the QRS complex. You may need to check another lead to clearly see them.

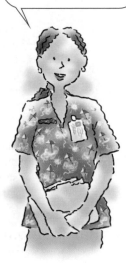

Cardioversion is the treatment of choice for atrial flutter.

normal sinus rhythm. Although stimulation of the vagus nerve may temporarily increase the block ratio and slow the ventricular rate, the effects won't last. For that reason, cardioversion remains the treatment of choice.

A shocking solution

Synchronized cardioversion delivers an electrical stimulus during depolarization. The stimulus makes part of the myocardium refractory to ectopic impulses and terminates circuit reentry movements.

Become a convert

Drug therapy includes digoxin and calcium channel blockers, which decrease AV conduction time. Quinidine may be given to convert flutter to fibrillation, an easier arrhythmia to treat. If digoxin and quinidine therapy is used, the patient must first be given a loading dose of digoxin. Ibutilide (Corvert) may be used to convert recent-onset atrial flutter to sinus rhythm. If possible, the underlying cause of the atrial flutter should be treated.

Keeping watch

Because atrial flutter may be an indication of intrinsic cardiac disease, monitor the patient closely for signs and symptoms of low cardiac output. If cardioversion is indicated, prepare the patient for I.V. administration of a sedative or anesthetic as ordered. Keep resuscitative equipment at the bedside. Be alert to the effects of digoxin, which depresses the SA node. Also be alert for bradycardia because cardioversion can decrease the heart rate.

Atrial fibrillation

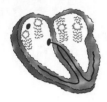

Atrial fibrillation, sometimes called *A-fib*, is defined as chaotic, asynchronous, electrical activity in atrial tissue. The ectopic impulses may fire at a rate of 400 to 600 times/minute, causing the atria to quiver instead of contract.

The ventricles respond only to those impulses that make it through the AV node. On an ECG, atrial activity is no longer represented by P waves but by erratic baseline waves called *fibrillatory waves*, or *F waves*. This rhythm may either be sustained or paroxysmal (occurring in bursts). It can be preceded by, or result from, PACs.

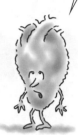

Sometimes my atria get so wired I just can't beat straight.

How it happens

Atrial fibrillation occurs more commonly than atrial flutter or atrial tachycardia. It stems from the firing of several impulses in circuit reentry pathways. (See *Causes of atrial fibrillation*.)

What to look for

In atrial fibrillation, small sections of the atria are activated individually. This situation causes the atrial muscle to quiver instead of contract. On an ECG, you'll see uneven baseline F waves rather than clearly distinguishable P waves. Also, when several ectopic sites in the atria fire impulses, depolarization can't spread in an organized manner, which causes an irregular ventricular response. (See *Recognizing atrial fibrillation*.)

That fabulous filter

The AV node protects the ventricles from the 400 to 600 erratic atrial impulses that occur each minute by acting as a filter and

---

Causes of atrial fibrillation

Atrial fibrillation may be caused by:
- cardiac surgery
- heart conditions, such as mitral insufficiency, mitral stenosis, hyperthyroidism, infection, coronary artery disease, acute myocardial infarction, pericarditis, hypoxia, and atrial septal defects
- coffee, alcohol, or cigarette use
- fatigue or stress
- certain drugs, such as aminophylline and digoxin (Lanoxin)
- catecholamine release during exercise.

Recognizing atrial fibrillation

Take a look at this example of how atrial fibrillation appears on a rhythm strip. Notice its distinguishing characteristics.

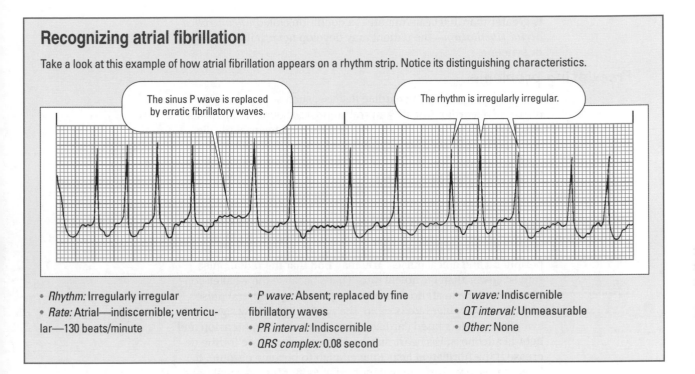

The sinus P wave is replaced by erratic fibrillatory waves.

The rhythm is irregularly irregular.

- *Rhythm:* Irregularly irregular
- *Rate:* Atrial—indiscernible; ventricular—130 beats/minute
- *P wave:* Absent; replaced by fine fibrillatory waves
- *PR interval:* Indiscernible
- *QRS complex:* 0.08 second
- *T wave:* Indiscernible
- *QT interval:* Unmeasurable
- *Other:* None

blocking some of the impulses. The AV node itself doesn't receive all the impulses, however. If muscle tissue around the AV node is in a refractory state, impulses from other areas of the atria can't reach the AV node, which further reduces the number of atrial impulses conducted through to the ventricles. These two factors help explain the characteristic wide variation in R-R intervals in atrial fibrillation.

Fast and furious

The atrial rate is almost indiscernible but is usually greater than 400 beats/minute. The ventricular rate usually varies from 100 to 150 beats/minute but can be lower. Atrial fibrillation is called *coarse* if the F waves are pronounced; the fibrillation is called *fine* if they aren't. Atrial fibrillation and flutter may also occur simultaneously. Look for a configuration that varies between fibrillatory waves and flutter waves.

As with other atrial arrhythmias, atrial fibrillation eliminates atrial systole (also known as *atrial kick*). That loss, combined with the decreased filling times associated with rapid rates, can lead to clinically significant problems. If the ventricular response

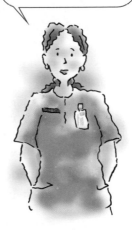

The AV node blocks erratic atrial impulses to protect the ventricles.

is greater than 100 beats/minute—a condition called *uncontrolled atrial fibrillation*—the patient may develop heart failure, angina, or syncope.

Preexisting problems

Patients with preexisting cardiac disease, such as hypertrophic obstructive cardiomyopathy, mitral stenosis, rheumatic heart disease, and mitral prosthetic valves, tend to tolerate atrial fibrillation poorly and may develop shock and severe heart failure.

Left untreated, atrial fibrillation can lead to cardiovascular collapse, thrombus formation, and systemic arterial or pulmonary embolism.

How you intervene

When assessing a patient with atrial fibrillation, assess both the peripheral and apical pulses. You may find that the radial pulse rate is slower than the apical rate. That's because the weaker contractions of the heart don't produce a palpable peripheral pulse.

If the ventricular rate is rapid, the patient may show signs and symptoms of decreased cardiac output, including hypotension and light-headedness. His heart may be able to compensate for the decrease if the fibrillation lasts long enough to become chronic. In those cases, however, the patient is at a greater-than-normal risk for developing pulmonary, cerebral, or other emboli and may exhibit signs of those conditions.

Goal: Reduce the rate

The major therapeutic goal in treating atrial fibrillation is to reduce the ventricular response rate to less than 100 beats/minute. When the onset of atrial fibrillation is acute and the patient can cooperate, vagal maneuvers or carotid sinus massage may slow the ventricular response but won't convert the arrhythmia.

The ventricular rate may be controlled with such drugs as diltiazem (Cardizem), verapamil (Isoptin), digoxin, and beta-adrenergic blockers. Ibutilide may be used to convert new-onset atrial fibrillation to sinus rhythm. Quinidine and procainamide (Pronestyl) can also convert atrial fibrillation to normal sinus rhythm, usually after anticoagulation.

A jolting recovery

If the patient is symptomatic, immediate synchronized cardioversion is necessary. Cardioversion is most successful if used within the first 3 days of treatment and less successful if the rhythm has existed for a long time. If possible, anticoagulants should be administered first because conversion to normal sinus rhythm causes forceful atrial contractions to resume abruptly. If a thrombus has formed in the atria, the resumption of contractions can result in systemic emboli.

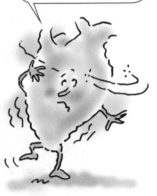

If all those other impulses would calm down, my SA node could resume control.

Resuming a commanding role

Drugs, such as digoxin, procainamide, propranolol (Inderal), quinidine, amiodarone, and verapamil can be given after successful cardioversion to maintain normal sinus rhythm and to control the ventricular rate in chronic atrial fibrillation. Some of these drugs prolong the atrial refractory period, giving the SA node an opportunity to reestablish its role as the heart's pacemaker, whereas others primarily slow AV node conduction, controlling the ventricular rate.

If drug therapy is used, monitor serum drug levels and observe the patient for evidence of toxicity. Tell the patient to report pulse rate changes, syncope or dizziness, chest pain, or signs of heart failure, such as increasing dyspnea and peripheral edema.

Radio blackout

Symptom-producing atrial fibrillation that doesn't respond to routine treatment may be treated with *radiofrequency ablation therapy*. In this invasive procedure, a transvenous catheter is used to locate the area within the heart that participates in initiating or perpetuating certain tachyarrhythmias.

Radiofrequency energy is then delivered to the myocardium through this catheter to produce a small area of necrosis. The damaged tissue can no longer cause or participate in the tachyarrhythmia. If the energy is delivered close to the AV node, bundle of His, or bundle branches, a block can occur.

Atrial tachycardia

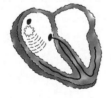

Atrial tachycardia is a supraventricular tachycardia, which means the impulses driving the rapid rhythm originate above the ventricles. Atrial tachycardia is characterized by an atrial rate of 150 to 250 beats/minute. The rapid rate shortens diastole, resulting in a loss of atrial kick, reduced cardiac output, reduced coronary perfusion, and ischemic myocardial changes.

Three types of atrial tachycardia exist: atrial tachycardia with block, multifocal atrial tachycardia (MAT) (or chaotic atrial rhythm), and paroxysmal atrial tachycardia (PAT).

How it happens

In a healthy person, atrial tachycardia is usually benign. However, this rhythm may be a forerunner of a more serious ventricular arrhythmia, especially if it occurs in a patient with an underlying heart condition. (See *Causes of atrial tachycardia*.)

The increased ventricular rate of atrial tachycardia decreases the time allowed for the ventricles to fill, increases myocardial oxygen consumption, and decreases oxygen supply. Angina, heart failure, ischemic myocardial changes, and even MI can result.

What to look for

Atrial tachycardia is characterized by three or more successive ectopic atrial beats at a rate of 140 to 250 beats/minute. The P wave is usually upright, if visible, and followed by a QRS complex.

Keep in mind that atrial beats may be conducted on a 1:1 basis into the ventricles (meaning that each P wave has a QRS complex), so atrial and ventricular rates will be equal. In other cases, atrial beats may be conducted only periodically, meaning there's a block in the AV conduction system. The block keeps the ventricles from receiving every impulse.

Hold it right there!

Think of the AV node as a gatekeeper or doorman. Sometimes it lets atrial impulses through to the ventricles regularly (every other impulse, for instance), and sometimes it lets them in irregularly (two impulses might get through, for instance, and then three, and then one).

Fast but regular

When assessing a rhythm strip for atrial tachycardia, you'll see that atrial rhythm is always regular, and ventricular rhythm is regular when the block is constant and irregular when it isn't. The rate consists of three or more successive ectopic atrial beats at a rate of 140 to 250 beats/minute. The ventricular rate varies according to the AV conduction ratio. (See *Recognizing atrial tachycardia*.)

The P wave has a 1:1 ratio with the QRS complex unless a block is present. The P wave may not be discernible because of the rapid rate and may be hidden in the previous ST segment or T wave. You may not be able to measure the PR interval if the P wave can't be distinguished from the preceding T wave.

The QRS complex is usually normal, unless the impulses are being conducted abnormally through the ventricles. The T wave may be normal or inverted if ischemia is present. The QT interval is usually within normal limits but may be shorter because of the rapid rate. ST-segment and T-wave changes may appear if ischemia occurs with a prolonged arrhythmia. (See *Identifying types of atrial tachycardia*, pages 168 and 169.)

Causes of atrial tachycardia

Atrial tachycardia can occur in patients with normal hearts. In those cases, the condition is commonly related to excessive use of caffeine or other stimulants, marijuana use, electrolyte imbalances, hypoxia, and physical or psychological stress. Atrial tachycardia may also be a component of sick sinus syndrome.

Other causes may include:
• digoxin toxicity (most common cause)
• myocardial infarction, cardiomyopathy, congenital anomalies, Wolff-Parkinson-White syndrome, and valvular disease
• cor pulmonale
• hyperthyroidism
• systemic hypertension.

Recognizing atrial tachycardia

Take a look at this example of how atrial tachycardia appears on a rhythm strip. Notice its distinguishing characteristics.

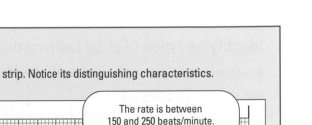

The P wave may hide in the preceding T wave.

The rate is between 150 and 250 beats/minute.

- *Rhythm:* Regular
- *Rate:* 200 beats/minute
- *P wave:* Abnormal

- *PR interval:* 0.12 second
- *QRS complex:* 0.10 second
- *T wave:* Distorted by P wave

- *QT interval:* 0.20 second
- *Other:* None

Feel the rhythm

Atrial tachycardia is characterized by a rapid apical or peripheral pulse rate. The rhythm may be regular or irregular, depending on the type of atrial tachycardia. A patient with PAT may complain that his heart suddenly starts to beat faster or that he suddenly feels palpitations. Persistent tachycardia and rapid ventricular rate cause decreased cardiac output, which can lead to blurred vision, syncope, and hypotension.

How you intervene

Treatment depends on the type of tachycardia and the severity of the patient's symptoms. Because one of the most common causes of atrial tachycardia is digoxin toxicity, monitor levels of the drug. (See *Signs of digoxin toxicity,* page 170.)

Measures to produce vagal stimulation, such as Valsalva's maneuver and carotid sinus massage, may be used to treat PAT. Vagal maneuvers are particularly effective when the tachycardia is caused by circuit reentry, which is signaled by frequent PACs. (See *Understanding carotid sinus massage,* page 171.)

(Text continues on page 170.)

Identifying types of atrial tachycardia

Atrial tachycardia comes in three varieties. Here's a quick rundown of each.

Atrial tachycardia with block

Atrial tachycardia with block is caused by increased automaticity of the atrial tissue. As atrial rate speeds up and the atrioventricular conduction becomes impaired, a 2:1 block typically occurs. Occasionally a type 1 (Wenckebach) second-degree heart block may be seen.

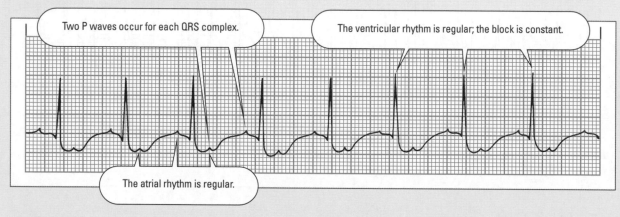

Two P waves occur for each QRS complex.

The ventricular rhythm is regular; the block is constant.

The atrial rhythm is regular.

Interpretation
• *Rhythm:* Atrial—regular; ventricular—regular if block is constant, irregular if block is variable

• *Rate:* Atrial—140 to 250 beats/minute, multiple of ventricular rate; ventricular—varies with block
• *P wave:* Slightly abnormal

• *PR interval:* Usually normal; may be hidden
• *QRS complex:* Usually normal
• *Other:* More than one P wave for each QRS

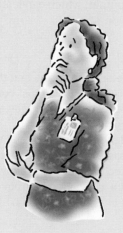

Multifocal atrial tachycardia

In multifocal atrial tachycardia (MAT), atrial tachycardia occurs with numerous atrial foci firing intermittently. MAT produces varying P waves on the strip and occurs most commonly in patients with chronic pulmonary disease. The irregular baseline in this strip is caused by movement of the chest wall.

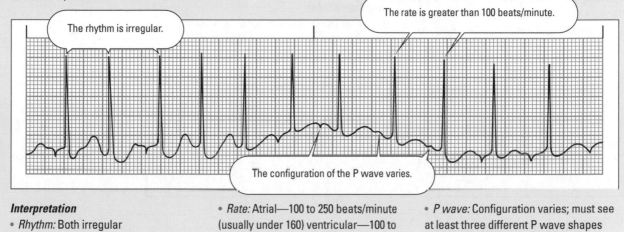

The rhythm is irregular.

The rate is greater than 100 beats/minute.

The configuration of the P wave varies.

Interpretation
- *Rhythm:* Both irregular

- *Rate:* Atrial—100 to 250 beats/minute (usually under 160) ventricular—100 to 250 beats/minute

- *P wave:* Configuration varies; must see at least three different P wave shapes
- *PR interval:* Varies
- *Other:* None

Paroxysmal atrial tachycardia

A type of paroxysmal supraventricular tachycardia, paroxysmal atrial tachycardia (PAT) features brief periods of tachycardia that alternate with periods of normal sinus rhythm. PAT starts and stops suddenly as a result of rapid firing of an ectopic focus. It commonly follows frequent premature atrial contractions (PACs), one of which initiates the tachycardia.

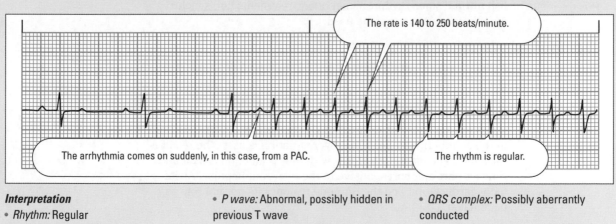

The rate is 140 to 250 beats/minute.

The arrhythmia comes on suddenly, in this case, from a PAC.

The rhythm is regular.

Interpretation
- *Rhythm:* Regular
- *Rate:* 140 to 250 beats/minute

- *P wave:* Abnormal, possibly hidden in previous T wave
- *PR interval:* Identical for each cycle

- *QRS complex:* Possibly aberrantly conducted
- *Other:* One P wave for each QRS complex

Signs of digoxin toxicity

With digoxin toxicity, atrial tachycardia isn't the only change you might see in your patient. Be alert for the following signs and symptoms, especially if the patient is taking digoxin (Lanoxin) and his potassium level is low or he's also taking amiodarone (Cordarone). Both combinations can increase the risk of digoxin toxicity.

Central nervous system
• Fatigue and general muscle weakness
• Agitation
• Hallucinations

Eyes, ears, nose, and throat
• Yellow-green halos around visual images
• Blurred vision

GI
• Anorexia
• Nausea and vomiting

Cardiovascular
• Arrhythmias (most commonly, conduction disturbances with or without atrioventricular block, premature ventricular contractions, and supraventricular arrhythmias)
• Increased severity of heart failure
• Hypotension (digoxin's toxic effects on the heart may be life-threatening and always require immediate attention)

Making a bigger block

Other treatment options include drugs that increase the degree of AV block, which in turn decreases the ventricular response and slows the rate. Such drugs include digoxin, beta-adrenergic blockers, and calcium channel blockers.

In addition, adenosine (Adenocard) may be used to stop atrial tachycardia, and quinidine or procainamide may be used to establish normal sinus rhythm. When other treatments fail, synchronized cardioversion may be used.

Going into overdrive

Atrial overdrive pacing (also called *burst pacing* or *rapid atrial pacing*) may be used to stop the arrhythmia. In this procedure, the patient's atrial rate is electronically paced slightly higher than the intrinsic arterial rate. With some patients, the atria are paced using much faster bursts or are paced prematurely at a critical time in the conduction cycle. Whichever variation is used, the result is the same. The pacing interferes with the conduction circuit and renders part of it unresponsive to the reentrant impulse. Atrial tachycardia stops, and the SA node resumes its normal role as pacemaker.

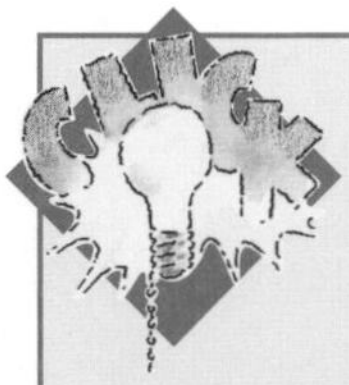

Now I get it!

Understanding carotid sinus massage

Carotid sinus massage (shown below) may be used to stop paroxysmal atrial tachycardia. Massaging the carotid sinus stimulates the vagus nerve, which then inhibits firing of the sinoatrial (SA) node and slows atrioventricular node conduction. As a result, the SA node can resume its job as primary pacemaker. Risks of carotid sinus massage include decreased heart rate, vasodilation, ventricular arrhythmias, stroke, and cardiac standstill.

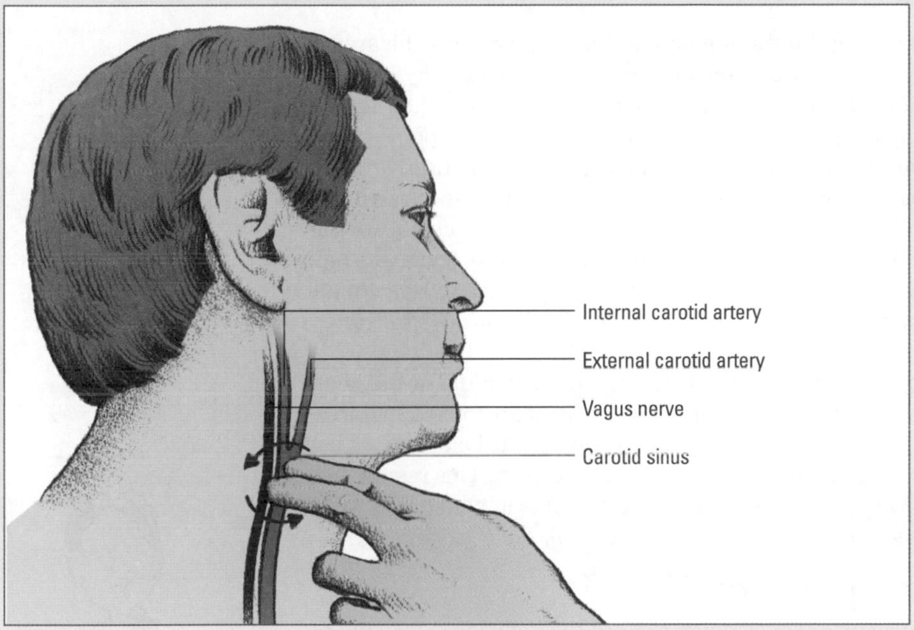

Internal carotid artery

External carotid artery

Vagus nerve

Carotid sinus

If the arrhythmia is associated with Wolff-Parkinson-White syndrome, radiofrequency ablation therapy may be used to control recurrent episodes of PAT. Because MAT commonly occurs in patients with chronic obstructive pulmonary disease, the rhythm may not respond to treatment. Treatment attempts to correct severe hypoxia when possible.

Keeping tabs on troublemakers

When caring for a patient with atrial tachycardia, carefully monitor the patient's rhythm strips. Doing so may provide information about the cause of atrial tachycardia, which in turn can facilitate treatment. Also monitor the patient for chest pain, indications of decreased cardiac output, and signs and symptoms of heart failure or myocardial ischemia.

Junctional arrhythmias

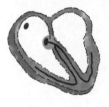

Junctional arrhythmias originate in the AV junction—the area around the AV node and the bundle of His. These arrhythmias occur when the SA node is suppressed and fails to conduct impulses or when a block occurs in conduction. Electrical impulses may then be initiated by pacemaker cells in the AV junction.

In normal impulse conduction, the AV node slows transmission of the impulse from the atria to the ventricles, which allows the atria to pump as much blood as they can into the ventricles before the ventricles contract. However, impulses aren't always conducted normally. (See *Conduction in Wolff-Parkinson-White syndrome.*)

Because the AV junction is located in the middle of the heart, impulses generated in this area cause the heart to be depolarized in an abnormal way. The impulse moves upward and causes backward, or retrograde, depolarization of the atria. This results in inverted P waves in leads II, III, and aV$_F$, leads in which you would usually see upright P waves. (See *Finding the P wave*, page 174.)

Which way did the impulse go?

The impulse also moves down toward the ventricles, causing forward, or antegrade, depolarization of the ventricles and an upright QRS complex. Arrhythmias that cause inverted P waves on an ECG may be atrial or junctional in origin.

Junctional mimic

Atrial arrhythmias are sometimes mistaken for junctional arrhythmias because impulses are generated so low in the atria that they cause retrograde depolarization and inverted P waves. Looking at the PR interval helps you determine whether an arrhythmia is atrial or junctional.

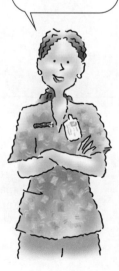

Don't mistake an atrial arrhythmia for a junctional arrhythmia. Check the PR interval.

Now I get it!

Conduction in Wolff-Parkinson-White syndrome

Conduction doesn't always take place in a normal way. In Wolff-Parkinson-White syndrome, for example, a conduction bypass develops outside the atrioventricular (AV) junction and connects the atria with the ventricles, as shown at right Wolff-Parkinson-White syndrome is typically a congenital rhythm disorder that occurs mainly in young children and in adults ages 20 to 35.

Rapidly conducted

The bypass formed in Wolff-Parkinson-White syndrome, known as *Kent's bundle,* conducts impulses to the atria or the ventricles. Impulses aren't delayed at the AV node, so conduction is abnormally fast. Retrograde conduction, reentry, and reentrant tachycardia can result.

Checking the ECG

Wolff-Parkinson-White syndrome causes a shortened PR interval (less than 0.10 second) and a widened QRS complex (greater than 0.10 second). The beginning of the QRS complex may look slurred because of altered ventricular depolarization. The hallmark sign of this syndrome is called a *delta wave,* shown in the inset above.

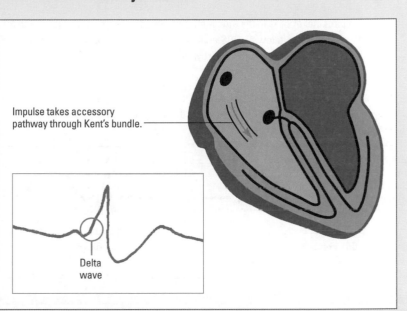

Impulse takes accessory pathway through Kent's bundle.

Delta wave

Bad PR

An arrhythmia with an inverted P wave before the QRS complex and a normal PR interval (0.12 to 0.20 second) originated in the atria. An arrhythmia with a PR interval less than 0.12 second originated in the AV junction.

Junctional arrhythmias include premature junctional contractions (PJCs), junctional escape rhythm, accelerated junctional rhythm, and junctional tachycardia.

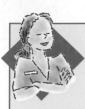

Peak technique

Finding the P wave

When the pacemaker fires in the atrioventricular junction, the impulse may reach the atria or the ventricles first. Therefore, the inverted P wave and the following QRS complex won't have a consistent relationship. These rhythm strips show the various positions the P wave can take in junctional rhythms.

Atria first
If the atria are depolarized first, the P wave will occur before the QRS complex.

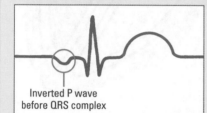

Inverted P wave
before QRS complex

Ventricles first
If the ventricles are depolarized first, the QRS complex will come before the P wave.

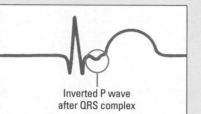

Inverted P wave
after QRS complex

Simultaneous
If the ventricles and atria are depolarized simultaneously, the P wave will be hidden in the QRS complex.

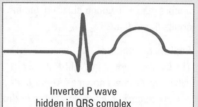

Inverted P wave
hidden in QRS complex

Premature junctional contraction

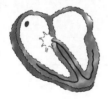

A PJC is a beat that occurs before a normal beat and causes an irregular rhythm. This ectopic beat occurs when an irritable location within the AV junction acts as a pacemaker and fires either prematurely or out of sequence.

As with all beats produced by the AV junction, the atria depolarize in retrograde fashion, causing an inverted P wave on the ECG. The ventricles depolarize normally.

How it happens

PJCs commonly occur in a normal heart and are rarely dangerous. In fact, they usually cause no symptoms and can go unrecognized for years. (See *Causes of PJCs.*)

What to look for

A PJC appears on a rhythm strip as an early beat causing an irregularity. The rest of the strip may show regular atrial and ventricular rhythms, depending on the patient's underlying rhythm.

Causes of PJCs

Premature junctional contractions (PJCs) may be caused by:
• toxic levels of digoxin (Lanoxin) (level greater than 2.5 ng/ml)
• excessive caffeine intake
• inferior-wall myocardial infarction
• rheumatic heart disease
• valvular disease
• swelling of the atrioventricular junction after heart surgery.

When upside down is right-side up

Look for an inverted P wave in leads II, III, and aV$_F$. Depending on when the impulse occurs, the P wave may fall before, during, or after the QRS complex. If it falls during the QRS complex, it's hidden. If it comes before the QRS complex, the PR interval is less than 0.12 second. (See *Recognizing a PJC*.)

Because the ventricles usually depolarize normally, the QRS complex has a normal configuration and a normal duration of less than 0.12 second. The T wave and the QT interval are usually normal.

That quickening feeling

The patient may be asymptomatic or he may complain of palpitations or a feeling of quickening in the chest. Palpation may reveal an irregular pulse. If the PJCs are frequent, the patient may have hypotension from a transient decrease in cardiac output.

How you intervene

Although PJCs themselves usually aren't dangerous, you'll need to monitor the patient carefully and assess him for other signs of intrinsic pacemaker failure. If digoxin toxicity is the culprit, check

Recognizing a PJC

Take a look at this example of how a premature junctional contraction (PJC)—a junctional beat that occurs before a normal sinus beat—appears on a rhythm strip. Notice its distinguishing characteristics.

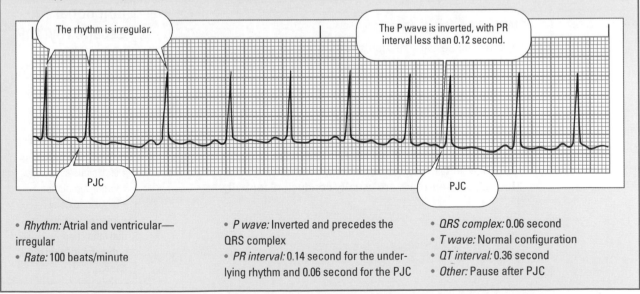

The rhythm is irregular.

The P wave is inverted, with PR interval less than 0.12 second.

PJC

PJC

• *Rhythm:* Atrial and ventricular—irregular
• *Rate:* 100 beats/minute

• *P wave:* Inverted and precedes the QRS complex
• *PR interval:* 0.14 second for the underlying rhythm and 0.06 second for the PJC

• *QRS complex:* 0.06 second
• *T wave:* Normal configuration
• *QT interval:* 0.36 second
• *Other:* Pause after PJC

with the patient's doctor about discontinuing the medication and monitoring serum drug levels.

You should also monitor the patient for hemodynamic instability. If ectopic beats are frequent, the patient should decrease or eliminate his caffeine intake.

Junctional escape rhythm

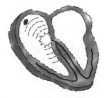

A junctional escape rhythm is a string of beats that occurs after a conduction delay from the atria. The normal intrinsic firing rate for cells in the AV junction is 40 to 60 beats/minute.

Remember that the AV junction can take over as the heart's pacemaker if higher pacemaker sites slow down or fail to fire or conduct. The junctional escape beat is an example of this compensatory mechanism. Because junctional escape beats prevent ventricular standstill, they should never be suppressed.

Backward and upside-down

In a junctional escape rhythm, as in all junctional arrhythmias, the atria are depolarized by means of retrograde conduction. The P waves are inverted, and impulse conduction through the ventricles is normal.

How it happens

A junctional escape rhythm can be caused by any condition that disturbs SA node function or enhances AV junction automaticity. (See *Causes of junctional escape rhythm.*)

What to look for

A junctional escape rhythm shows a regular rhythm of 40 to 60 beats/minute on an ECG strip. Look for inverted P waves in leads II, III, and aV$_F$.

The P waves will occur before, after, or hidden within the QRS complex. The PR interval is less than 0.12 second and is measurable only if the P wave comes before the QRS complex. (See *Recognizing junctional escape rhythm.*)

The rest of the ECG waveform—including the QRS complex, T wave, and QT interval—should appear normal because impulses through the ventricles are usually conducted normally.

Causes of junctional escape rhythm

Junctional escape rhythm can be caused by any condition that disturbs sinoatrial node function or enhances atrioventricular junction automaticity, including:
• sick sinus syndrome
• vagal stimulation
• digoxin toxicity
• inferior-wall myocardial infarction
• rheumatic heart disease.

Recognizing junctional escape rhythm

Take a look at this example of how junctional escape rhythm appears on a rhythm strip. Note the inverted P wave.

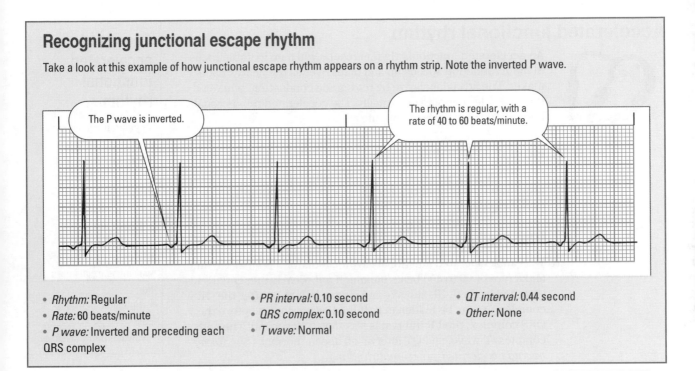

The P wave is inverted.

The rhythm is regular, with a rate of 40 to 60 beats/minute.

- *Rhythm:* Regular
- *Rate:* 60 beats/minute
- *P wave:* Inverted and preceding each QRS complex
- *PR interval:* 0.10 second
- *QRS complex:* 0.10 second
- *T wave:* Normal
- *QT interval:* 0.44 second
- *Other:* None

I may be slow, but at least I'm regular

A patient with a junctional escape rhythm has a slow, regular pulse rate of 40 to 60 beats/minute. The patient may be asymptomatic. Whether junctional escape rhythm harms the patient depends on how well the patient's heart tolerates a decreased heart rate and decreased cardiac output. Typically, pulse rates less than 60 beats/minute may lead to inadequate cardiac output, causing hypotension, syncope, or blurred vision.

How you intervene

Treatment of a junctional escape rhythm involves correcting the underlying cause. Atropine may be given to increase the heart rate, or a temporary or permanent pacemaker may be inserted.

Nursing care includes monitoring the patient's serum digoxin and electrolyte levels and watching for signs of decreased cardiac output, such as hypotension, syncope, or blurred vision. If the patient is hypotensive, lower the head of his bed as far as he can tolerate and keep atropine at the bedside.

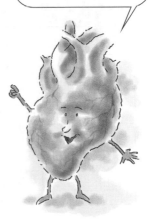

If I can tolerate a low heart rate and cardiac output, I can handle a junctional escape rhythm.

Accelerated junctional rhythm

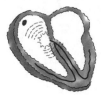

An accelerated junctional rhythm results when an irritable focus in the AV junction speeds up and takes over as the heart's pacemaker. The atria depolarize by retrograde conduction, whereas the ventricles depolarize normally. The accelerated rate is usually between 60 and 100 beats/minute.

How it happens

Conditions that affect SA node or AV node automaticity can cause accelerated junctional rhythm. (See *Causes of accelerated junctional rhythm.*)

What to look for

With an accelerated junctional rhythm, look for a regular rhythm and a rate of 60 to 100 beats/minute. If a P wave is present, it's inverted in leads II, III, and aV$_F$ and occurs before or after the QRS complex or may be hidden in it. If the P wave comes before the QRS complex, the PR interval is less than 0.12 second. The QRS complex, T wave, and QT interval all appear normal. (See *Recognizing accelerated junctional rhythm*)

Causes of accelerated junctional rhythm

Accelerated junctional rhythm can be caused by conditions that affect sinoatrial node or atrioventricular node automaticity, including:
- digoxin toxicity
- hypokalemia
- inferior- or posterior-wall myocardial infarction
- rheumatic heart disease
- valvular heart disease.

Recognizing accelerated junctional rhythm

Take a look at this example of how an accelerated junctional rhythm appears on a rhythm strip. Notice its distinguishing characteristics.

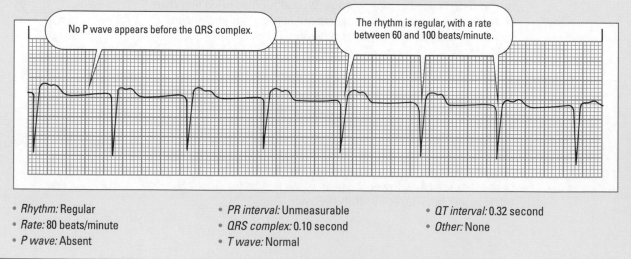

No P wave appears before the QRS complex.

The rhythm is regular, with a rate between 60 and 100 beats/minute.

- *Rhythm:* Regular
- *Rate:* 80 beats/minute
- *P wave:* Absent
- *PR interval:* Unmeasurable
- *QRS complex:* 0.10 second
- *T wave:* Normal
- *QT interval:* 0.32 second
- *Other:* None

Low-down, dizzy, and confused

The patient may be asymptomatic because accelerated junctional rhythm has the same rate as sinus rhythm. This arrhythmia is significant if the patient has symptoms of decreased cardiac output—hypotension, syncope, and blurred vision. These can occur if the atria are depolarized after the QRS complex, which prevents blood ejection from the atria into the ventricles, or atrial kick.

How you intervene

Treatment of accelerated junctional arrhythmia involves correcting the underlying cause. Nursing interventions include observing the patient for signs of decreased cardiac output and monitoring his vital signs for hemodynamic instability. You should also assess the levels of potassium and other electrolytes and administer supplements as ordered. Finally, monitor the patient's digoxin level and withhold his digoxin dose as ordered.

Junctional tachycardia

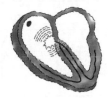

In junctional tachycardia, three or more PJCs occur in a row. The rate is usually 100 to 200 beats/minute.

How it happens

This supraventricular tachycardia occurs when an irritable focus from the AV junction has enhanced automaticity, overriding the SA node's ability to function as the heart's pacemaker. In this arrhythmia, the atria are depolarized by retrograde conduction; however, conduction through the ventricles remains normal. (See *Causes of junctional tachycardia.*)

What to look for

When assessing a rhythm strip for junctional tachycardia, look for a rate of 100 to 200 beats/minute. The P wave is inverted in leads II, III, and aV_F and can occur before, during (hidden P wave), or after the QRS complex. If it comes before the QRS complex, the only time the PR interval can be measured, it's always less than 0.12 second. (See *Recognizing junctional tachycardia*, page 180.)

The QRS complexes look normal, as does the T wave, unless a P wave occurs in it or the rate is so fast that the T wave can't be detected. (See *Junctional and supraventricular tachycardia*, page 181.)

Causes of junctional tachycardia

The most common cause of junctional tachycardia is digoxin toxicity, which can be enhanced by hypokalemia.

Other possible causes include:
• inferior- or posterior-wall myocardial infarction or ischemia
• congenital heart disease in children
• swelling of the atrioventricular junction after heart surgery.

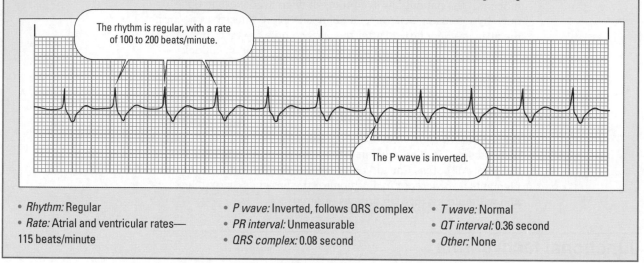

Recognizing junctional tachycardia

Take a look at this example of how junctional tachycardia appears on a rhythm strip. Notice its distinguishing characteristics.

The rhythm is regular, with a rate of 100 to 200 beats/minute.

The P wave is inverted.

- *Rhythm:* Regular
- *Rate:* Atrial and ventricular rates— 115 beats/minute

- *P wave:* Inverted, follows QRS complex
- *PR interval:* Unmeasurable
- *QRS complex:* 0.08 second

- *T wave:* Normal
- *QT interval:* 0.36 second
- *Other:* None

Compromisin' rhythm

The significance of junctional tachycardia depends on the rate, underlying cause, and severity of the accompanying cardiac disease. At higher ventricular rates, junctional tachycardia may compromise cardiac output by decreasing the amount of blood filling the ventricles with each beat. Higher rates also result in the loss of atrial kick. As a result, the patient may exhibit signs and symptoms of decreased cardiac output, such as a rapid pulse, low blood pressure, and dizziness.

How you intervene

The underlying cause of junctional tachycardia should be treated. If the cause is digoxin toxicity, digoxin should be discontinued. Vagal maneuvers and such medications as verapamil may slow the heart rate for the symptomatic patient.

Setting the pace

If the patient recently had an MI or heart surgery, he may need a temporary pacemaker to reset the heart's rhythm. Children with permanent arrhythmias may be resistant to drug therapy and require surgery. Patients with recurrent junctional tachycardia may be treated with ablation therapy, followed by permanent pacemaker insertion.

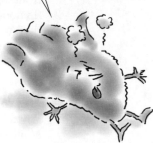

A higher ventricular rate means more problems for me!

Junctional and supraventricular tachycardia

If a tachycardia has a narrow QRS complex, you may have trouble deciding whether its source is junctional or atrial. When the rate approaches 150 beats/minute, a formerly visible P wave is hidden in the previous T wave, so you won't be able to use the P wave to figure out where the rhythm originated.

In these cases, call the rhythm *supraventricular tachycardia,* a general term that refers to the origin as being above the ventricles. Examples of supraventricular tachycardia include atrial flutter, multifocal atrial tachycardia, and junctional tachycardia.

Monitor patients with junctional tachycardia for signs of decreased cardiac output. You should also check digoxin and potassium levels and administer potassium supplements, as ordered. If symptoms are severe and digoxin is the culprit, the doctor may order digoxin immune fab (DigiFab), a digoxin-binding drug.

Ventricular arrhythmias

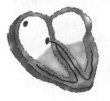

Ventricular arrhythmias originate in the ventricles below the bundle of His. They occur when electrical impulses depolarize the myocardium using a different pathway from normal impulses.

Ventricular arrhythmias appear on an ECG in characteristic ways. The QRS complex is wider than normal because of the prolonged conduction time through the ventricles. The T wave and the QRS complex deflect in opposite directions because of the difference in the action potential during ventricular depolarization and repolarization. Also, the P wave is absent because atrial depolarization doesn't occur.

You've lost your kick

When electrical impulses originate in the ventricles instead of the atria, atrial kick is lost and cardiac output decreases by as much as 30%. As a result, patients with ventricular arrhythmias may show signs and symptoms of cardiac decompensation, including hypotension, angina, syncope, and respiratory distress.

Potential to kill

Although ventricular arrhythmias may be benign, they're potentially deadly because the ventricles are ultimately responsible for cardiac output. Rapid recognition and treatment of ventricular arrhythmias increases the chance for successful resuscitation.

Ventricular arrhythmias include premature ventricular contractions (PVCs), ventricular tachycardia, ventricular fibrillation, and idioventricular rhythms. This section also discusses asystole, which is the lack of ventricular movement.

Premature ventricular contraction

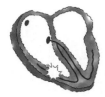

A PVC is an ectopic beat originating low in the ventricles and occurring earlier than normal. PVCs may occur in healthy people without causing problems. PVCs may occur singly, in clusters of two or more, or in repeating patterns, such as bigeminy or trigeminy. When PVCs occur in patients with underlying heart disease, they may indicate impending lethal ventricular arrhythmias.

How it happens

PVCs are usually caused by electrical irritability in the ventricular conduction system or muscle tissue. This irritability may be provoked by anything that disrupts normal electrolyte shifts during cell depolarization and repolarization. (See *Causes of PVCs*.)

This could get serious

PVCs are significant for two reasons. First, they can lead to more serious arrhythmias, such as ventricular tachycardia or ventricular fibrillation. The risk of developing a more serious arrhythmia increases in patients with ischemic or damaged hearts.

PVCs also decrease cardiac output, especially if the ectopic beats are frequent or sustained. Decreased cardiac out-

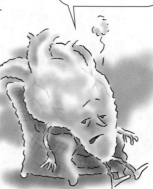

Because I'm weak, I'm at greater risk for developing a serious arrhythmia.

Causes of PVCs

Premature ventricular contractions (PVCs) may be caused by conditions that provoke electrical irritability in the ventricular conduction system or muscle tissue, including anything that disrupts normal electrolyte shifts during cell depolarization and repolarization. Conditions that may disrupt electrolyte shifts include:
• electrolyte imbalances, such as hypokalemia, hyperkalemia, hypomagnesemia, and hypocalcemia

• metabolic acidosis
• hypoxia
• myocardial ischemia
• drug intoxication, particularly cocaine, amphetamines, and tricyclic antidepressants
• enlargement of the ventricular chambers
• increased sympathetic stimulation
• myocarditis.

put is caused by reduced ventricular diastolic filling time and a loss of atrial kick. The clinical impact of PVCs hinges on how well perfusion is maintained and how long the abnormal rhythm lasts.

What to look for

On the ECG strip, PVCs look wide and bizarre and appear as early beats causing atrial and ventricular irregularity. The rate follows the underlying rhythm, which is usually regular. (See *Recognizing PVCs*.)

The P wave is usually absent. A PVC may trigger retrograde P waves, which can distort the ST segment. The PR interval and QT interval aren't measurable on a premature beat, only on the normal beats.

Complex configuration

The QRS complex occurs early. Configuration of the QRS complex is usually normal in the underlying rhythm. The duration of the QRS complex in the premature beat exceeds 0.12 second. The

Recognizing PVCs

This rhythm strip shows premature ventricular contractions (PVCs) on beats 1, 6, and 11. Note the wide and bizarre appearance of the QRS complex.

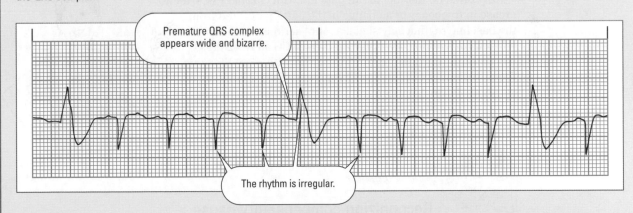

- *Rhythm:* Atrial and ventricular—irregular
- *Rate:* 120 beats/minute
- *P wave:* None with PVC, but P wave present with other QRS complexes

- *PR interval:* 0.12 second in underlying rhythm
- *QRS complex:* Early, with bizarre configuration and duration of 0.14 second in PVC; QRS complexes are 0.08 second in underlying rhythm

- *T wave:* Normal; opposite direction from QRS complex
- *QT interval:* 0.28 second with underlying rhythm
- *Other:* None

T wave in the premature beat has a deflection opposite that of the QRS complex.

When a PVC strikes on the downslope of the preceding normal T wave—the R-on-T phenomenon—it can trigger more serious rhythm disturbances.

The pause that compensates

A horizontal baseline called a *compensatory pause* may follow the T wave of the PVC. When a compensatory pause appears, the interval between two normal sinus beats containing a PVC equals two normal sinus intervals. (See *Recognizing compensatory pause*.) This pause occurs because the ventricle is refractory and can't respond to the next regularly timed P wave from the sinus node. When a compensatory pause doesn't occur, the PVC is referred to as *interpolated*.

PVCs all in a row

PVCs that look alike are called *unifocal* and originate from the same ectopic focus. These beats may also appear in patterns that can progress to more lethal arrhythmias. (See *When PVCs spell danger*, pages 186 and 187.)

Ruling out trouble

To help determine the seriousness of PVCs, ask yourself these questions:
• How often do they occur? In patients with chronic PVCs, an increase in frequency or a change in the pattern of PVCs from the baseline rhythm may signal a more serious condition.
• What pattern do they occur in? If the ECG shows a dangerous pattern—such as paired PVCs, PVCs with more than one focus, bigeminy, or R-on-T phenomenon—the patient may require immediate treatment.

> When evaluating PVCs, remember that an increase in frequency, a change in pattern, or a dangerous pattern may indicate a more serious condition.

Peak technique

Recognizing compensatory pause

You can determine if a compensatory pause exists by using calipers to mark off two normal P-P intervals. Place one leg of the calipers on the sinus P wave that comes just before the premature ventricular contraction. If the pause is compensatory, the other leg of the calipers will fall precisely on the P wave that comes after the pause.

• Are they really PVCs? Make sure the complex you see is a PVC, not another, less dangerous arrhythmia. Don't delay treatment, however, if the patient is unstable.

Outward signs tell a story

The patient with PVCs has a much weaker pulse wave after the premature beat and a longer-than-normal pause between pulse waves. At times, you won't be able to palpate any pulse after the PVC. If the carotid pulse is visible, however, you may see a weaker pulse wave after the premature beat. When auscultating for heart sounds, you'll hear an abnormally early heart sound and a diminished amplitude with each premature beat.

Patients with frequent PVCs may complain of palpitations and may also experience hypotension or syncope.

How you intervene

If the patient is asymptomatic and doesn't have heart disease, the arrhythmia probably won't require treatment. If he has symptoms or a dangerous form of PVCs, the type of treatment depends on the cause of the problem.

If the PVCs have a cardiac origin, the doctor may order drugs to suppress ventricular irritability such as procainamide or lidocaine. Procainamide may be given in an infusion at a maintenance dose of 1 to 4 mg/minute. After an I.V. bolus of 1 to 1.5 mg/kg of lidocaine, you may give an infusion of 1 to 4 mg/minute.

When PVCs have a noncardiac origin, treatment aims to correct the cause, which may include adjusting drug therapy or correcting acidosis, electrolyte imbalances, hypothermia, or hypoxia.

Stat patient stats

Patients who have recently developed PVCs need prompt assessment, especially if they have underlying heart disease or complex medical problems. Those with chronic PVCs should be observed closely for the development of more frequent PVCs or more dangerous PVC patterns.

Until effective treatment begins, patients with PVCs accompanied by serious symptoms should have continuous ECG monitoring and ambulate only with assistance. If the patient is discharged from the hospital on antiarrhythmic medications, make sure family members know how to contact the emergency medical system and how to perform cardiopulmonary resuscitation (CPR).

When PVCs spell danger

Here are some examples of patterns of dangerous premature ventricular contractions (PVCs).

Paired PVCs

Two PVCs in a row are called a *pair* or *couplet* (see highlighted areas). A pair can produce ventricular tachycardia because the second contraction usually meets refractory tissue. A salvo—three or more PVCs in a row—is considered a run of ventricular tachycardia.

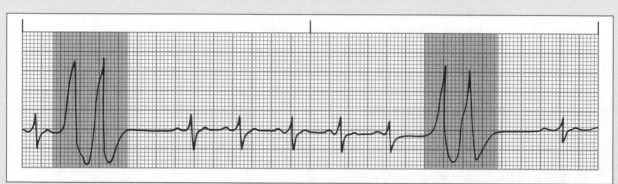

Multiform PVCs

PVCs that look different from one another arise from different sites or from the same site with abnormal conduction (see highlighted areas). Multiform PVCs may indicate severe heart disease or digoxin toxicity.

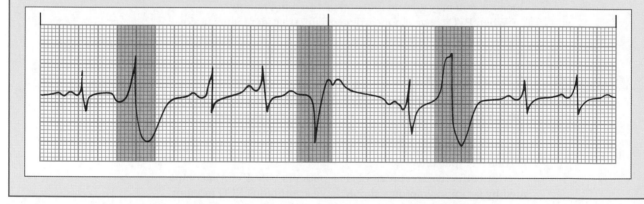

Ventricular tachycardia

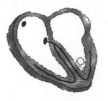

In ventricular tachycardia, commonly called *V-tach*, three or more PVCs occur in a row and the ventricular rate exceeds 100 beats/minute. This arrhythmia usually precedes ventricular fibrillation and sudden cardiac death, especially in patients who aren't in the hospital.

Bigeminy and trigeminy

PVCs that occur every other beat (bigeminy) or every third beat (trigeminy) can result in ventricular tachycardia or ventricular fibrillation (see highlighted areas).

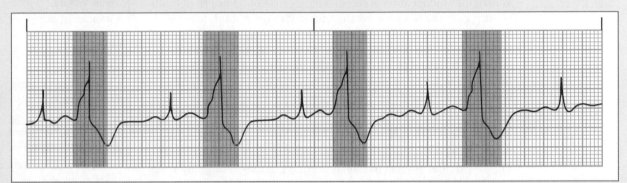

R-on-T phenomenon

In R-on-T phenomenon, the PVC occurs so early that it falls on the T wave of the preceding beat (see highlighted area). Because the cells haven't fully repolarized, ventricular tachycardia or ventricular fibrillation can result.

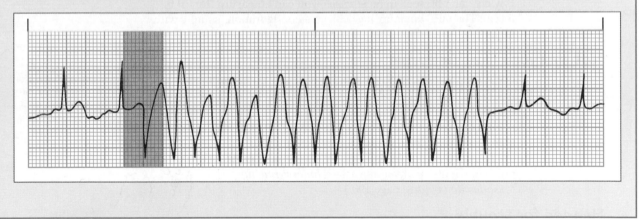

Ventricular tachycardia is an extremely unstable rhythm. It can occur in short, paroxysmal bursts lasting fewer than 30 seconds and causing few or no symptoms. Alternatively, it can be sustained, requiring immediate treatment to prevent death, even in patients initially able to maintain adequate cardiac output.

How it happens

Ventricular tachycardia usually results from increased myocardial irritability, which may be triggered by enhanced automaticity or reentry within the Purkinje system or by PVCs initiating the R-on-T phenomenon. (See *Causes of ventricular tachycardia*.)

Running on empty

Ventricular tachycardia is significant because of its unpredictability and potential to cause death. A patient may be stable with a normal pulse and adequate hemodynamics or unstable with hypotension and no detectable pulse. Because of reduced ventricular filling time and the drop in cardiac output, the patient's condition can quickly deteriorate to ventricular fibrillation and complete cardiac collapse.

What to look for

On the ECG strip, the atrial rhythm and rate can't be determined. The ventricular rhythm is usually regular but may be slightly irregular. The ventricular rate is usually rapid—100 to 200 beats/minute.

The P wave is usually absent but may be obscured by the QRS complex. Retrograde P waves may be present. Because the P wave can't be seen in most cases, you can't measure the PR interval. The QRS complex has a bizarre configuration, usually with an increased amplitude and a duration of longer than 0.14 second.

Not everyone likes uniforms

QRS complexes in monomorphic ventricular tachycardia have a uniform shape. In polymorphic ventricular tachycardia, the shape of the QRS complex constantly changes. If the T wave is visible, it occurs opposite the QRS complex. The QT interval isn't measurable. (See *Recognizing ventricular tachycardia*.)

Torsades de pointes is a special variation of polymorphic ventricular tachycardia. (See *Understanding torsades de pointes*, page 190.)

Headed for trouble

Although some patients have only minor symptoms at first, the arrhythmia can quickly lead to cardiac collapse. Most patients with ventricular tachycardia have weak or absent pulses. Low cardiac output leads to hypotension and a decreased LOC, causing unresponsiveness. Ventricular tachycardia may precipitate angina, heart failure, or a substantial decrease in organ perfusion.

Causes of ventricular tachycardia

Conditions that can cause ventricular tachycardia include:
- myocardial ischemia
- myocardial infarction
- coronary artery disease
- valvular heart disease
- heart failure
- cardiomyopathy
- electrolyte imbalances such as hypokalemia
- drug intoxication from digoxin (Lanoxin), procainamide (Pronestyl), quinidine, or cocaine.

I'll soon shake my configuration and rattle my waves for the QRS complex is a-changin'.

Polymorphic Records

Recognizing ventricular tachycardia

Take a look at this example of how ventricular tachycardia appears on a rhythm strip. Notice its distinguishing characteristics.

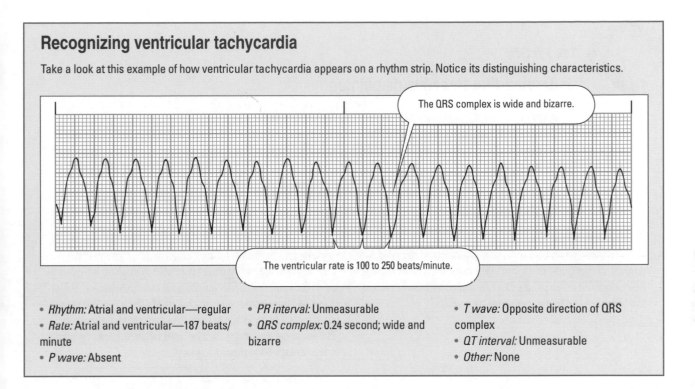

The QRS complex is wide and bizarre.

The ventricular rate is 100 to 250 beats/minute.

- *Rhythm:* Atrial and ventricular—regular
- *Rate:* Atrial and ventricular—187 beats/minute
- *P wave:* Absent

- *PR interval:* Unmeasurable
- *QRS complex:* 0.24 second; wide and bizarre

- *T wave:* Opposite direction of QRS complex
- *QT interval:* Unmeasurable
- *Other:* None

How you intervene

Treatment depends on whether the patient's pulse is detectable or undetectable. Patients with pulseless ventricular tachycardia require immediate resuscitation, using the pulseless arrest algorithm. (See *Treating pulseless arrest*, pages 194 and 195.)

Looking for some stability

Treatment of patients with a detectable pulse depends on whether their condition is stable or unstable. Unstable patients generally have heart rates greater than 150 beats/minute. They may also have hypotension, shortness of breath, an altered LOC, heart failure, angina, or MI—conditions that indicate cardiac decompensation. These patients are treated immediately with direct-current synchronized cardioversion.

A stable patient with a wide QRS complex tachycardia and no signs of cardiac decompensation is treated differently. First, if the patient has monomorphic ventricular tachycardia, amiodarone is given. If the patient becomes unstable, immediate synchronized cardioversion is performed. If the patient has polymorphic ventricular tachycardia, amiodarone or magnesium may be given. Stop medications that cause prolonged QT intervals and correct

Now I get it!

Understanding torsades de pointes

Torsades de pointes, which means "twisting about the points," is a special form of polymorphic ventricular tachycardia. The hallmark characteristics of this rhythm, shown below, are QRS complexes that rotate about the baseline, deflecting downward and upward for several beats. The rate is 150 to 250 beats/ minute, usually with an irregular rhythm, and the QRS complexes are wide. The P wave is usually absent.

Paroxysmal rhythm

This arrhythmia may be paroxysmal, starting and stopping suddenly, and may deteriorate into ventricular fibrillation. It should be considered when ventricular tachycardia doesn't respond to antiarrhythmic therapy or other treatments.

Reversible causes

The cause of this form of ventricular tachycardia is usually reversible. The most common causes are drugs that lengthen the QT interval, such as the antiarrhythmics quinidine, procainamide (Pronestyl), and sotalol (Betapace). Other causes include myocardial ischemia and electrolyte abnormalities, such as hypokalemia, hypomagnesemia, and hypocalcemia.

Going into overdrive

Torsades de pointes is treated by correcting the underlying cause, especially if the cause is related to specific drug therapy. The doctor may order mechanical overdrive pacing, which overrides the ventricular rate and breaks the triggered mechanism for the arrhythmia. Magnesium may also be effective. Electrical cardioversion may be used when torsades de pointes doesn't respond to other treatment.

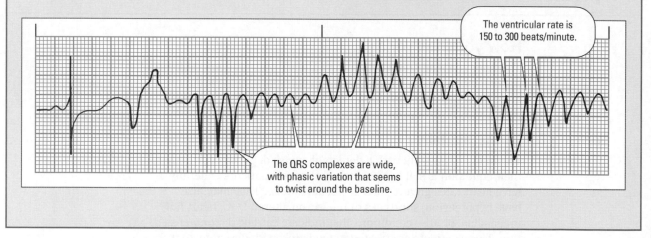

The ventricular rate is 150 to 300 beats/minute.

The QRS complexes are wide, with phasic variation that seems to twist around the baseline.

electrolyte imbalances. If the patient becomes clinically unstable immediately perform synchronized cardioversion.

A permanent relationship

Patients with chronic, recurrent episodes of ventricular tachycardia who are unresponsive to drug therapy may have a cardioverter-defibrillator implanted. This device is a more permanent solution for this type of arrhythmia.

Assume the worst

Any wide QRS complex tachycardia should be treated as ventricular tachycardia until definitive evidence is found to establish another diagnosis, such as supraventricular tachycardia with abnormal ventricular conduction. Always assume that the patient has ventricular tachycardia and treat him accordingly. Rapid intervention will prevent cardiac decompensation or the onset of more lethal arrhythmias.

Teacher, teacher

Be sure to teach patients and their families about the serious nature of this arrhythmia and the need for prompt treatment. If your patient is undergoing cardioversion, tell him he'll be given an analgesic or a sedative to help prevent discomfort.

If a patient will be discharged with an implanted defibrillator or a prescription for long-term antiarrhythmic medications, teach family members how to contact the emergency medical system and how to perform CPR.

Family members of patients with ventricular tachycardia should know how to perform CPR.

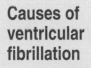

Ventricular fibrillation

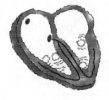

Ventricular fibrillation, commonly called *V fib*, is a chaotic pattern of electrical activity in the ventricles in which electrical impulses arise from many different foci. It produces no effective muscular contraction and no cardiac output. Untreated ventricular fibrillation causes most cases of sudden cardiac death in people outside of a hospital.

How it happens

With ventricular fibrillation, the ventricles quiver instead of contracting, so cardiac output falls to zero. If fibrillation continues, it leads to ventricular standstill and death. (See *Causes of ventricular fibrillation*.)

What to look for

On the ECG strip, ventricular activity appears as fibrillatory waves with no recognizable pattern. Atrial rate and rhythm can't be determined, nor can ventricular rhythm because no pattern or regularity occurs. As a result, the ventricular rate, P wave, PR interval, QRS complex, T wave, and QT interval can't be determined. Larger, or coarse, fibrillatory waves are easier to convert to a normal rhythm than are smaller waves because larger waves indicate a

---

Causes of ventricular fibrillation

Ventricular fibrillation can be caused by:
• myocardial ischemia
• myocardial infarction
• untreated ventricular tachycardia
• underlying heart disease
• acid-base imbalance
• electric shock
• severe hypothermia
• electrolyte imbalances, such as hypokalemia, hyperkalemia, and hypercalcemia.

greater degree of electrical activity in the heart. (See *Recognizing ventricular fibrillation.*)

911 emergency

The patient in ventricular fibrillation is in full cardiac arrest, unresponsive, and without a detectable blood pressure or carotid or femoral pulse. Whenever you see a pattern resembling ventricular fibrillation, check the patient immediately, check the rhythm in another lead, and start treatment.

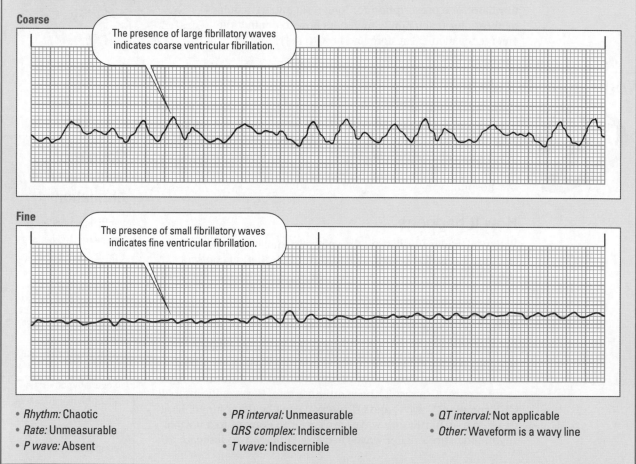

Recognizing ventricular fibrillation

The first rhythm strip shows coarse ventricular fibrillation, the second shows fine ventricular fibrillation. Fine ventricular fibrillation sometimes resembles asystole.

Coarse

The presence of large fibrillatory waves indicates coarse ventricular fibrillation.

Fine

The presence of small fibrillatory waves indicates fine ventricular fibrillation.

- *Rhythm:* Chaotic
- *Rate:* Unmeasurable
- *P wave:* Absent
- *PR interval:* Unmeasurable
- *QRS complex:* Indiscernible
- *T wave:* Indiscernible
- *QT interval:* Not applicable
- *Other:* Waveform is a wavy line

How you intervene

Defibrillation is the most effective treatment for ventricular fibrillation. (See *Treating pulseless arrest*, pages 194 and 195.) CPR must be performed until the defibrillator arrives to preserve oxygen supply to the brain and other vital organs. Drugs such as epinephrine or vasopressin may help the heart respond better to defibrillation. Amiodarone and magnesium may be given to decrease heart irritability and prevent a recurrence of ventricular fibrillation.

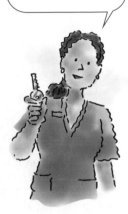

Defibrillation is the key to getting the heart back on track.

Jump start

During defibrillation, electrode paddles direct an electric current through the patient's heart. The current causes the myocardium to depolarize, which, in turn, encourages the SA node to resume normal control of the heart's electrical activity. One paddle is placed to the right of the upper sternum, and one is placed over the fifth or sixth intercostal space at the left anterior axillary line. During cardiac surgery, internal paddles are placed directly on the myocardium.

ABCs of AEDs

Automated external defibrillators (AEDs) are increasingly being used to provide early defibrillation. In this method, electrode pads are placed on the patient's chest and a microcomputer in the unit interprets the cardiac rhythm, providing the caregiver with step-by-step instructions on how to proceed. These defibrillators can be used by people without medical experience.

Speedy delivery

For the patient with ventricular fibrillation, successful resuscitation requires rapid recognition of the problem and prompt defibrillation. Many health care facilities and emergency medical systems have established protocols to help health care workers initiate prompt treatment. Make sure you know where your facility keeps its emergency equipment and how to recognize and deal with potentially lethal arrhythmias.

You'll also need to teach your patient and his family how to contact the emergency medical system. Family members need instruction in CPR. Teach them about long-term therapies that prevent recurrent episodes of ventricular fibrillation, including chronic antiarrhythmic drugs and implantation of a cardioverter-defibrillator.

(Text continues on page 196.)

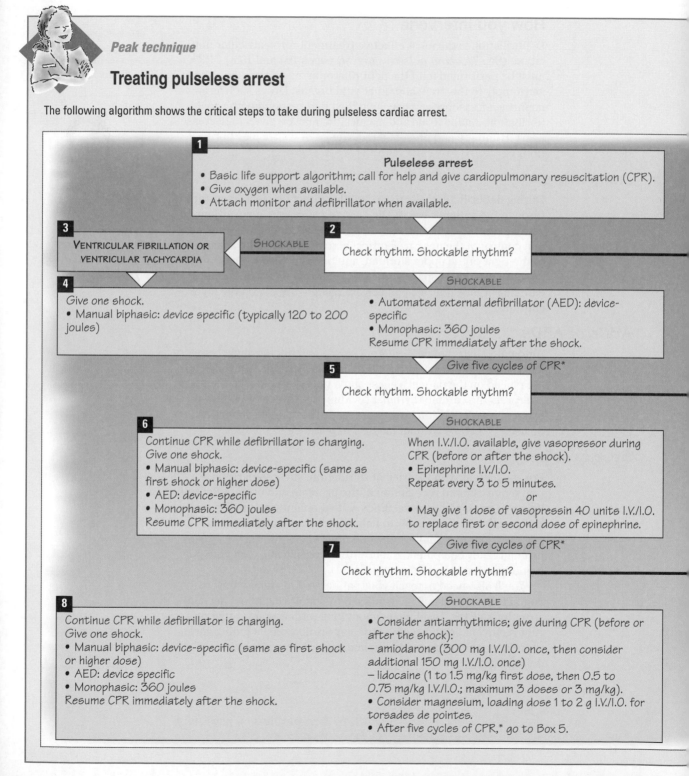

Peak technique

Treating pulseless arrest

The following algorithm shows the critical steps to take during pulseless cardiac arrest.

1

Pulseless arrest
- Basic life support algorithm; call for help and give cardiopulmonary resuscitation (CPR).
- Give oxygen when available.
- Attach monitor and defibrillator when available.

2 Check rhythm. Shockable rhythm?

SHOCKABLE →

3 VENTRICULAR FIBRILLATION OR VENTRICULAR TACHYCARDIA

SHOCKABLE

4
Give one shock.
- Manual biphasic: device specific (typically 120 to 200 joules)

- Automated external defibrillator (AED): device-specific
- Monophasic: 360 joules
Resume CPR immediately after the shock.

Give five cycles of CPR*

5 Check rhythm. Shockable rhythm?

SHOCKABLE

6
Continue CPR while defibrillator is charging. Give one shock.
- Manual biphasic: device-specific (same as first shock or higher dose)
- AED: device-specific
- Monophasic: 360 joules
Resume CPR immediately after the shock.

When I.V./I.O. available, give vasopressor during CPR (before or after the shock).
- Epinephrine I.V./I.O.
Repeat every 3 to 5 minutes.
or
- May give 1 dose of vasopressin 40 units I.V./I.O. to replace first or second dose of epinephrine.

Give five cycles of CPR*

7 Check rhythm. Shockable rhythm?

SHOCKABLE

8
Continue CPR while defibrillator is charging. Give one shock.
- Manual biphasic: device-specific (same as first shock or higher dose)
- AED: device specific
- Monophasic: 360 joules
Resume CPR immediately after the shock.

- Consider antiarrhythmics; give during CPR (before or after the shock):
– amiodarone (300 mg I.V./I.O. once, then consider additional 150 mg I.V./I.O. once)
– lidocaine (1 to 1.5 mg/kg first dose, then 0.5 to 0.75 mg/kg I.V./I.O.; maximum 3 doses or 3 mg/kg).
- Consider magnesium, loading dose 1 to 2 g I.V./I.O. for torsades de pointes.
- After five cycles of CPR,* go to Box 5.

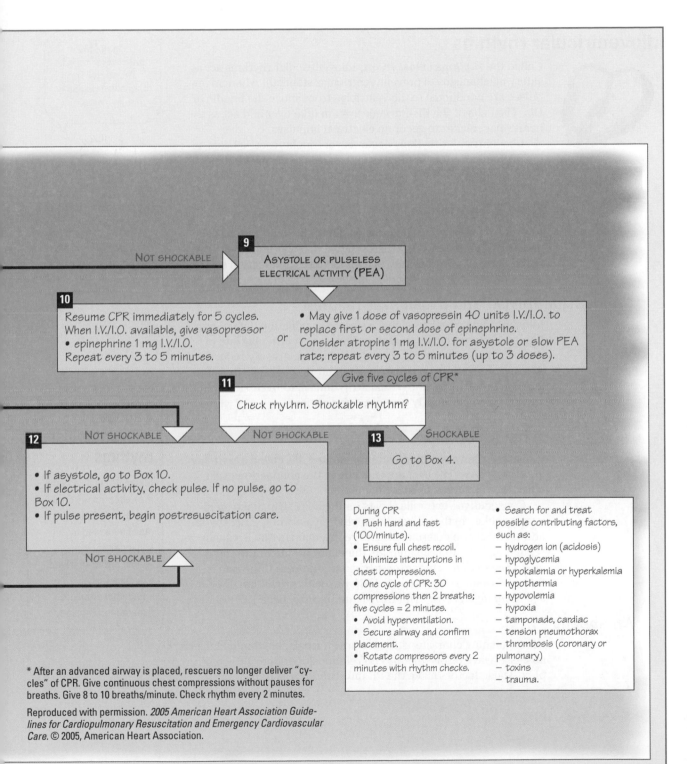

9 ASYSTOLE OR PULSELESS ELECTRICAL ACTIVITY (PEA)

NOT SHOCKABLE

10
Resume CPR immediately for 5 cycles. When I.V./I.O. available, give vasopressor
• epinephrine 1 mg I.V./I.O. Repeat every 3 to 5 minutes.

or

• May give 1 dose of vasopressin 40 units I.V./I.O. to replace first or second dose of epinephrine.
Consider atropine 1 mg I.V./I.O. for asystole or slow PEA rate; repeat every 3 to 5 minutes (up to 3 doses).

Give five cycles of CPR*

11
Check rhythm. Shockable rhythm?

NOT SHOCKABLE   NOT SHOCKABLE   SHOCKABLE

13
Go to Box 4.

12
• If asystole, go to Box 10.
• If electrical activity, check pulse. If no pulse, go to Box 10.
• If pulse present, begin postresuscitation care.

NOT SHOCKABLE

During CPR
• Push hard and fast (100/minute).
• Ensure full chest recoil.
• Minimize interruptions in chest compressions.
• One cycle of CPR: 30 compressions then 2 breaths; five cycles = 2 minutes.
• Avoid hyperventilation.
• Secure airway and confirm placement.
• Rotate compressors every 2 minutes with rhythm checks.

• Search for and treat possible contributing factors, such as:
– hydrogen ion (acidosis)
– hypoglycemia
– hypokalemia or hyperkalemia
– hypothermia
– hypovolemia
– hypoxia
– tamponade, cardiac
– tension pneumothorax
– thrombosis (coronary or pulmonary)
– toxins
– trauma.

* After an advanced airway is placed, rescuers no longer deliver "cycles" of CPR. Give continuous chest compressions without pauses for breaths. Give 8 to 10 breaths/minute. Check rhythm every 2 minutes.

Idioventricular rhythms

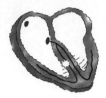

Called the *rhythms of last resort*, idioventricular rhythms act as safety mechanisms to prevent ventricular standstill when no impulses are conducted to the ventricles from above the bundle of His. The cells of the His-Purkinje system take over and act as the heart's pacemaker to generate electrical impulses.

Idioventricular rhythms occur as ventricular escape beats, idioventricular rhythm (a term used to designate a specific type of idioventricular rhythm), or accelerated idioventricular rhythm.

How it happens

Idioventricular rhythms occur when all of the heart's other pacemakers fail to function or when supraventricular impulses can't reach the ventricles because of a block in the conduction system. (See *Causes of idioventricular rhythms*.)

Conduction foibles and pacemaker failures

Idioventricular rhythms signal a serious conduction defect with a failure of the primary pacemaker. The slow ventricular rate of these arrhythmias and the loss of atrial kick markedly reduce cardiac output. Patients require close monitoring because this problem can progress to more lethal arrhythmias. Idioventricular rhythms also commonly occur in dying patients.

What to look for

If just one idioventricular beat is generated, it's called a *ventricular escape beat*. The beat appears late in the conduction cycle, when the rate drops to 40 beats/minute.

Consecutive ventricular beats on the ECG strip make up idioventricular rhythm. When this arrhythmia occurs, atrial rhythm and rate can't be determined. The ventricular rhythm is usually regular at 20 to 40 beats/minute, the inherent rate of the ventricles. (See *Recognizing idioventricular rhythm*.) If the rate is faster, it's called an *accelerated idioventricular rhythm*. (See *Recognizing accelerated idioventricular rhythm*, page 198.)

An absent P...

Distinguishing characteristics of idioventricular rhythm include an absent P wave or one that has no relationship to the QRS complex. These factors make the PR interval unmeasurable.

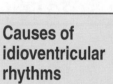

Oh no! My pacemaker failed. I'm at risk for idioventricular rhythms.

Causes of idioventricular rhythms

Idioventricular rhythms may accompany third-degree heart block or may be caused by:
- myocardial ischemia
- myocardial infarction
- digoxin toxicity
- pacemaker failure
- metabolic imbalances.

Recognizing idioventricular rhythm

Take a look at this example of how an idioventricular rhythm appears on a rhythm strip. Notice its distinguishing characteristics.

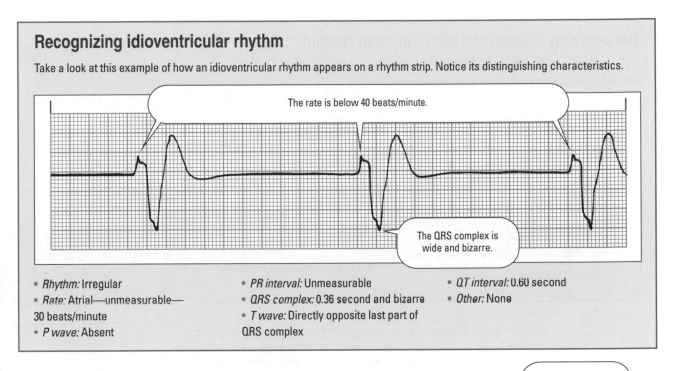

The rate is below 40 beats/minute.

The QRS complex is wide and bizarre.

- *Rhythm:* Irregular
- *Rate:* Atrial—unmeasurable—30 beats/minute
- *P wave:* Absent
- *PR interval:* Unmeasurable
- *QRS complex:* 0.36 second and bizarre
- *T wave:* Directly opposite last part of QRS complex
- *QT interval:* 0.60 second
- *Other:* None

...and a bizarre QRS...

Because of abnormal ventricular depolarization, the QRS complex has a duration of longer than 0.12 second, with a wide and bizarre configuration. The T-wave deflection may be opposite the QRS complex. The QT interval is usually prolonged, indicating delayed depolarization and repolarization.

...make for one dizzy patient

The patient may complain of palpitations, dizziness, or light-headedness, or he may have a syncopal episode. If the arrhythmia persists, hypotension, weak peripheral pulses, decreased urine output, or confusion can occur.

How you intervene

Treatment should be initiated immediately to increase the patient's heart rate, improve cardiac output, and establish a normal rhythm. Atropine may be prescribed to increase the heart rate. If atropine isn't effective or if the patient develops hypotension or

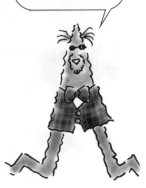

Bizarre QRS complexes characterize idioventricular rhythms.

Recognizing accelerated idioventricular rhythm

An accelerated idioventricular rhythm has the same characteristics as an idioventricular rhythm except that it's faster. The rate shown here varies between 40 and 100 beats/minute.

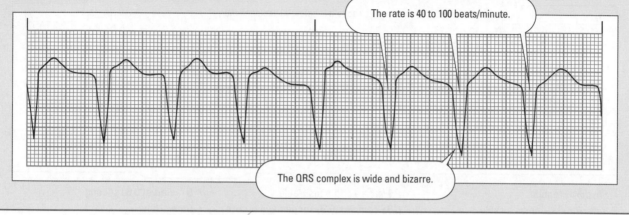

The rate is 40 to 100 beats/minute.

The QRS complex is wide and bizarre.

other signs of instability, a pacemaker may be needed to reestablish a heart rate that provides enough cardiac output to perfuse organs properly. A transcutaneous pacemaker may be used in an emergency until a temporary or permanent transvenous pacemaker can be inserted. (See *Transcutaneous pacemaker*.)

Remember that the goal of treatment doesn't include suppressing the idioventricular rhythm because it acts as a safety mechanism to protect the heart from standstill. Idioventricular rhythm should never be treated with lidocaine or other antiarrhythmics that would suppress that safety mechanism.

Electronic surveillance

Patients with idioventricular rhythms need continuous ECG monitoring and constant assessment until treatment restores hemodynamic stability. Keep atropine and pacemaker equipment at the bedside. Enforce bed rest until a permanent system is in place for maintaining an effective heart rate.

Be sure to tell the patient and his family members about the serious nature of this arrhythmia and all aspects of treatment. If a permanent pacemaker is inserted, teach the patient and his family how it works, how to recognize problems, when to contact the doctor, and how pacemaker function will be monitored.

Never give lidocaine to a patient with an idioventricular rhythm. Doing so could suppress the rhythm and lead to cardiac standstill.

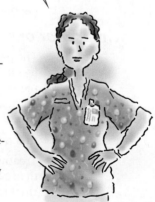

Asystole

Asystole is ventricular standstill. The patient is completely unresponsive, with no electrical activity in the heart and no cardiac

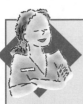

Peak technique

Transcutaneous pacemaker

In life-threatening situations, in which time is critical, a transcutaneous pacemaker may be used to regulate the heart rate. This device sends an electrical impulse from the pulse generator to the heart by way of two pacing electrodes placed on the patient's chest and back, as shown at right.

The pacing electrodes are placed at heart level, on either side of the heart, so the electrical stimulus has only a short distance to travel to the heart. Transcutaneous pacing is quick and effective, but it's used only until transvenous pacing can be started.

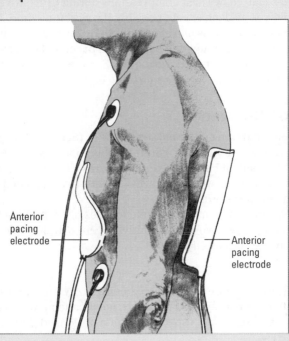

Anterior pacing electrode

Anterior pacing electrode

output. This arrhythmia results most commonly from a prolonged period of cardiac emergency, such as ventricular fibrillation, without effective resuscitation.

Asystole has been called the *arrhythmia of death*. The patient is in cardiopulmonary arrest. Without rapid initiation of CPR and appropriate treatment, the situation quickly becomes irreversible.

How it happens

Without ventricular electrical activity, ventricular contractions can't occur. As a result, cardiac output drops to zero and vital organs are no longer perfused. Asystole is typically considered to be a confirmation of death, rather than an arrhythmia to be treated. (See *Causes of asystole*, page 200.)

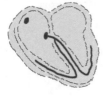

Asystole is sometimes called the arrhythmia of death because without immediate initiation of CPR it's deadly.

What to look for

A patient in asystole is unresponsive, without any discernible pulse or blood pressure.

On the ECG strip, asystole looks like a nearly flat line (except for changes caused by chest compressions during CPR). No electrical activity is evident, except possibly P waves for a time. Atrial and ventricular activity is at a standstill, so no intervals can be measured. In the patient with a pacemaker, pacer spikes may be evident on the strip, but no P wave or QRS complex occurs in response to the stimulus. (See *Recognizing asystole*.)

How you intervene

The immediate treatment for asystole is CPR. (See *Treating pulseless arrest*, pages 194 and 195.) Start CPR as soon as you determine that the patient has no pulse. Then verify the presence of asystole by checking two different ECG leads. Give repeated doses of epinephrine as ordered.

Subsequent treatment for asystole focuses on identifying and either treating or removing the underlying cause. Transcutaneous pacing may also be considered.

Start me up

Your job is to recognize this life-threatening arrhythmia and start resuscitation right away. Unfortunately, most patients with asystole can't be resuscitated, especially after a prolonged period of cardiac arrest.

Causes of asystole

Anything that causes inadequate blood flow to the heart may lead to asystole, including:
• myocardial infarction
• severe electrolyte disturbances such as hyperkalemia
• massive pulmonary embolism
• prolonged hypoxemia
• severe, uncorrected acid-base disturbances
• electric shock
• drug intoxication such as cocaine overdose.

Recognizing asystole

This rhythm strip shows asystole, the absence of electrical activity in the ventricles. Except for a few P waves or pacer spikes, nothing appears on the waveform and the line is almost flat.

The absence of electrical activity in the ventricles results in a nearly flat line.

Now I get it!

Pulseless electrical activity

In pulseless electrical activity, the heart muscle loses its ability to contract even though electrical activity is preserved. As a result, the patient goes into cardiac arrest.

On an electrocardiogram, you'll see evidence of organized electrical activity, but you won't be able to palpate a pulse or measure the blood pressure.

Causes

This condition requires rapid identification and treatment. Causes include hypovolemia, hypoxia, acidosis, tension pneumothorax, cardiac tamponade, massive pulmonary embolism, hypothermia, hyperkalemia, massive acute myocardial infarction, and an overdose of drugs such as tricyclic antidepressants.

Treatment

Cardiopulmonary resuscitation is the immediate treatment, along with epinephrine. Atropine may be given to patients with bradycardia. Subsequent treatment focuses on identifying and correcting the underlying cause.

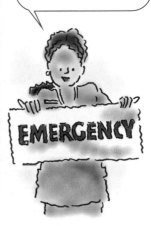

Treat any situation where you can't find the patient's pulse as an emergency—even if the monitor shows a waveform.

EMERGENCY

You should also be aware that pulseless electrical activity can lead to asystole. Know how to recognize this problem and treat it. (See *Pulseless electrical activity*.)

Atrioventricular blocks

AV heart block results from an interruption in the conduction of impulses between the atria and ventricles. AV block can be total or partial or it may delay conduction. The block can occur at the AV node, the bundle of His, or the bundle branches.

The heart's electrical impulses normally originate in the SA node, so when those impulses are blocked at the AV node, atrial rates are commonly normal (60 to 100 beats/minute). The clinical effect of the block depends on how many impulses are completely blocked, how slow the ventricular rate is as a result, and how the block ultimately affects the heart. A slow ventricular rate can decrease cardiac output, possibly causing light-headedness, hypotension, and confusion.

A troubled relationship

Various factors may lead to AV block, including underlying heart conditions, use of certain drugs, congenital anomalies, and conditions that disrupt the cardiac conduction system. Here are some typical examples:

• *Myocardial ischemia* impairs cellular function so cells repolarize more slowly or incompletely. The injured cells, in turn, may conduct impulses slowly or inconsistently. Relief of the ischemia can restore normal function to the AV node.

• In *MI*, cell death occurs. If the necrotic cells are part of the conduction system, they no longer conduct impulses and a permanent AV block occurs.

• *Excessive dosage* of or an *exaggerated response* to a drug can cause AV block or increase the likelihood that a block will develop. Although many antiarrhythmic medications can have this effect, the drugs more commonly known to cause or exacerbate AV blocks include digoxin, beta-adrenergic blockers, and calcium channel blockers.

• *Congenital anomalies* such as congenital ventricular septal defect may involve cardiac structures and affect the conduction system. Anomalies of the conduction system, such as an AV node that doesn't conduct impulses, may occur in the absence of structural defects.

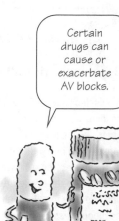

Certain drugs can cause or exacerbate AV blocks.

Under the knife

AV block may also be caused by inadvertent damage to the heart's conduction system during cardiac surgery. Damage is most likely to occur in operations involving the mitral or tricuspid valve or in the closure of a ventricular septal defect. If the injury involves tissues adjacent to the surgical site and the conduction system isn't physically disrupted, the block may be only temporary. If a portion of the conduction system itself is severed, a permanent block results. Similar disruption of the conduction system may occur from radiofrequency ablation therapy.

Class consciousness

AV blocks are classified according to their severity, not their location. That severity is measured according to how well the node conducts impulses and is separated by degrees—first, second, and third. In this section, we'll look at all four types of AV blocks.

First-degree AV block

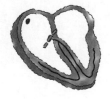

First-degree AV block occurs when impulses from the atria are consistently delayed during conduction through the AV node. Conduction eventually occurs; it just takes longer than normal. It's as if people are walking in a line through a doorway, but each person hesitates before crossing the threshold.

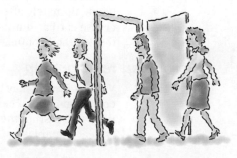

How it happens

First-degree AV block may be temporary, particularly if it stems from medications or ischemia early in the course of an MI. The presence of first-degree block, the least dangerous type of AV block, indicates some kind of problem in the conduction system. Because first-degree AV block can progress to a more severe block, it should be monitored for changes. (See *Causes of first-degree AV block.*)

What to look for

In general, a rhythm strip with this block looks like a normal sinus rhythm except that the PR interval is longer than normal. The rhythm is regular, with one normal P wave for every QRS complex. The PR interval is greater than 0.20 second and is consistent for each beat. The QRS complex is usually normal, although sometimes a bundle-branch block may occur along with first-degree AV block and cause a widening of the QRS complex. (See *Recognizing first-degree AV block.*)

> ### Causes of first-degree AV block
>
> First-degree atrioventricular (AV) block may appear normally in a healthy person or may result from:
> - myocardial ischemia or infarction
> - myocarditis
> - degenerative changes in the heart
> - medications, such as digoxin (Lanoxin), calcium channel blockers, and beta-adrenergic blockers.

Recognizing first-degree AV block

Take a look at this example of how first-degree atrioventricular (AV) block appears on a rhythm strip. Notice its distinguishing characteristics.

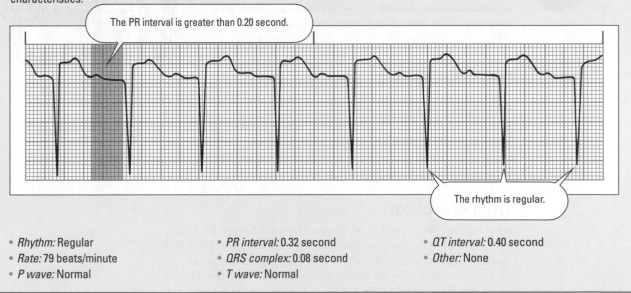

The PR interval is greater than 0.20 second.

The rhythm is regular.

- *Rhythm:* Regular
- *Rate:* 79 beats/minute
- *P wave:* Normal
- *PR interval:* 0.32 second
- *QRS complex:* 0.08 second
- *T wave:* Normal
- *QT interval:* 0.40 second
- *Other:* None

Blocked but not bothered

Most patients with first-degree AV block show no symptoms of the block because cardiac output isn't significantly affected. If the PR interval is extremely long, a longer interval between S_1 and S_2 may be noted on cardiac auscultation.

How you intervene

Usually, just the underlying cause is treated, not the conduction disturbance itself. For example, if a medication is causing the block, the dosage may be reduced or the medication discontinued. Close monitoring helps to detect progression of first-degree AV block to a more serious form of block.

When caring for a patient with first-degree AV block, evaluate him for underlying causes that can be corrected, such as medications he may be taking or ischemia. Observe the ECG for progression of the block to a more severe form of block. Administer digoxin, calcium channel blockers, or beta-adrenergic blockers cautiously.

Type I second-degree AV block

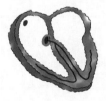

Also called *Wenckebach* or *Mobitz type I block,* type I second-degree AV block occurs when each successive impulse from the SA node is delayed slightly longer than the previous impulse. That pattern continues until an impulse fails to be conducted to the ventricles, and the cycle then repeats. It's like a line of people trying to get through a doorway, each one taking longer and longer until finally one can't get through.

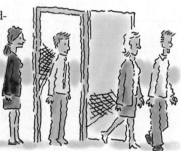

How it happens

Type I second-degree AV block may occur normally in an otherwise healthy person. Almost always temporary, this type of block resolves when the underlying condition is corrected. Although an asymptomatic patient with this block has a good prognosis, the block may progress to a more serious form, especially if it occurs early during an MI. (See *Causes of type I second-degree AV block.*)

What to look for

When monitoring a patient with type I second-degree AV block, you'll note that because the SA node isn't affected by this lower block, it continues its normal activity. As a result, the atrial rhythm is normal. The PR interval gets gradually longer with each successive beat until finally a P wave fails to conduct to the ventricles. This lack of conduction makes the ventricular rhythm ir-regular, with a repeating pattern of groups of QRS complexes fol-lowed by a dropped beat in which the P wave isn't followed by a QRS complex. The QRS complexes are usually normal because the delays occur in the AV node. (See *Recognizing type I second-degree AV block* and *Following the footprints*, page 206.)

When you're trying to identify type I second-degree AV block, think of the phrase "longer, longer, drop," which describes the pro-gressively prolonged PR intervals and the missing QRS complex.

Lonely Ps, light-headed patients

A patient with type I second-degree AV block is usually asympto-matic, although he may show signs and symptoms of decreased cardiac output, such as light-headedness and hypotension. Symp-toms may be especially pronounced if ventricular rate is slow.

How you intervene

No treatment is needed for type I AV block if the patient is asymp-tomatic. For a symptomatic patient, atropine may improve AV node conduction. A temporary pacemaker may be required for long-term relief of symptoms until the rhythm resolves.

Causes of type I second-degree AV block

Causes of type I second-degree atrioventricular (AV) block include:
- coronary artery dis-ease
- inferior-wall myocar-dial infarction
- rheumatic fever
- cardiac medications, such as beta-adrenergic blockers, digoxin (Lanox-in), and calcium channel blockers
- increased vagal stimu-lation.

Recognizing type I second-degree AV block

Take a look at this example of how type I second-degree atrioventricular (AV) block appears on a rhythm strip. Notice its distin-guishing characteristics.

The PR interval gets progressively longer…

…until a QRS complex is dropped.

- *Rhythm:* Atrial—regular; ventricular—irregular
- *Rate:* Atrial—80 beats/minute; ventricu-lar—50 beats/minute
- *P wave:* Normal
- *PR interval:* Progressively prolonged
- *QRS complex:* 0.08 second
- *T wave:* Normal
- *QT interval:* 0.46 second
- *Other:* Wenckebach pattern of grouped beats

Following the footprints

The pattern of grouped beating that accompanies type I second-degree atrioventricular (AV) block is sometimes referred to as the *footprints of Wenckebach*. Karel Frederik Wenckebach was a Dutch internist who, at the turn of the century and long before the introduction of the electrocardiogram (ECG), described the two forms of what's now known as second-degree AV block by analyzing waves in the jugular venous pulse. Following the introduction of the ECG, German cardiologist Woldemar Mobitz clarified Wenckebach's findings as type I and type II.

When caring for a patient with this block, assess his tolerance for the rhythm and the need for treatment to improve cardiac output. Evaluate the patient for possible causes of the block, including the use of certain medications or the presence of ischemia.

Keep an eye on the ECG

Check the ECG frequently to see if a more severe type of AV block develops. Make sure the patient has a patent I.V. line. Teach him about his temporary pacemaker if indicated.

Type II second-degree AV block

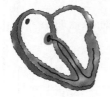

Type II second-degree AV block, also known as *Mobitz type II block*, is less common than type I but more serious. It occurs when occasional impulses from the SA node fail to conduct to the ventricles.

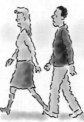
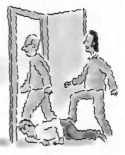

On an ECG, you won't see the PR interval lengthen before the impulse fails to conduct, as you do with type I second-degree AV block. You'll see, instead, consistent AV node conduction and an occasional dropped beat. This block is like a line of people passing through a doorway at the same speed, except that, periodically, one of them just can't get through.

How it happens

Type II second-degree AV block indicates a problem at the level of the bundle of His or bundle branches. (See *Causes of type II second-degree AV block*.)

Type II block is more serious than type I because the ventricular rate tends to be slower and the cardiac output is diminished. It's also more likely to cause symptoms, particularly if the sinus rhythm is slow and the ratio of conducted beats to dropped beats is low, such as 2:1. Usually chronic, type II second-degree AV block may progress to a more serious form of block. (See *Recognizing high-grade AV block.*)

What to look for

When monitoring a rhythm strip, look for an atrial rhythm that's regular and a ventricular rhythm that may be regular or irregular, depending on the block. (See *Recognizing type II second-degree AV block*, page 208.) If the block is intermittent, the rhythm is irregular. If the block is constant, such as 2:1 or 3:1, the rhythm is regular.

Overall, the strip will look as if someone erased some QRS complexes. The PR interval will be constant for all conducted beats but may be prolonged in some cases. The QRS complex is usually wide, but normal complexes may occur. (See *2:1 second-degree AV block*, page 209.)

Causes of type II second-degree AV block

Type II second-degree atrioventricular (AV) block is usually caused by:
• anterior-wall myocardial infarction
• degenerative changes in the conduction system
• severe coronary artery disease.

Recognizing high-grade AV block

When two or more successive atrial impulses are blocked, the conduction disturbance is called *high-grade atrioventricular (AV) block.* Expressed as a ratio of atrial-to-ventricular beats, this block is at least 3:1. With the prolonged refractory period of this block, latent pacemakers can discharge. As a result, escape rhythms commonly develop.

Complications

High-grade AV block causes severe complications. For instance, decreased cardiac output and reduced heart rate can combine to cause Stokes-Adams syncopal attacks. In addition, high-grade AV block usually progresses quickly to third-degree block.

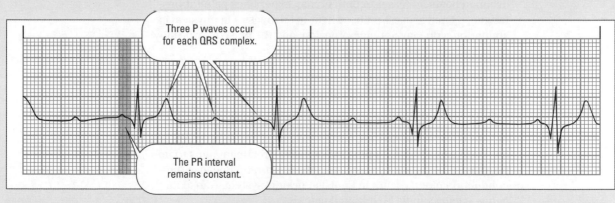

Three P waves occur for each QRS complex.

The PR interval remains constant.

• *Rhythm:* Atrial—usually regular; ventricular—usually irregular
• *Rate:* Atrial rate exceeds ventricular rate, usually below 40 beats/minute
• *P wave:* Usually normal but some not followed by a QRS complex
• *PR interval:* Constant but may be normal or prolonged
• *QRS complex:* Usually normal, periodically absent
• *Other:* Rhythm has appearance of complete AV block except for occasional conducted beat

Recognizing type II second-degree AV block

Take a look at this example of how type II second-degree atrioventricular (AV) block appears on a rhythm strip. Notice its distinguishing characteristics.

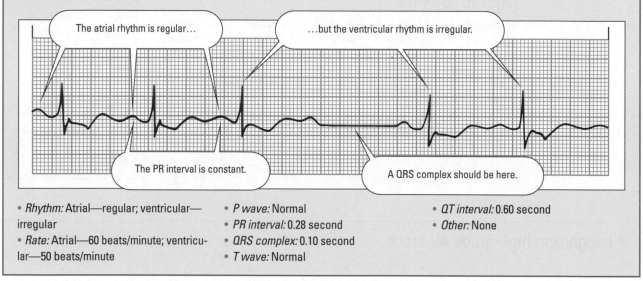

The atrial rhythm is regular...

...but the ventricular rhythm is irregular.

The PR interval is constant.

A QRS complex should be here.

- *Rhythm:* Atrial—regular; ventricular—irregular
- *Rate:* Atrial—60 beats/minute; ventricular—50 beats/minute
- *P wave:* Normal
- *PR interval:* 0.28 second
- *QRS complex:* 0.10 second
- *T wave:* Normal
- *QT interval:* 0.60 second
- *Other:* None

Jumpin' palpitations!

Most patients who experience a few dropped beats remain asymptomatic as long as cardiac output is maintained. As the number of dropped beats increases, a patient may experience palpitations, fatigue, dyspnea, chest pain, or light-headedness. On physical examination, you may note hypotension, and the pulse may be slow and regular or irregular.

How you intervene

If the dropped beats are infrequent and the patient shows no symptoms of decreased cardiac output, the doctor may choose only to observe the rhythm, particularly if the cause is thought to be reversible. If the patient is hypotensive, treatment aims to improve cardiac output by increasing the heart rate. Because the conduction block occurs in the His-Purkinje system, transcutaneous pacing should be initiated quickly.

Pick up the pace

Type II second-degree AV block commonly requires placement of a pacemaker. A temporary pacemaker may be used until a permanent pacemaker can be placed.

When caring for a patient with type II second-degree block, assess his tolerance for the rhythm and the need for treatment to im-

Advice from the experts

2:1 second-degree AV block

In 2:1 second-degree atrioventricular (AV) block, every other QRS complex is dropped, so there are always two P waves for every QRS complex. The resulting ventricular rhythm is regular.

Type I or type II?
To help determine whether a rhythm is type I or type II block, look at the width of the QRS complexes. If they're wide and a short PR interval is present, the block is probably type II.

Keep in mind that type II block is more likely to impair cardiac output, lead to symptoms such as syncope, and progress to a more severe form of block. Be sure to monitor the patient carefully.

prove cardiac output. Evaluate for possible correctable causes such as ischemia.

Keep the patient on bed rest, if indicated, to reduce myocardial oxygen demands. Administer oxygen therapy as ordered. Observe the patient for progression to a more severe form of AV block. If the patient receives a pacemaker, teach him and his family about its use.

Third-degree AV block

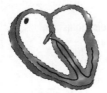

Also called *complete heart block*, third-degree AV block occurs when impulses from the atria are completely blocked at the AV node and can't be conducted to the ventricles. Maintaining our doorway analogy, this form of block is like a line of people waiting to go through a doorway, but no one can go through.

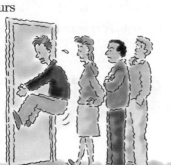

Beats of different drummers

Acting independently, the atria, generally under the control of the SA node, tend to maintain a regular rate of 60 to 100 beats/minute. The ventricular rhythm can originate from the AV node and maintain a rate of 40 to 60 beats/ minute or from the Purkinje system in the ventricles and maintain a rate of 20 to 40 beats/minute.

How it happens

Third-degree AV block that originates at the level of the AV node is most commonly a congenital condition. (See *Causes of third-degree AV block*, page 210.) It may be temporary or permanent.

Loss of productivity

Because the ventricular rate is so slow, third-degree AV block presents a potentially life-threatening situation because cardiac output can drop dramatically. In addition, the patient loses his atrial kick—that extra 30% of blood flow pushed into the ventricles by atrial contraction—as a result of the loss of synchrony between the atrial and ventricular contractions. The loss of atrial kick further decreases cardiac output. Any exertion on the part of the patient can worsen symptoms.

What to look for

When analyzing an ECG for this rhythm, you'll note regular atrial and ventricular rhythms. However, because the atria and ventricles beat independently of each other, PR intervals vary with no pattern or regularity.

Mixing up your Ps and Qs

Some P waves may be buried in QRS complexes or T waves. In fact, the rhythm strip of a patient with third-degree AV block looks like a strip of P waves laid independently over a strip of QRS complexes. (See *Recognizing third-degree AV block.*)

Causes of third-degree AV block

In addition to congenital causes, third-degree atrioventricular (AV) block may be caused by:
• coronary artery disease
• an anterior- or inferior-wall myocardial infarction
• degenerative changes in the heart
• digoxin toxicity
• calcium channel blockers
• beta-adrenergic blockers
• surgical injury.

Recognizing third-degree AV block

Take a look at this example of how third-degree atrioventricular (AV) block appears on a rhythm strip. Notice its distinguishing characteristics.

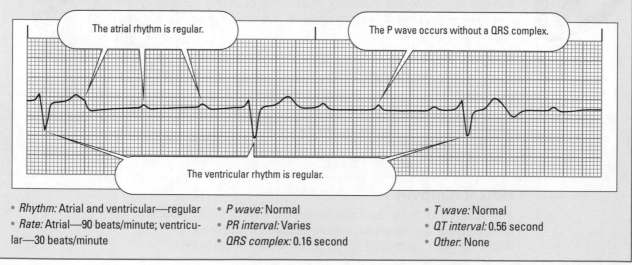

The atrial rhythm is regular.

The P wave occurs without a QRS complex.

The ventricular rhythm is regular.

• *Rhythm:* Atrial and ventricular—regular
• *Rate:* Atrial—90 beats/minute; ventricular—30 beats/minute
• *P wave:* Normal
• *PR interval:* Varies
• *QRS complex:* 0.16 second
• *T wave:* Normal
• *QT interval:* 0.56 second
• *Other:* None

The site of the escape rhythm determines the appearance of the QRS complex. If it originates in the AV node, the QRS complex is normal and the ventricular rate is 40 to 60 beats/minute. If the escape rhythm originates in the Purkinje system, the QRS complex is wide, with a ventricular rate below 40 beats/minute.

Third-degree block is a similar rhythm to complete AV dissociation; however, there are some key differences. (See *Recognizing complete AV dissociation*.)

Sinking spell

Most patients with third-degree AV block experience significant symptoms, including severe fatigue, dyspnea, chest pain, lightheadedness, changes in mental status, and loss of consciousness.

Recognizing complete AV dissociation

With third-degree atrioventricular (AV) block and complete AV dissociation, the atria and ventricles beat independently, each controlled by its own pacemaker.

However, there's a key difference between these two arrhythmias: In third-degree AV block, the atrial rate is faster than the ventricular rate. With complete AV dissociation, the two rates are usually about the same, with the ventricular rate slightly faster.

Rhythm disturbances

Never the primary problem, complete AV dissociation results from one of three underlying rhythm disturbances:
• slowed or impaired sinus impulse formation or sinoatrial conduction, as in sinus bradycardia or sinus arrest

• accelerated impulse formation in the AV junction or the ventricular pacemaker, as in junctional or ventricular tachycardia
• AV conduction disturbance, as in complete AV block.

When to treat

The clinical significance of complete AV dissociation—as well as treatment for the arrhythmia—depends on the underlying cause and its effects on the patient. If the underlying rhythm decreases cardiac output, the patient needs treatment to correct the arrhythmia.

Depending on the underlying cause, the patient may be treated with an antiarrhythmic, such as atropine or isoproterenol, to restore synchrony. Alternatively, the patient may be given a pacemaker to support a slow ventricular rate. If drug toxicity caused the original disturbance, the drug should be discontinued.

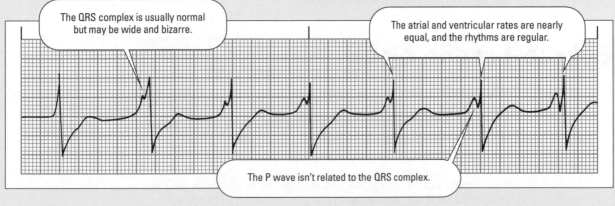

You may note hypotension, pallor, diaphoresis, bradycardia, and a variation in the intensity of the pulse.

A few patients will be relatively free from symptoms, complaining only that they can't tolerate exercise and that they're often tired for no apparent reason. The severity of symptoms depends to a great extent on the resulting ventricular rate.

How you intervene

When caring for a patient with third-degree heart block, immediately assess the patient's tolerance of the rhythm and the need for treatment to support cardiac output and relieve symptoms. Make sure the patient has a patent I.V. line. Administer oxygen therapy as ordered. Evaluate for possible correctable causes of the arrhythmia, such as medications or ischemia. Minimize the patient's activity and maintain his bed rest.

If cardiac output isn't adequate or the patient's condition seems to be deteriorating, therapy aims to improve the ventricular rate. Atropine may be given, or a temporary pacemaker may be used to restore adequate cardiac output. Temporary pacing may continue until the cause of the block resolves or until a permanent pacemaker can be inserted. A permanent block requires placement of a permanent pacemaker.

A pacemaker may be just what I need to get me out of this slump.

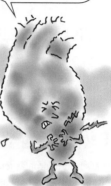

Bundles of troubles

The patient with an anterior-wall MI is more likely to have permanent third-degree AV block if the MI involved the bundle of His or the bundle branches than if it involved other areas of the myocardium. Those patients commonly require prompt placement of a permanent pacemaker.

An AV block in a patient with an inferior-wall MI is more likely to be temporary, as a result of injury to the AV node. Placement of a permanent pacemaker is usually delayed in such cases to evaluate recovery of the conduction system.

Bundle-branch block

Bundle-branch block is a potential complication of MI. In this disorder, either the left or the right bundle branch fails to conduct impulses. A bundle-branch block that occurs low in the left bundle, in the posterior or anterior fasciculus, is called a *hemiblock*.

Impulsive behavior

In a bundle-branch block, the impulse travels down the unaffected bundle branch and then from one myocardial cell to the next to depolarize the ventricle. Because this cell-to-cell conduction progresses much slower than the conduction along the specialized cells of the conduction system, ventricular depolarization is prolonged.

Wide world of complexes

Prolonged ventricular depolarization means that the QRS complex will be widened. The normal width of the complex is 0.06 to 0.10 second. If the width increases to greater than 0.12 second, a bundle-branch block is present.

After you identify a bundle-branch block, examine lead V_1, which lies to the right of the heart, and lead V_6, which lies to the left of the heart. You'll use these leads to determine whether the block is in the right or the left bundle.

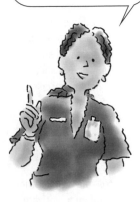

Use leads V_1 and V_6 to determine whether a block is in the right or the left bundle.

Right bundle-branch block

When the right bundle branch fails to conduct impulses, the patient has a right bundle-branch block (RBBB).

How it happens

RBBB may occur in patients with CAD or pulmonary embolism or patients who have recently had an anterior-wall MI. However, it can also occur without the presence of cardiac disease. If this block develops as the heart rate increases, it's called *rate-related RBBB*. (See *How RBBB occurs*, page 214.)

What to look for

On an ECG, RBBB is characterized by a QRS complex that's greater than 0.12 second and has a different configuration, sometimes resembling rabbit ears or the letter "M." Septal depolarization isn't affected in lead V_1, so the initial small R wave remains. The R wave is followed by an S wave, which represents left ventricular depolarization, and a tall R wave (called *R prime*, or *R'*), which represents late right ventricular depolarization. The T wave is negative in this lead. However, that deflection is called a *secondary T-wave change* and is of no clinical significance.

Opposing moves

The opposite occurs in lead V_6. A small Q wave is followed by depolarization of the left ventricle, which produces a tall R wave. Depolarization of the right ventricle then causes a broad S wave. In lead V_6, the T wave should be positive. (See *Recognizing RBBB*, page 215.)

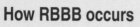

How RBBB occurs

In right bundle-branch block (RBBB), the initial impulse activates the interventricular septum from left to right, just as in normal activation (arrow 1). Next, the left bundle branch activates the left ventricle (arrow 2). The impulse then crosses the interventricular septum to activate the right ventricle (arrow 3).

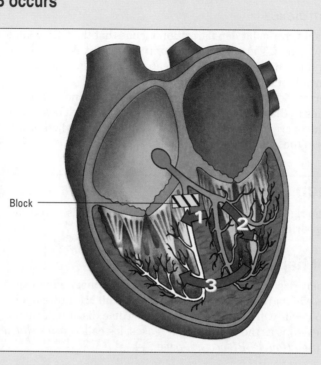

Block

How you intervene

Some blocks require treatment with a temporary pacemaker. Others are monitored only to detect whether they progress to a more complete block.

Left bundle-branch block

When the left bundle branch fails to conduct, the patient has a left bundle-branch block (LBBB).

How it happens

LBBB never occurs normally. This block is usually caused by hypertensive heart disease, aortic stenosis, degenerative changes of the conduction system, or CAD. (See *How LBBB occurs*, page 216.)

Recognizing RBBB

This 12-lead electrocardiogram shows the characteristic changes of right bundle-branch block (RBBB). In lead V_1, note the rsR′ pattern and T-wave inversion. In lead V_6, see the widened S wave and the upright T wave. Also note the prolonged QRS complexes.

Lead I **Lead II** **Lead III**

Lead aV_R **Lead aV_L** **Lead aV_F**

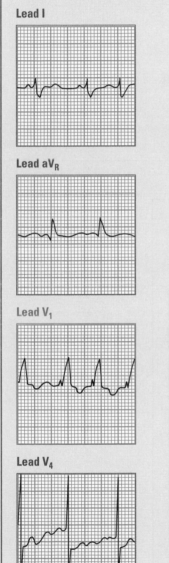

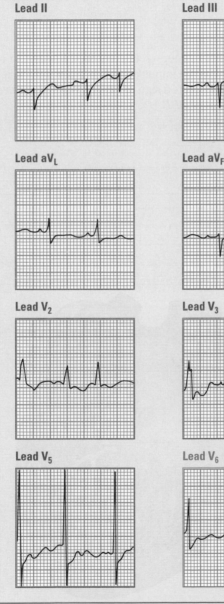

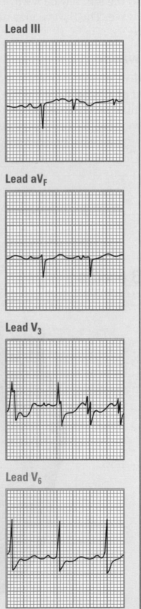

Lead V_1 **Lead V_2** **Lead V_3**

Lead V_4 **Lead V_5** **Lead V_6**

What to look for

In LBBB, the QRS complexes on an ECG are greater than 0.12 second because the ventricles are activated sequentially, not simultaneously. As the wave of depolarization spreads from the right ventricle to the left, a wide S wave is produced in lead V_1, with a positive T wave. The S wave may be preceded by a Q wave or a small R wave.

Slurring your R waves

In lead V_6, no initial Q wave occurs. A tall, notched R wave, or a slurred one, is produced as the impulse spreads from right to left. This initial positive deflection is a sign of LBBB. The T wave is negative. (See *Recognizing LBBB*.)

Now I get it!

How LBBB occurs

In left bundle-branch block (LBBB), the impulse first travels down the right bundle branch (arrow 1). Then the impulse activates the interventricular septum from right to left (arrow 2), the opposite of normal activation. Finally, the impulse activates the left ventricle (arrow 3).

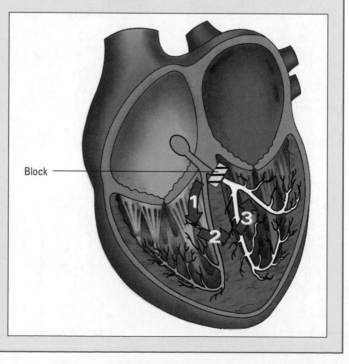

Block

Recognizing LBBB

This 12-lead electrocardiogram shows characteristic changes of left bundle-branch block (LBBB). All leads have prolonged QRS complexes. In lead V_1, note the QS wave pattern. In lead V_6, you'll see the slurred R wave and T-wave inversion. The elevated ST segments and upright T waves in leads V_1 to V_4 are also common in LBBB.

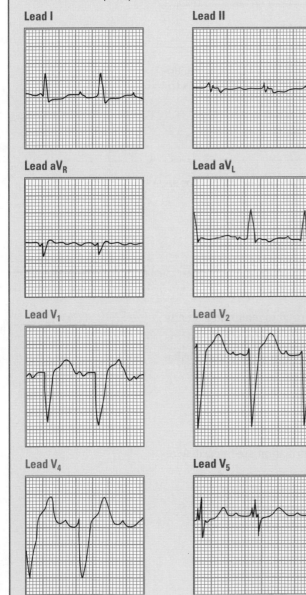

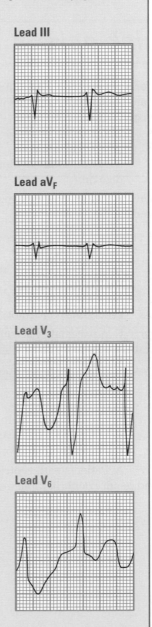

How you intervene

When LBBB occurs along with an anterior-wall MI, it usually signals complete heart block, which requires insertion of a pacemaker.

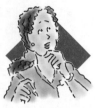

Quick quiz

1. For a patient with symptom-producing sinus bradycardia, appropriate nursing interventions include establishing I.V. access to administer:

A.   atropine.
B.   anticoagulants.
C.   a calcium channel blocker.
D.   digoxin.

Answer: A. Atropine or epinephrine is standard treatment for sinus bradycardia.

2. Treatment for symptom-producing sick sinus syndrome includes:

A.   beta-adrenergic blockers.
B.   ventilatory support.
C.   pacemaker insertion.
D.   synchronized cardioversion.

Answer: C. A pacemaker is commonly used to maintain a steady heart rate in patients with sick sinus syndrome.

3. The treatment of choice for a patient with ventricular fibrillation is:

A.   defibrillation.
B.   transesophageal pacing.
C.   synchronized cardioversion.
D.   digoxin administration.

Answer: A. Patients with ventricular fibrillation are in cardiac arrest and require defibrillation.

4. The term pulseless electrical activity refers to a condition in which there's:
- A.   a ventricular rate exceeding 100 beats/minute.
- B.   asystole on a monitor or rhythm strip.
- C.   an extremely slow heart rate but no pulse.
- D.   electrical activity in the heart but no actual contraction.

Answer: D. Pulseless electrical activity is electrical activity without mechanical contraction. The patient is in cardiac arrest, with no blood pressure or pulse.

5. In type I second-degree AV block, the PR interval:
- A.   varies according to the ventricular response rate.
- B.   progressively lengthens until a QRS complex is dropped.
- C.   remains constant despite an irregular ventricular rhythm.
- D.   can't be determined.

Answer: B. Progressive lengthening of the PR interval creates an irregular ventricular rhythm with a repeating pattern of groups of QRS complexes. Those groups are followed by a dropped beat in which the P wave isn't followed by a QRS complex.

6. In atrial flutter, the key consideration in determining treatment is the:
- A.   atrial rate.
- B.   ventricular rate.
- C.   configuration of the flutter waves.
- D.   PR interval.

Answer: B. If the ventricular rate is too fast or too slow, cardiac output will be compromised. A rapid ventricular rate may require immediate cardioversion.

Scoring

☆☆☆ If you answered all six questions correctly, sensational! Don't get a complex, but we think you have QRS complexes and P waves down pat.

☆☆ If you answered four or five questions correctly, great job! It may seem impulsive, but we think that at this junction, you're ready to move on.

☆ If you answered fewer than four questions correctly, don't worry. It can take a while to get into the rhythm of understanding arrhythmias. Take a break and then try the Quick quiz again.

Inflammatory and valvular disorders

Just the facts

In this chapter, you'll learn:

♦ disorders that affect the lining or valves of the heart

♦ pathophysiology and treatments related to these disorders

♦ diagnostic tests, assessment findings, and nursing interventions for each disorder.

A look at inflammatory disorders

Inflammatory cardiac disorders include endocarditis, myocarditis, and pericarditis. With these conditions, scar formation and otherwise normal healing processes can cause debilitating structural damage to the heart.

Endocarditis

Endocarditis is an infection of the endocardium, the heart valves, or a cardiac prosthesis. It typically results from bacterial invasion. In I.V. drug abusers, it may also result from fungal invasion.

Green growth

This invasion produces vegetative growths on the heart valves, the endocardial lining of a heart chamber, or the endothelium of a blood vessel that may embolize to the spleen, kidneys, central nervous system (CNS), extremities, and lungs. (See *Effects of endocarditis*, page 222.)

> Endocarditis occurs when bacteria invade the inner lining of the heart.

Effects of endocarditis

This illustration shows vegetative growths on the endocardium produced by fibrin and platelet deposits on infection sites.

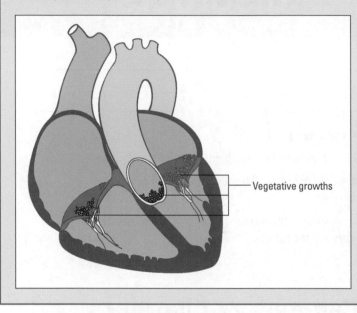

Vegetative growths

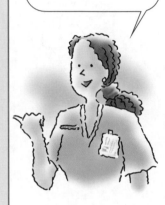

Not all vegetative growths are good. Just look at those formed by fibrin and platelet deposits in endocarditis.

Type talk

There are three types of endocarditis:

Acute infective endocarditis usually results from bacteremia that follows septic thrombophlebitis, open-heart surgery involving prosthetic valves, or skin, bone, and pulmonary infections. This form of endocarditis also occurs in I.V. drug abusers.

Subacute infective endocarditis typically occurs in individuals with acquired valvular or congenital cardiac lesions. It can also follow dental, genitourinary, gynecologic, and GI procedures.

Rheumatic endocarditis commonly affects the mitral valve; less frequently, the aortic or tricuspid valve; and rarely, the pulmonic valve. Preexisting rheumatic endocardial lesions are a common predisposing factor.

Treat, or else

Untreated endocarditis usually proves fatal; however, with proper treatment, 70% of patients recover. Prognosis becomes much worse when endocarditis causes severe valvular damage (leading to insufficiency and heart failure) or when it involves a prosthetic valve.

Other complications include cerebrovascular or peripheral vascular ischemia, thrombosis, and renal failure.

What causes it

In acute infective endocarditis, infecting organisms include:
• group A nonhemolytic streptococcus (rheumatic endocarditis)
• pneumococcus
• staphylococcus
• enterococcus
• gonococcus (rare).

Causes of acute endocarditis in I.V. drug users include *Staphylococcus aureus, Pseudomonas* bacteria, *Candida* fungi, and skin saprophytes that are typically harmless.

In subacute infective endocarditis, infecting organisms include:
• *Streptococcus viridans,* which normally inhabits the upper respiratory tract
• *Streptococcus faecalis* (enterococcus), usually found in GI and perineal flora.

How it happens

In endocarditis, fibrin and platelets cluster on valve tissue and engulf circulating bacteria or fungi. This process produces vegetation, which in turn may cover the valve surfaces, causing deformities and destruction of valvular tissue. The destruction may then extend to the chordae tendineae (threadlike bands of fibrous tissue that attach the tricuspid and mitral valves to the papillary muscles), causing them to rupture. This rupturing then leads to valvular insufficiency. Vegetative growth on the heart valves, the endocardial lining of a heart chamber, or the endothelium of a blood vessel may embolize to the spleen, kidneys, CNS, extremities, and lungs.

What to look for

Early clinical features of endocarditis are usually nonspecific and include:
• weakness and fatigue
• weight loss
• anorexia
• arthralgia
• night sweats
• intermittent fever (may recur for weeks).

A loud, regurgitant murmur may also be present. This murmur is typical of the underlying rheumatic or congenital heart disease.

A sudden change in an existing murmur or the discovery of a new murmur along with fever is a classic sign of endocarditis.

What else?

Other signs include:
• petechiae on the skin (especially common on the upper anterior trunk); the buccal, pharyngeal, or conjunctival mucosa; and the nails (splinter hemorrhages)
• Osler's nodes (small, raised, swollen tender areas that most commonly occur on the hands and feet)
• Roth's spots (round, white retina spots surrounded by hemorrhage)
• Janeway lesions (irregular, painless, erythematous lesions on the soles of the feet, the palms, and the fingers).

Subacute signs

In subacute endocarditis, embolization from vegetating lesions or diseased valve tissue may produce:
• splenic infarction (abdominal rigidity and pain in the left upper quadrant that radiates to the left shoulder)
• renal infarction (hematuria, pyuria, flank pain, and decreased urine output and renal function)
• cerebral infarction (hemiparesis, aphasia, or other neurologic deficits)
• pulmonary infarction (cough, pleuritic pain, pleural friction rub, dyspnea, and hemoptysis; most common in right-sided endocarditis, which commonly occurs among I.V. drug abusers and after cardiac surgery)
• peripheral vascular occlusion (severe pain, limb pallor and coldness, absent pulse, diminished sensation, and paralysis, a late sign of impending peripheral gangrene).

What tests tell you

• Three or more blood cultures drawn at least 1 hour apart during a 24-hour period identify the causative organism in up to 90% of patients. The remaining 10% may have negative blood cultures, possibly suggesting fungal infection.
• Echocardiography, including transesophageal echocardiography (TEE), may identify vegetations and valvular damage.
• Electrocardiogram (ECG) readings may show atrial fibrillation and other arrhythmias that accompany valvular disease.
• Abnormal laboratory results include elevated white blood cell (WBC) count; abnormal histocytes (macrophages); elevated erythrocyte sedimentation rate (ESR); normocytic, normochromic anemia (in subacute bacterial endocarditis); and rheumatoid factor (occurs in about 50% of patients).

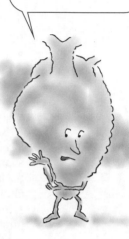

A fever plus a new or changed heart murmur are classic signs of endocarditis.

How it's treated

Treatment seeks to eradicate the infecting organism. It should start promptly and continue over several weeks. The doctor bases antibiotic selection on sensitivity studies of the infecting organism—or the probable organism, if blood cultures are negative. I.V. antibiotic therapy usually lasts 4 to 6 weeks and may be followed by oral antibiotics.

Be supportive

Supportive treatment includes bed rest, antipyretics for fever and aches, and sufficient fluid intake. Severe valvular damage, especially aortic insufficiency, or infection of a cardiac prosthesis may require corrective surgery if refractory heart failure develops.

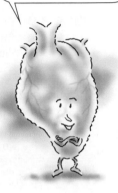

Treatment for endocarditis focuses on eradicating the infecting organism.

What to do

• Collaborate with a skilled team, which may include a cardiologist, an infectious disease specialist, a cardiothoracic surgeon, a nephrologist, and a cardiac and stroke rehabilitation team.
• Obtain the patient's allergy history.
• Administer antibiotics on time to maintain consistent blood levels. Check dilutions for compatibility with other patient medications, and use a compatible solution (for example, add methicillin to a buffered solution).

Check progress

• Evaluate the patient. The patient has recovered from endocarditis if he maintains a normal temperature, clear lungs, stable vital signs, and adequate tissue perfusion and can tolerate activity for a reasonable period and maintain normal weight.
• Teach the patient about the anti-infective medication that he'll continue to take. Stress the importance of taking the medication and restricting activity for as long as recommended.
• Tell the patient to watch for and report signs of embolization and to watch closely for fever, anorexia, and other signs of relapse that could occur about 2 weeks after treatment stops.

Stay the course

• Discuss the importance of completing the full course of antibiotics, even if he's feeling better. Make sure a susceptible patient understands the need for prophylactic antibiotics before, during, and after dental work, childbirth, and genitourinary, GI, or gynecologic procedures.
• Document vital signs, cardiac and respiratory status, and response to treatment.

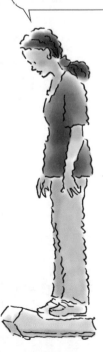

Signs of improved endocarditis include maintaining a normal weight.

Myocarditis

Myocarditis is a focal or diffuse inflammation of the cardiac muscle (myocardium). It may be acute or chronic and can strike at any age.

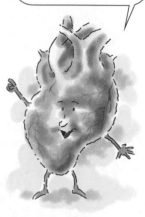

A spontaneous recovery from myocarditis isn't unusual.

Vague signs, sudden recovery

In many cases, myocarditis fails to produce specific cardiovascular symptoms or ECG abnormalities. The patient commonly experiences spontaneous recovery without residual defects.

And to complicate matters...

Occasionally, myocarditis is complicated by heart failure and, rarely, it leads to cardiomyopathy. Other complications include arrhythmias, pulmonary edema, respiratory distress, and multiple-organ-dysfunction syndrome (MODS).

What causes it

Potential causes of myocarditis include:
• viral infections (most common cause in the United States), such as coxsackievirus A and B strains and, possibly, poliomyelitis, influenza, rubeola, rubella, adenoviruses, and echoviruses
• bacterial infections, such as diphtheria, tuberculosis, typhoid fever, tetanus, and staphylococcal, pneumococcal, and gonococcal infections
• hypersensitivity reactions, such as acute rheumatic fever and postcardiotomy syndrome
• radiation therapy to the chest
• chronic alcoholism
• parasitic infections, such as toxoplasmosis and, especially, South American trypanosomiasis (Chagas' disease) in infants and immunosuppressed adults
• intestinal parasitic infections such as trichinosis.

How it happens

The myocardium may become damaged when an infectious organism triggers an autoimmune, cellular, or humoral reaction or when a noninfectious cause leads to toxic inflammation. In either case, the resulting inflammation may lead to hypertrophy, fibrosis, and inflammatory changes of the myocardium and conduction system.

Feeling the flab

Because of this damage, the heart muscle weakens and contractility is reduced. The heart muscle becomes flabby and dilated, and pinpoint hemorrhages may develop.

What to look for

Signs and symptoms of myocarditis include:
- dyspnea and fatigue
- palpitations and fever
- mild, continuous pressure or soreness in the chest
- signs and symptoms of heart failure (with advanced disease).

What tests tell you

- Laboratory tests may reveal elevated cardiac enzymes, such as creatine kinase (CK) and CK-MB, increased WBC count and ESR, and elevated antibody titers (such as antistreptolysin-O titer; which indicates a recent streptococcal infection in rheumatic fever).
- ECG changes provide the most reliable diagnostic information. Typically, the ECG shows diffuse ST-segment and T-wave abnormalities such as occur with pericarditis, conduction defects (prolonged PR interval), and other supraventricular ectopic arrhythmias.
- Stool and throat cultures may allow identification of bacteria.
- Endomyocardial biopsy provides a definitive diagnosis.

How it's treated

Treatment for myocarditis includes antibiotics for bacterial infection, modified bed rest to decrease heart workload, and careful management of complications. If a thromboembolism occurs, anticoagulant therapy is required. If heart failure occurs, inotropic drugs, such as amrinone, dobutamine, or dopamine, may be necessary. Nitroprusside (Nitropress) and nitroglycerin may be administered to reduce preload and afterload.

Upping the ante

Treatment with immunosuppressive drugs or steroids is controversial but may be helpful after the acute inflammation has passed. Patients with low cardiac output may benefit from intra-aortic balloon pulsation and ventricular assist devices. Heart transplantation is performed as a last resort.

What to do

- Collaborate with a skilled team, which may include a cardiologist, an infectious disease specialist, a cardiothoracic surgeon, a nephrologist, and a cardiac and stroke rehabilitation team.
- Assess cardiovascular status frequently, watching for such signs of heart failure as dyspnea, hypotension, and tachycardia.

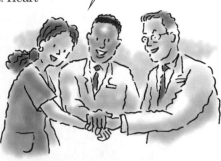

Collaboration is key when treating myocarditis.

• Assist the patient with activities such as bathing as necessary. Encourage use of a bedside commode because this activity stresses the heart less than using a bedpan.

• Evaluate the patient. After successful treatment, the patient's cardiac output should be adequate, as evidenced by normal blood pressure; warm, dry skin; normal level of consciousness; and absence of dizziness. He should be able to tolerate a normal level of activity, his temperature should be normal, and he shouldn't be dyspneic. Tests such as echocardiography help confirm myocardial recovery.

• Teach the patient about anti-infective drugs. Stress the importance of taking the prescribed drug as ordered.

It's only for a while

• Reassure the patient that activity limitations are temporary. Offer diversional activities that are physically undemanding.

• Stress the importance of bed rest. During recovery, recommend that the patient resume normal activities slowly and avoid competitive sports.

• Document vital signs, cardiac and respiratory status, and response to treatment. Document all patient teaching and the patient's understanding of the information.

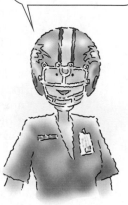

When recovering from myocarditis, the patient should avoid competitive sports.

Pericarditis

Pericarditis is an inflammation of the pericardium, the fibroserous sac that envelops, supports, and protects the heart. It occurs in acute and chronic forms:

• Acute pericarditis can be fibrinous or effusive, with purulent, serous, or hemorrhagic exudate.

• Chronic constrictive pericarditis is characterized by dense fibrous pericardial thickening.

Complications of pericarditis include pericardial effusion, heart failure, cardiac tamponade, respiratory distress, and MODS.

What causes it

Pericarditis may result from:

• bacterial, fungal, or viral infection (infectious pericarditis)

• neoplasms (primary disease or metastasis)

• high-dose radiation to the chest

• uremia

• hypersensitivity or autoimmune disease, such as acute rheumatic fever (the most common cause of pericarditis in children), systemic lupus erythematosus, and rheumatoid arthritis

• drugs, such as hydralazine or procainamide (Procanbid)

• idiopathic factors (most common in acute pericarditis)

• myocardial infarction (Dressler's syndrome), trauma, or surgery (postcardiotomy syndrome) that leaves the pericardium intact but causes blood to leak into the pericardial cavity
• aortic aneurysm with pericardial leakage (less common)
• myxedema with cholesterol deposits in the pericardium (less common).

How it happens

Pericardial tissue damaged by bacteria or other substances results in the release of chemical mediators of inflammation (prostaglandins, histamines, bradykinins, and serotonin) into the surrounding tissue, thereby initiating the inflammatory process.

There's the rub

Friction occurs as the inflamed pericardial layers rub against each other. Histamines and other chemical mediators dilate vessels and increase vessel permeability. Vessel walls then leak fluids and protein (including fibrinogen) into tissues, causing extracellular edema, and macrophages already present in the tissue begin to phagocytose the invading bacteria and are joined by neutrophils and monocytes.

A short time later...

After several days, the pericardial cavity (the space bewteen the epicardium and the fibrous pericardium) fills with an exudate composed of necrotic issue and dead and dying bacteria, neutrophils, and macrophages. Eventually, the contents of the cavity autolyze and are gradually reabsorbed into healthy tissue.

Then what?

When this occurs, there are several possible results:
• If fluid accumulates in the pericardial cavity, a pericardial effusion develops. This effusion may produce heart failure effects, such as dyspnea, orthopnea, and tachyarrhythmias. It may also produce ill-defined substernal chest pain and a feeling of chest fullness.
• If fluid rapidly accumulates in the pericardial space, cardiac tamponade results. This condition compresses the heart and prevents it from filling during diastole, causing a drop in cardiac output. Heart failure results, causing symptoms such as pallor, clammy skin, hypotension, pulsus paradoxus, jugular vein distention and, eventually, cardiovascular collapse and death.

- If the pericardium becomes thick and stiff from chronic or recurrent pericarditis, chronic constrictive pericarditis develops. The heart becomes encased in a stiff shell, which prevents proper filling during diastole. Left- and right-sided filling pressures increase, leading to a drop in stroke volume and diminished cardiac output.

What to look for

A patient with acute pericarditis typically complains of sharp, sudden pain, usually starting over the sternum and radiating to the neck, shoulders, back, and arms.

Forward feels better

The pain is usually pleuritic, increasing with deep inspiration and decreasing when the patient sits up and leans forward. This decrease occurs because leaning forward pulls the heart away from the diaphragmatic pleurae of the lungs.

What tests tell you

- ECG may reveal diffuse ST-segment elevation in the limb leads and most precordial leads that reflects the inflammatory process. Upright T waves are present in most leads. QRS segments may be diminished when pericardial effusion exists. Arrhythmias may occur. In chronic constrictive pericarditis, low-voltage QRS complexes, T-wave inversion or flattening, and P mitral waves (wide P waves) may occur in leads I, II, and V_6.
- Laboratory testing may reveal an elevated ESR as a result of the inflammatory process or a normal or elevated WBC count, especially in infectious pericarditis. An elevated blood urea nitrogen level and elevated creatinine levels may point to uremia as a cause of pericarditis.
- Blood cultures may be used to identify an infectious cause.
- Antistreptolysin-O titers may be positive if pericarditis is caused by rheumatic fever.
- A purified protein derivative skin test may be positive if pericarditis is caused by tuberculosis.

Where's the echo?

- Echocardiography may show an echo-free space between the ventricular wall and the pericardium and reduced pumping action.
- Chest X-rays may be normal with acute pericarditis. The cardiac silhouette may be enlarged, with a water bottle shape caused by fluid accumulation, if pleural effusion is present.

How it's treated

The goals of treatment for a patient with pericarditis are to relieve symptoms, prevent or correct pericardial effusion and cardiac tamponade, and manage the underlying disease.

In idiopathic pericarditis, post–myocardial infarction pericarditis, and postthoracotomy pericarditis, treatment includes:
• bed rest as long as fever and pain persist
• nonsteroidal anti-inflammatory drugs (NSAIDs), such as aspirin and indomethacin (Indocin SR), to relieve pain and reduce inflammation.

If symptoms continue, the doctor may prescribe corticosteroids to provide rapid and effective relief. Corticosteroids must be used cautiously because pericarditis may recur when drug therapy stops.

Going in

When infectious pericarditis results from disease of the left pleural space, mediastinal abscesses, or septicemia, the patient requires antibiotics, surgical drainage, or both.

If cardiac tamponade develops, the doctor may perform emergency pericardiocentesis and may inject antibiotics directly into the pericardial sac. (See *Understanding pericardiocentesis.*)

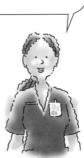

Treatment for pericarditis starts with bed rest and drugs to reduce inflammation...

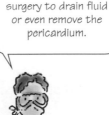

...but can involve surgery to drain fluid or even remove the pericardium.

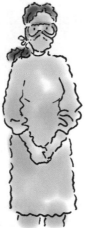

Understanding pericardiocentesis

Typically performed at the bedside in an intensive care unit, pericardiocentesis involves needle aspiration of excess fluid from the pericardial sac. It may be the treatment of choice for life-threatening cardiac tamponade (except when fluid accumulates rapidly, in which case immediate surgery is usually preferred). Pericardiocentesis may also be used to aspirate fluid in such subacute conditions as viral or bacterial infection and pericarditis. What's more, it can be used to obtain a sample for laboratory analysis to confirm diagnosis and identify the cause of pericardial effusion.

Complications

Pericardiocentesis carries some risk of potentially fatal complications, such as inadvertent puncture of internal organs (particularly the heart, lungs, stomach, and liver) or laceration of the myocardium or a coronary artery. Emergency equipment should be readily available during the procedure in case of such complications.

Heavy-duty treatments

If pericarditis is recurrent, a partial pericardiectomy may be indicated. In this procedure, a window is created that allows fluid to drain into the pleural space. In constrictive pericarditis, total pericardiectomy may be necessary to permit the heart to fill and contract adequately.

What to do

• Collaborate with a skilled team, which may include a cardiologist, an infectious disease specialist, a cardiothoracic surgeon, a respiratory therapist, and a physical therapist.
• Maintain the patient on bed rest until fever and pain diminish. Provide a bedside commode to reduce myocardial oxygen demand.
• Assist the patient with bathing, if necessary.
• Place the patient in an upright position to relieve dyspnea and chest pain. Auscultate lung sounds at least every 2 hours. Administer supplemental oxygen as needed, based on oxygen saturation or mixed venous oxygen saturation levels.
• Administer analgesics to relieve pain and NSAIDs, as ordered, to reduce inflammation. Administer steroids if the patient doesn't respond to NSAIDs.
• If your patient has a pulmonary artery catheter, monitor hemodynamic status. Assess the patient's cardiovascular status frequently, watching for signs of cardiac tamponade.

Watch the clock

• Administer antibiotics on time to maintain consistent drug levels in the blood.
• Institute continuous cardiac monitoring to evaluate for changes in the ECG. Look for the return of ST segments to baseline with T-wave flattening by the end of the first 7 days.
• Keep a pericardiocentesis set and emergency equipment available if pericardial effusion is suspected, and prepare the patient for pericardiocentesis as indicated.
• Provide appropriate postoperative care, similar to that given after cardiothoracic surgery.

Class begins

• Explain tests and treatments to the patient.
• Instruct him to resume his daily activities slowly and to schedule rest periods into his daily routine.
• Show him how to position himself to relieve pain.
• Document vital signs and hemodynamic measurements. Note cardiac and respiratory status and response to treatment. Document teaching and the patient's understanding of the information.

A look at valvular heart disease

In valvular heart disease, three types of disruption can occur:
- stenosis (tissue thickening that narrows the valvular opening)
- incomplete closure of the valve
- prolapse of the valve.

The nature and severity of associated symptoms determine treatment in valvular heart disease. The patient may need to restrict activities to avoid extreme fatigue and dyspnea.

Memory jogger

To remember the three types of disruption that can occur in valvular heart disease, just think **SIP**:

Stenosis

Insufficiency

Prolapse.

Mitral insufficiency

Mitral insufficiency occurs when the mitral valve doesn't close completely, allowing blood to flow back through the valve.

What causes it

Mitral insufficiency can result from rheumatic fever, hypertrophic cardiomyopathy, mitral valve prolapse, myocardial infarction, severe left-sided heart failure, or ruptured chordae tendineae. It's also associated with congenital anomalies such as transposition of the great arteries and past use of the appetite suppressants fenfluramine or dexfenfluramine for more than 4 months. It's rare in children unless other congenital anomalies are present.

How it happens

In mitral insufficiency, blood from the left ventricle flows back into the left atrium during systole, causing the atrium to enlarge to accommodate the backflow. As a result, the left ventricle also dilates to accommodate the increased volume of blood from the atrium and to compensate for diminished cardiac output.

System failure

Ventricular hypertrophy and increased end-diastolic pressure result in increased pulmonary artery pressure, eventually leading to left-sided and right-sided heart failure.

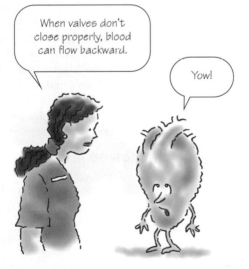

When valves don't close properly, blood can flow backward.

Yow!

What to look for

Signs and symptoms of mitral insufficiency include:
- orthopnea, dyspnea, or cough (particularly when lying down)
- fatigue

- angina and palpitations
- right-sided heart failure (jugular vein distention, peripheral edema, and hepatomegaly)
- systolic murmur
- cardiac arrhythmias.

What tests tell you

- Cardiac catheterization reveals mitral insufficiency with increased left ventricular end-diastolic volume and pressure, increased atrial pressure and pulmonary artery wedge pressure (PAWP), and decreased cardiac output.
- Chest X-rays show left atrial and ventricular enlargement and pulmonary venous congestion.
- Echocardiography and TEE show abnormal valve leaflet motion and left atrial enlargement.
- ECG may show left atrial and ventricular hypertrophy, sinus tachycardia, and atrial fibrillation.
- Holter monitoring can detect intermittent cardiac arrhythmias.

How it's treated

Heart failure caused by mitral insufficiency may require angiotensin-converting enzyme (ACE) inhibitors such as lisinopril (Zestril), beta-adrenergic blockers such as metoprolol (Lopressor), digoxin (Lanoxin), diuretics, a sodium-restricted diet and, in acute cases, oxygen. Atrial fibrillation or atrial flutter requires beta-adrenergic blockers or digoxin to slow the ventricular rate. Other appropriate measures include anticoagulant therapy to prevent thrombus formation around diseased or replaced valves and prophylactic antibiotics before and after surgery or dental care to prevent endocarditis.

If the patient has severe signs and symptoms that can't be managed medically, he may need open-heart surgery with cardiopulmonary bypass for valve replacement.

For the not so young at heart

Valvuloplasty may be used in elderly patients who have end-stage disease and can't tolerate general anesthesia.

Complications of treatment may include arrhythmias, heart failure, pulmonary edema, respiratory distress, endocarditis, myocardial ischemia, renal failure and MODS.

What to do

• Provide periods of rest between periods of activity to prevent excessive fatigue.
• Keep the patient on a low-sodium diet; consult with a dietitian to ensure that the patient receives as many favorite foods as possible during the restriction.
• Monitor for left-sided heart failure, pulmonary edema, and adverse reactions to drug therapy. Provide oxygen to prevent tissue hypoxia, as needed.
• If the patient undergoes surgery, monitor postoperatively for hypotension, arrhythmias, and thrombus formation.
• Monitor the patient's vital signs, arterial blood gas (ABG) levels, intake and output, daily weights, blood chemistry studies, chest X-rays, and pulmonary artery catheter readings.
• Teach the patient about diet and activity restrictions, medications, symptoms that should be reported to the doctor, and the importance of consistent follow-up care.
• Make sure the patient and his family understand the need to comply with prolonged antibiotic therapy and follow-up care. In addition, explain the possible need for prophylactic antibiotics during dental surgery or other invasive procedures.

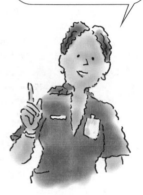

When teaching a patient, stress the importance of complying with antibiotic therapy.

Mitral stenosis

Mitral stenosis is hardening or narrowing of the mitral valve.

Trouble ahead

Complications of mitral stenosis include pulmonary hypertension, left atrial enlargement, arrhythmias (particularly of atrial origin), endocarditis, right- and left-sided heart failure, pulmonary edema, and hemoptysis.

What causes it

Most commonly resulting from rheumatic fever, mitral stenosis typically occurs in females. It may also be associated with other congenital anomalies and radiation treatments to the chest. Rarely, blood clots and tumors can block the valve, preventing it from opening properly.

How it happens

In mitral stenosis, the valve narrows as a result of valvular abnormalities, fibrosis, calcification, or other factors. This narrowing obstructs blood flow from the left atrium to the left ventricle. Consequently, left atrial volume and pressure increase and the chamber dilates.

Not going with the flow

Greater resistance to blood flow causes pulmonary hypertension, right ventricular hypertrophy, and right-sided heart failure. Also, inadequate filling of the left ventricle produces low cardiac output.

What to look for

Signs and symptoms of mitral stenosis include:
• dyspnea on exertion, paroxysmal nocturnal dyspnea, and orthopnea
• fatigue and weakness
• right-sided heart failure and cardiac arrhythmias
• crackles on auscultation
• heart murmur.

What tests tell you

• Cardiac catheterization reveals elevated left atrial pressure and PAWP greater than 15 mm Hg with severe pulmonary hypertension, elevated right-sided heart pressure with decreased cardiac output, and abnormal contraction of the left ventricle.
• Echocardiography and TEE show thickened mitral valve leaflets and left atrial enlargement.
• Chest X-rays show left atrial and ventricular enlargement, enlarged pulmonary arteries, and mitral valve calcification.
• ECG shows left atrial hypertrophy, atrial fibrillation, right ventricular hypertrophy, and right axis deviation.
• Holter monitoring detects intermittent cardiac arhythmias over a 24- to 48-hour period.

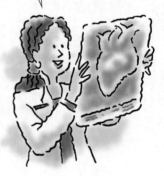

In mitral stenosis, chest X-rays reveal left atrial and ventricular enlargement, enlarged pulmonary arteries, and mitral valve calcification.

How it's treated

If the patient is symptomatic, treatment varies. Heart failure may require bed rest, digoxin, diuretics, ACE inhibitors, a sodium-restricted diet and, in acute cases, oxygen. Small doses of beta-adrenergic blockers may also be used to slow the ventricular rate when cardiac glycosides fail to control atrial fibrillation or flutter. Synchronized cardioversion may be used to correct atrial fibrillation in an unstable patient. Anticoagulants may be necessary to help prevent blood clots

If hemoptysis develops, the patient requires bed rest, sodium restriction, and diuretics to decrease pulmonary venous pressure.

Out of control

A patient with severe, medically uncontrollable symptoms may need open-heart surgery with cardiopulmonary bypass for commissurotomy or valve replacement.

In asymptomatic mitral stenosis in young patients, penicillin is an important prophylactic to prevent endocarditis. Percutaneous balloon valvuloplasty may be used in young patients who have no calcifications or subvalvular deformities, in symptomatic pregnant women, and in elderly patients with end-stage disease who can't withstand general anesthesia. This procedure is usually performed in the cardiac catheterization laboratory.

What to do

- If the patient is required to be on bed rest, stress its importance. Assist with activities of daily living (ADLs) as necessary.
- Watch closely for signs of heart failure, pulmonary edema, and adverse reactions to drug therapy.
- Place the patient in an upright position to relieve dyspnea, if needed. Administer oxygen to prevent tissue hypoxia, as needed.
- If the patient has had surgery, watch for hypotension, arrhythmias, and thrombus formation. Monitor vital signs, ABG levels, intake and output, daily weights, blood chemistry studies, chest X-rays, and pulmonary artery catheter readings.
- Keep the patient on a low-sodium diet, but provide as many favorite foods as possible. Restrict fluids as ordered.

Aortic insufficiency

Aortic insufficiency occurs when the aortic semilunar valve doesn't close completely, allowing blood to flow back through the valve into the left ventricle.

Consider the complications

Complications of aortic insufficiency include left ventricular hypertrophy, heart failure, pulmonary edema, arrhythmias, and endocarditis.

What causes it

Aortic insufficiency can result from rheumatic fever, syphilis, hypertension, or endocarditis, or it may be idiopathic. It's also associated with Marfan syndrome and with ventricular septal defect, even after surgical closure. It typically occurs in males.

How it happens

In aortic insufficiency, blood flows back into the left ventricle during diastole, causing fluid overload in the ventricle which, in turn, dilates and hypertrophies. The excess volume causes fluid overload in the left atrium and, finally, the pulmonary system. Left-sided heart failure and pulmonary edema eventually result.

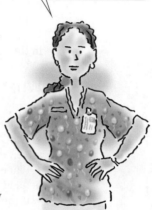

In aortic insufficiency, blood flows back into the left ventricle during diastole, causing fluid overload and, eventually, left-sided heart failure and pulmonary edema.

What to look for

Signs and symptoms of aortic insufficiency include dyspnea (especially with exertion), chest pain, syncope, arrhythmias, cough, left-sided heart failure, pulsus biferiens (rapidly rising and collapsing pulses), and blowing diastolic murmur or third heart sound.

What tests tell you

• Cardiac catheterization reveals a reduction in arterial diastolic pressure, aortic insufficiency, other valvular abnormalities, and increased left ventricular end-diastolic pressure.
• Chest X-rays show left ventricular enlargement and pulmonary venous congestion.
• Echocardiography and TEE show left ventricular enlargement, alterations in mitral valve movement (indirect indication of aortic valve disease), and mitral thickening.
• ECG shows sinus tachycardia; left ventricular hypertrophy may also be present in severe disease.

How it's treated

Valve replacement is the treatment of choice for aortic insufficiency and should be performed before significant ventricular dysfunction occurs. This may not be possible, however, because signs and symptoms seldom occur until after myocardial dysfunction develops.

ACE of spades

Cardiac glycosides, a low-sodium diet, diuretics, vasodilators, and especially ACE inhibitors are used to treat patients with left-sided heart failure. In acute episodes, supplemental oxygen may be necessary. Beta-adrenergic blockers are avoided because of their negative inotropic effects.

What to do

• If the patient is required to be on bed rest, stress its importance. Assist with ADLs as necessary.
• Alternate periods of activity and rest to prevent extreme fatigue and dyspnea.
• Keep the patient's legs elevated to improve venous return to the heart.
• Place the patient in an upright position to relieve dyspnea, if necessary, and administer oxygen to prevent tissue hypoxia.
• Keep the patient on a low-sodium diet. Consult a dietitian to make sure that the patient receives foods he likes.
• Monitor for signs of heart failure, pulmonary edema, and adverse reactions to drug therapy.
• If the patient undergoes surgery, watch for hypotension, arrhythmias, and thrombus formation. Monitor his vital signs, ABG levels, intake and output, daily weights, blood chemistry studies, chest X-rays, and pulmonary artery catheter readings.
• Teach the patient about diet and activity restrictions, medications, symptoms that should be reported to the doctor, and the importance of consistent follow-up care.

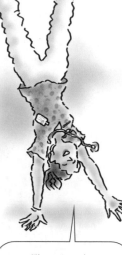

Elevating the patient's legs improves venous return to the heart.

Aortic stenosis

Aortic stenosis is hardening or narrowing of the aortic valve or of the aorta itself.

Complications of aortic stenosis include endocarditis, left ventricular hypertrophy, heart failure, myocardial infarction, pulmonary edema, and arrhythmias.

What causes it

Aortic stenosis results from a congenital aortic bicuspid valve (associated with coarctation of the aorta), congenital stenosis of valve cusps, rheumatic fever or, in elderly patients, atherosclerosis or calcification. It's most common in males older than age 60.

Aortic stenosis can really increase my workload, but sometimes I just can't take it.

How it happens

In aortic stenosis, elevated left ventricular pressure tries to overcome the resistance of the narrowed valvular opening. This added workload increases the demand for oxygen. Diminished cardiac output causes poor coronary artery perfusion, ischemia of the left ventricle, and left-sided heart failure.

What to look for

Signs and symptoms of aortic stenosis include:
- dyspnea on exertion and paroxysmal nocturnal dyspnea
- fatigue
- syncope or dizziness with exertion
- angina, palpitations, and cardiac arrhythmias
- left-sided heart failure
- systolic murmur at the base of the carotids
- decreased cardiac output
- chest pain.

What tests tell you

- Cardiac catheterization reveals increased ventricular end-diastolic pressure.
- Chest X-rays show valvular calcification, left ventricular enlargement, and pulmonary vein congestion.
- ECG shows left ventricular hypertrophy.
- Echocardiography and TEE show a thickened aortic valve and left ventricular wall, possibly with mitral wall stenosis.

How it's treated

Cardiac glycosides, a low-sodium diet, diuretics and, in acute cases, oxygen are used to treat patients with heart failure. Nitroglycerin helps to relieve angina. Prophylactic antibiotics may be necessary before invasive procedures to prevent endocarditis.

Surgical solutions

A Ross procedure may be performed. In this procedure, the pulmonic valve is used to replace the aortic valve and a cadaver pulmonic valve is inserted. This procedure allows longer valve life and anticoagulant therapy isn't necessary.

In children who don't have calcified valves, simple commissurotomy under direct visualization is usually effective. Adults with calcified valves need valve replacement when they become symptomatic or are at risk for developing left-sided heart failure. Patients with mechanical valve replacements require lifelong anticoagulant therapy.

Percutaneous balloon aortic valvuloplasty is useful in children and young adults who have congenital aortic stenosis and in elderly patients with severe calcifications. This procedure may improve left ventricular function so that the patient can tolerate valve replacement surgery.

What to do

• If the patient needs bed rest, stress its importance. Assist the patient with ADLs if necessary.
• Alternate periods of activity and rest to prevent extreme fatigue and dyspnea.
• To reduce anxiety, allow the patient to express his concerns about the effects of activity restrictions on his responsibilities and routines. Reassure him that the restrictions are temporary.
• Place the patient in an upright position to relieve dyspnea, if needed. Administer oxygen to prevent tissue hypoxia, as needed.
• Keep the patient on a low-sodium diet. Consult with a dietitian to ensure that the patient receives foods he likes while adhering to the diet restrictions.
• Monitor for signs of heart failure, pulmonary edema, and adverse reactions to drug therapy.
• If the patient has surgery, watch for hypotension, arrhythmias, and thrombus formation. Monitor his vital signs, ABG levels, intake and output, daily weights, blood chemistry studies, chest X-rays, and pulmonary artery catheter readings.
• Teach the patient about diet and activity restrictions, medications, symptoms that should be reported to the doctor, and the importance of consistent follow-up care.
• Make sure the patient and family understand the need to comply with prolonged antibiotic therapy and follow-up care and the possible need for prophylactic antibiotics during dental surgery or other invasive procedures.

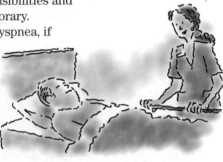

Activity restrictions may frustrate the patient. Remind him that they are temporary.

Pulmonic stenosis

Pulmonic stenosis is a hardening or narrowing of the opening between the pulmonary artery and the right ventricle. Complications of pulmonic stenosis include arrhythmias, right-sided heart failure, and right ventricular hypertrophy.

What causes it

Pulmonic stenosis is rare but can result from congenital stenosis of the valve cusp or from rheumatic heart disease. It's also associated with tetralogy of Fallot.

How it happens

In pulmonic stenosis, obstructed right ventricular outflow causes right ventricular hypertrophy in an attempt to overcome resistance to the narrow valvular opening. The ultimate result is right-sided heart failure.

What to look for

Although a patient with pulmonic stenosis may be asymptomatic, possible signs and symptoms include dyspnea on exertion, right-sided heart failure, arrhythmias or palpitations, periperhal edema, and a systolic murmur.

What tests tell you

• Cardiac catheterization reveals increased right ventricular pressure, decreased pulmonary artery pressure, and abnormal valve orifice.
• ECG may show right ventricular hypertrophy, right axis deviation, right atrial hypertrophy and atrial fibrillation.
• Echocardiography and TEE show stenotic blood flow through the valve, right ventricular hypertrophy, and right atrial enlargement.

How it's treated

A low-sodium diet and diuretics help reduce hepatic congestion before surgery. Antiarrhythmics may be necessary to control heart rhythm disturbances. Additionally, cardiac catheter balloon valvuloplasty is usually effective even with moderate to severe obstruction. Severe stenosis may require valve replacement surgery. Prophylactic antibiotics may be necessary before invasive procedures to prevent endocarditis.

What to do

• Alternate periods of activity and rest to prevent extreme fatigue and dyspnea.
• Keep the patient on a low-sodium diet and restrict fluids, if ordered. Consult with a dietitian to ensure that the patient receives foods he likes while adhering to the diet restrictions.
• Monitor for signs of heart failure, pulmonary edema, and adverse reactions to drug therapy.
• Teach the patient about diet restrictions, medications, signs and symptoms that should be reported to the doctor, and the importance of consistent follow-up care.

> You're working at a great pace. After this valvular disease, it's on to the Quick quiz!

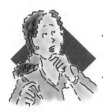

Quick quiz

1. Vegetation on the heart valves results from:
A.   bacterial invasion.
B.   poor diet.
C.   hypertension.
D.   diabetes mellitus.

Answer: A. Bacterial invasion produces vegetative growths on the heart valves, the endocardial lining of a heart chamber, or the endothelium of a blood vessel. These growths may embolize to the spleen, kidneys, CNS, extremities, and lungs.

2. A focal or diffuse inflammation of the cardiac muscle is known as:
A.   endocarditis.
B.   pericarditis.
C.   myocarditis.
D.   myocardial infarction.

Answer: C. Myocarditis is a focal or diffuse inflammation of the cardiac muscle (myocardium). It may be acute or chronic and can strike at any age.

3. Chest pain is described as pleuritic when it:
A.   resolves with sublingual nitroglycerin.
B.   occurs only during sleep.
C.   increases with deep inspiration and decreases when the patient sits up and leans forward.
D.   resolves with a deep breath.

Answer: C. Pleuritic pain increases with deep inspiration and decreases when the patient sits up and leans forward. This decrease occurs because leaning forward pulls the heart away from the diaphragmatic pleurae of the lungs.

4. Surgical treatment of a valvular disorder includes:
A.   coronary bypass surgery.
B.   balloon angioplasty.
C.   cardiac stents.
D.   balloon valvuloplasty.

Answer: D. A balloon valvuloplasty may be done to enlarge the orifice of a stenotic mitral, aortic, or pulmonic valve. Other surgical treatments include annuloplasty or valvuloplasty to reconstruct or repair the valve in mitral insufficiency or valve replacement with a prosthetic valve for mitral and aortic valve disease.

Scoring

☆☆☆ If you answered all four questions correctly, fabulous! You've learned your linings and vetted your valves.

☆☆ If you answered three questions correctly, that's fine! You have these disorders under control.

☆ If you answered fewer than three questions correctly, don't get stuck. The sure way to open those valves is to reread the chapter.

8

Degenerative disorders

Just the facts

In this chapter, you'll learn:
♦ disorders that diminish coronary blood flow and cardiac function
♦ pathophysiology and treatments related to these disorders
♦ diagnostic tests, assessment findings, and nursing interventions for each disorder.

A look at degenerative disorders

Degenerative disorders, which cause damage over time, are the most common cardiovascular ailments. The onset of these disorders may be insidious, triggering symptoms only after the disease has progressed. Degenerative cardiac disorders include acute coronary syndromes, cardiomyopathy, heart failure, hypertension, and pulmonary hypertension.

Acute coronary syndromes

Patients with acute coronary syndromes have some degree of coronary artery occlusion. Depending on the degree of occlusion, the syndrome is defined as unstable angina, ST-segment elevation myocardial infarction (STEMI), or non-ST-segment elevation myocardial infarction (NSTEMI).

Plaque's place

The development of any acute coronary syndrome begins with a rupture or erosion of plaque—an unstable and lipid-rich substance. The rupture results in platelet adhesions, fibrin clot formation, and activation of thrombin.

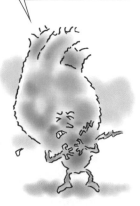

Owww! An MI is just one kind of acute coronary syndrome.

What you want to avoid

Complications of acute coronary syndromes include heart failure, chronic chest pain, chronic activity intolerance, and death.

What causes it

Patients with certain risk factors appear to face a greater likelihood of developing an acute coronary syndrome. These factors include:
- family history of heart disease
- obesity
- smoking
- high-fat, high-carbohydrate diet
- hyperlipoproteinemia
- sedentary lifestyle
- menopause
- stress
- diabetes
- hypertension.

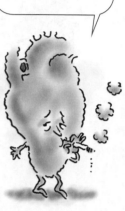

Smoking is a risk factor for acute coronary syndromes. I better quit!

How it happens

An acute coronary syndrome most commonly results when plaque ruptures inside a coronary artery and a resulting thrombus occludes blood flow. (A plaque deposit in a coronary artery doesn't necessarily block blood flow significantly.) The effect is an imbalance in myocardial oxygen supply and demand.

The two Ds

The degree and duration of blockage dictate the type of ischemia or infarct that occurs:
- If the patient has unstable angina, a thrombus partially occludes a coronary vessel. This thrombus is full of platelets. The partially occluded vessel may have distal microthrombi that cause necrosis in some myocytes. The patient typically experiences symptoms.
- STEMI results when reduced blood flow through one of the coronary arteries causes myocardial ischemia, injury, and necrosis. The damage extends through all myocardial layers.
- If smaller vessels infarct, the patient is at higher risk for MI, which may progress to an NSTEMI. Usually, only the innermost layer of the heart is damaged.

What to look for

A patient with angina typically experiences:
- burning
- squeezing

Atypical chest pain in women

Women with coronary artery disease may experience classic chest pain, which may occur without any relationship to activity or stress. However, they also commonly experience atypical chest pain, vague chest pain, or a lack of chest pain.

Location, location, location

Whereas men tend to complain of crushing pain in the center of the chest, women are more likely to experience arm or shoulder pain; jaw, neck, or throat pain; toothache; back pain; or pain under the breastbone or in the stomach.

Other signs and symptoms women may experience include nausea or dizziness; shortness of breath; unexplained anxiety, weakness, or fatigue; palpitations; cold sweat; or paleness.

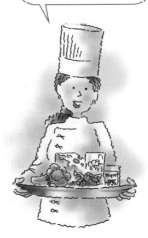

Angina can follow exercise, excitement, exposure to cold—or even a large meal.

• crushing tightness in the substernal or precordial chest that may radiate to the left arm, neck, jaw, or shoulder blade.

Any patient may experience atypical chest pain, but it's more common in women. (See *Atypical chest pain in women.*)

It hurts when I do this

Angina most frequently follows physical exertion but may also follow emotional excitement, exposure to cold, or a large meal. Angina symptoms may be relieved by nitroglycerin. It's less severe and shorter-lived than the pain of acute MI.

Four forms

Angina has four major forms:

stable—predictable pain, in frequency and duration, that can be relieved with nitrates and rest

unstable—easily induced, increased pain or change in pain pattern that may occur at rest

Prinzmetal's or a variant—pain from unpredictable coronary artery spasm

microvascular—angina-like chest pain due to impairment of vasodilator reserve (ability of the arteries to dilate) in a patient with normal coronary arteries.

My, my, MI pain

A patient with MI may experience severe, persistent chest pain that isn't relieved by rest or sublingual nitroglycerin. He may describe the pain as pressure, crushing, or squeezing. The pain is usually substernal but may radiate to the left arm, jaw, neck, or shoulder blades.

And many more

Other signs and symptoms of MI include:
- a feeling of impending doom
- fatigue
- nausea and vomiting
- shortness of breath
- cool extremities
- perspiration
- anxiety
- hypotension or hypertension
- palpable precordial pulse
- muffled heart sounds
- pallor or cyanosis.

What tests tell you

These tests are used to diagnose acute coronary syndromes:
- Electrocardiography (ECG) during an anginal episode may show ischemia. Serial 12-lead ECGs may be normal or inconclusive during the first few hours after an MI. Abnormalities include serial ST-segment depression in an NSTEMI and ST-segment elevation and Q waves, representing scarring and necrosis, in a STEMI. (See *Pinpointing infarction.*)
- Coronary angiography reveals coronary artery stenosis or occlusion and collateral circulation and shows the condition of the arteries beyond the narrowing.
- Myocardial perfusion imaging with thallium-201 during treadmill exercise discloses ischemic areas of the myocardium, visualized as "cold spots."
- With MI, serial serum cardiac marker measurements show elevated creatine kinase (CK), especially the CK-MB isoenzyme (the cardiac muscle fraction of CK), troponin T and I, and myoglobin.
- With a STEMI, echocardiography shows ventricular wall dyskinesia.

How it's treated

For patients with angina, the goal of treatment is to reduce myocardial oxygen demand or increase oxygen supply.

These treatments are used to manage angina:
- Nitrates reduce myocardial oxygen consumption.
- Beta-adrenergic blockers may be administered to reduce the workload and oxygen demands of the heart.
- If angina is caused by coronary artery spasm, calcium channel blockers may be given.
- Antiplatelet drugs decrease platelet aggregation and the danger of coronary artery occlusion.

Now I get it!

Pinpointing infarction

The site of myocardial infarction (MI) depends on the vessels involved:
- Occlusion of the circumflex branch of the left coronary artery causes a lateral wall infarction.
- Occlusion of the anterior descending branch of the left coronary artery leads to an anterior wall infarction.
- True posterior or inferior wall infarctions generally result from occlusion of the right coronary artery or one of its branches.
- Right ventricular infarctions can also result from right coronary artery occlusion, can accompany inferior infarctions, and may cause right-sided heart failure.
- In an ST-segment elevation MI, tissue damage extends through all myocardial layers; in a non-ST-segment elevation MI, damage occurs only in the innermost layer.

- Antilipemic drugs can reduce elevated serum cholesterol or triglyceride levels.
- Obstructive lesions may necessitate coronary artery bypass grafting (CABG) or percutaneous transluminal coronary angioplasty (PTCA). Other alternatives include laser angioplasty, minimally invasive surgery, rotational atherectomy, or stent placement.
- Enhanced external counterpulsation may be used to treat anginal pain when other therapies are unsuccessful.

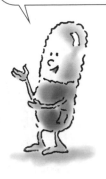

Drug therapy for angina may include nitrates, beta-adrenergic blockers, calcium channel blockers, antiplatelet drugs, and antilipemics.

MI relief

The goals of treatment for MI are to relieve pain, stabilize heart rhythm, revascularize the coronary artery, preserve myocardial tissue, and reduce cardiac workload.

Here are some guidelines for treatment:
- Emergency medical service providers or emergency department staff should give 160 to 325 mg of aspirin unless the patient has a history of aspirin allergy or signs of active or recent GI bleeding.
- Thrombolytic therapy should be started within 3 hours of the onset of symptoms (unless contraindications exist). Thrombolytic therapy involves administration of streptokinase (Streptase), alteplase (Activase), or reteplase (Retavase).
- PTCA is an option for opening blocked or narrowed arteries.
- Oxygen is administered to increase oxygenation of the blood.
- Nitroglycerin is administered sublingually to relieve chest pain, unless systolic blood pressure is less than 90 mm Hg or heart rate is less than 50 beats/minute or greater than 100 beats/minute.
- Morphine is administered as analgesia because pain stimulates the sympathetic nervous system, leading to an increase in heart rate and vasoconstriction. Additionally, morphine is a venodilator that reduces ventricular preload and oxygen requirements.
- I.V. heparin is given to patients who have received tissue plasminogen activator to increase the chances of patency in the affected coronary artery.
- Physical activity is limited for the first 12 hours to reduce cardiac workload, thereby limiting the area of necrosis.
- Lidocaine, amiodarone (Pacerone), transcutaneous pacing patches (or a transvenous pacemaker), defibrillation, or epinephrine may be necessary if arrhythmias are present.
- I.V. nitroglycerin is administered for 24 to 48 hours in patients without hypotension, bradycardia, or excessive tachycardia to reduce afterload and preload and to relieve chest pain.
- Glycoprotein IIb/IIIa inhibitors (such as abciximab [ReoPro]) are administered to patients with continued unstable angina or acute chest pain to reduce platelet aggregation. They're also administered after invasive cardiac procedures.
- An I.V. beta-adrenergic blocker is administered early to patients with evolving acute MI; it's followed by oral therapy to reduce

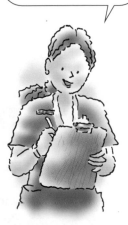

Treatment for MI can take many forms, depending on the patient's symptoms and the extent of damage.

heart rate and contractility and to reduce myocardial oxygen requirements.
• Angiotensin-converting enzyme (ACE) inhibitors are administered to those with evolving MI with ST-segment elevation or left bundle-branch block to reduce afterload and preload and to prevent remodeling.
• Laser angioplasty, atherectomy, or stent placement may be initiated.
• Lipid-lowering drugs are administered to patients with elevated low-density lipoprotein and cholesterol levels.

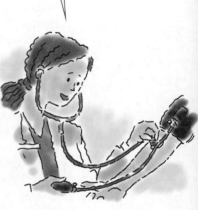

During anginal episodes, be sure to monitor blood pressure and heart rate.

What to do

• Collaborate care with a skilled team, which may include emergency medical personnel, a cardiologist, a cardiothoracic surgeon, a nutritionist, and a cardiac rehabilitation team.
• During anginal episodes, monitor blood pressure and heart rate. Take an ECG before administering nitroglycerin or other nitrates. Record the duration of pain, the amount of medication required to relieve it, and accompanying symptoms.
• On admission to the coronary care unit, monitor and record the patient's ECG, blood pressure, temperature, and heart and breath sounds. Also, assess and record the severity, location, type, and duration of pain.
• Obtain a 12-lead ECG and assess heart rate and blood pressure when the patient experiences acute chest pain.

Status checks

• Monitor the patient's hemodynamic status closely. Be alert for indicators suggesting decreased cardiac output, such as decreased blood pressure, increased heart rate, increased pulmonary artery pressure (PAP), increased pulmonary artery wedge pressure (PAWP), decreased cardiac output measurements, and decreased right atrial pressure.
• Assess urine output hourly.
• Monitor the patient's oxygen saturation levels, and notify the doctor if oxygen saturation falls below 90%.
• Check the patient's blood pressure after giving nitroglycerin, especially after the first dose.
• Frequently monitor ECG rhythm strips to detect heart rate changes and arrhythmias.

Things heat up

• During episodes of chest pain, monitor ECG, blood pressure, and pulmonary artery (PA) catheter readings (if applicable) to determine changes.

- Obtain serial measurements of cardiac enzyme levels as ordered.
- Be aware that a serum B-type natriuretic peptide (BNP) assay may be ordered to determine if the patient is developing heart failure.
- Watch for crackles, cough, tachypnea, and edema—signs of impending left-sided heart failure. Carefully monitor daily weight, intake and output, respiratory rate, serum enzyme levels, ECG waveforms, and blood pressure. Auscultate for third or fourth heart sound (S_3 or S_4) gallops.
- Prepare the patient for reperfusion therapy as indicated.
- Administer and titrate medications as ordered. Avoid giving I.M. injections; I.V. administration provides more rapid symptom relief.
- Organize patient care and activities to allow rest periods. If the patient is immobilized, turn him often and use intermittent compression devices. Gradually increase the patient's activity level as tolerated.
- Provide a clear-liquid diet until nausea subsides. Anticipate a possible order for a low-cholesterol, low-sodium diet without caffeine.
- Provide a stool softener to prevent straining during defecation.

Teach, review, document

- Teach the patient about signs and symptoms to report to the doctor.
- Review medications and their proper administration and possible adverse effects.
- Teach about risk factors and how to reduce them, as appropriate.
- Encourage family members to learn cardiopulmonary resuscitation.
- Document the patient's response to treatment, vital signs, cardiac rhythm, episodes of pain and pain relief, and understanding of teaching.

Cardiomyopathy

Cardiomyopathy generally refers to disease of the heart muscle fibers. It takes three main forms:
- dilated
- hypertrophic (obstructive and nonobstructive)
- restrictive (extremely rare).

Number two killer

Cardiomyopathy is the second most common direct cause of sudden death. (Coronary artery disease is first.) Because dilated car-

Memory jogger

The American Heart Association's acronym for saying goodbye to heart disease, **ALOHA**, can help you remember recommendations for your female patients who are at risk:

Assess your risk. Know important levels, such as cholesterol, weight, and blood pressure.

Lifestyle is the priority. Lifestyle changes such as smoking cessation, exercise, and a healthy diet can help prevent cardiovascular disease.

Other interventions may be necessary if lifestyle changes don't significantly reduce the risk of heart disease. Consult with a physician.

High-risk cases are serious and need to be addressed immediately and consistently.

Avoid hormone therapy, antioxidant vitamin supplements, and aspirin therapy because these treatments may do more harm than good, especially in low-risk patients.

diomyopathy usually isn't diagnosed until its advanced stages, the prognosis is generally poor.

Other complications include heart failure, arrhythmias, hypoxemia, pulmonary edema, valvular dysfunction, hepatomegaly, and multiple-organ-dysfunction syndrome (MODS) resulting from low cardiac output.

What causes it

Risk factors for cardiomyopathy include hypertension, pregnancy, viral infections, and alcohol use. Overall, males and blacks of both sexes are at greatest risk.

How it happens

Most patients with cardiomyopathy have idiopathic, or primary, disease, but some cases are secondary to identifiable causes. Obstructive hypertrophic cardiomyopathy is almost always inherited as a non-sex-linked autosomal dominant trait.

Dilated cardiomyopathy

Dilated cardiomyopathy primarily affects systolic function. It results from extensively damaged myocardial muscle fibers. Consequently, contractility in the left ventricle decreases.

Poor compensation

As systolic function declines, stroke volume, ejection fraction, and cardiac output decrease. As end-diastolic volumes increase, pulmonary congestion may occur. The elevated end-diastolic volume is a compensatory response to preserve stroke volume despite a reduced ejection fraction.

The sympathetic nervous system is stimulated to increase heart rate and contractility.

Kidneys kick in

The kidneys are stimulated to retain sodium and water to maintain cardiac output, and vasoconstriction occurs as the renin-angiotensin system is stimulated. When these compensatory mechanisms can no longer maintain cardiac output, the heart begins to fail.

Detrimental dilation

Left ventricular dilation occurs as venous return and systemic vascular resistance increase. Eventually, the atria also dilate because more work is required to pump blood into the full ventricles. Cardiomegaly is a consequence of dilation of the atria and ventricles. Blood pooling in the ventricles increases the risk of thrombus for-

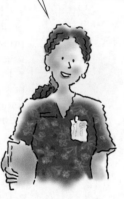

Cardiomyopathy commonly affects either systolic or diastolic function, but not both.

mation and emboli. Dilation of the left ventricle may lead to mitral valve dysfunction.

Hypertrophic cardiomyopathy

Hypertrophic cardiomyopathy primarily affects diastolic function. The features of hypertrophic cardiomyopathy include:
- asymmetrical left ventricular hypertrophy
- hypertrophy of the intraventricular septum (obstructive hypertrophic cardiomyopathy)
- rapid, forceful contractions of the left ventricle
- impaired relaxation
- obstruction of left ventricular outflow.

Fouled-up filling

The hypertrophied ventricle becomes stiff, noncompliant, and unable to relax during ventricular filling. Consequently, ventricular filling is reduced and left ventricular filling pressure rises, causing increases in left atrial and pulmonary venous pressures and leading to venous congestion and dyspnea.

Ventricular filling time is further reduced as a compensatory response to tachycardia. Reduced ventricular filling during diastole and obstruction of ventricular outflow lead to low cardiac output.

Hypertrophy hazards

If papillary muscles become hypertrophied and don't close completely during contraction, mitral insufficiency occurs. Moreover, intramural coronary arteries are abnormally small and may not be sufficient to supply the hypertrophied muscle with enough blood and oxygen to meet the increased needs of the hyperdynamic muscle.

Restrictive cardiomyopathy

Restrictive cardiomyopathy is characterized by stiffness of the ventricle caused by left ventricular hypertrophy and endocardial fibrosis and thickening. The ability of the ventricle to relax and fill during diastole is reduced. Furthermore, the rigid myocardium fails to contract completely during systole. As a result, cardiac output decreases.

What to look for

Generally, for patients with dilated or restrictive cardiomyopathy, the onset is insidious. As the disease progresses, exacerbations and hospitalizations are common regardless of the type of cardiomyopathy.

Symptoms of dilated cardiomyopathy tend to be overlooked until the patient's condition is very serious.

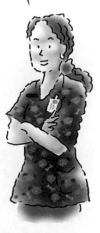

Dilated cardiomyopathy

For a patient with dilated cardiomyopathy, signs and symptoms may be overlooked until left ventricular failure occurs. Be sure to evaluate the patient's current condition and then compare it with his condition over the past 6 to 12 months.

Signs and symptoms of dilated cardiomyopathy may include:
• shortness of breath, orthopnea, dyspnea on exertion, paroxysmal nocturnal dyspnea, fatigue, and a dry cough at night due to left-sided heart failure
• peripheral edema, hepatomegaly, jugular vein distention, and weight gain caused by right-sided heart failure
• peripheral cyanosis
• tachycardia
• pansystolic murmur associated with mitral and tricuspid insufficiency
• S_3 and S_4 gallop murmurs
• irregular pulse, if atrial fibrillation exists
• fatigue and exercise intolerance.

Hypertrophic cardiomyopathy

Signs and symptoms vary widely among patients with hypertrophic cardiomyopathy. The presenting symptom is commonly syncope or sudden cardiac death. Other possible signs and symptoms include:
• angina
• dyspnea
• fatigue
• systolic ejection murmur along the left sternal border and apex
• peripheral pulse with a characteristic double impulse (pulsus biferiens)
• abrupt arterial pulse
• irregular pulse with atrial fibrillation.

Restrictive cardiomyopathy

A patient with restrictive cardiomyopathy presents with signs of heart failure and other signs and symptoms, including:
• fatigue
• dyspnea
• orthopnea
• chest pain
• edema
• liver engorgement
• peripheral cyanosis
• pallor
• S_3 or S_4 gallop rhythms
• systolic murmurs.

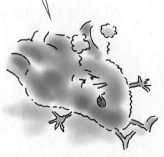

Yikes! The presenting symptom of hypertrophic cardiomyopathy is commonly syncope or cardiac death.

What tests tell you

These tests are used to diagnose cardiomyopathy:
• Echocardiography confirms dilated cardiomyopathy.
• Chest X-ray may reveal cardiomegaly associated with any of the cardiomyopathies.
• Cardiac catheterization with possible heart biopsy can be definitive in diagnosing the causes of cardiomyopathy.

How it's treated

There's no known cure for cardiomyopathy. Treatment is individualized based on the type and cause of cardiomyopathy and the patient's condition.

Dilated cardiomyopathy

For a patient with dilated cardiomyopathy, treatment may involve:
• management of the underlying cause, if known
• ACE inhibitors, as first-line therapy, to reduce afterload through vasodilation
• diuretics, taken with ACE inhibitors, to reduce fluid retention
• digoxin, for patients not responding to ACE inhibitors and diuretic therapy, to improve myocardial contractility
• hydralazine and isosorbide dinitrate (Isordil), in combination, to produce vasodilation
• beta-adrenergic blockers for patients with mild or moderate heart failure
• antiarrhythmics, such as amiodarone, used cautiously to control arrhythmias
• cardioversion to convert atrial fibrillation to sinus rhythm
• pacemaker insertion to correct arrhythmias
• biventricular pacemaker insertion to improve heart function by synchronizing atrial and ventricular contractions
• anticoagulants to reduce the risk of emboli (controversial)
• revascularization, such as CABG surgery, if dilated cardiomyopathy is due to ischemia
• valvular repair or replacement, if dilated cardiomyopathy is due to valve dysfunction
• lifestyle modifications, such as smoking cessation; low-fat, low-sodium diet; physical activity; and abstinence from alcohol
• heart transplantation or left ventricular assist device (VAD) in patients resistant to medical therapy.

Hypertrophic cardiomyopathy

For a patient with hypertrophic cardiomyopathy, treatment may involve:

• beta-adrenergic blockers to slow the heart rate, reduce myocardial oxygen demands, and increase ventricular filling by relaxing the obstructing muscle, thereby increasing cardiac output
• antiarrhythmic drugs, such as amiodarone, to reduce arrhythmias
• cardioversion to treat atrial fibrillation
• anticoagulation therapy to reduce the risk of systemic embolism with atrial fibrillation
• verapamil (Calan) and diltiazem (Cardizem) to reduce ventricular stiffness and elevated diastolic pressures
• ablation of the atrioventricular node and implantation of a dual-chamber pacemaker (controversial) in patients with obstructive hypertrophic cardiomyopathy and ventricular tachycardias, to reduce the outflow gradient by altering the pattern of ventricular contraction
• implantable cardioverter-defibrillator to correct ventricular arrhythmias
• ventricular myotomy or myectomy (resection of the hypertrophied septum) to ease outflow tract obstruction and relieve symptoms
• mitral valve replacement to correct mitral insufficiency
• heart transplantation for intractable symptoms.

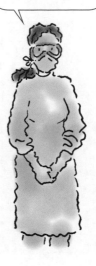

Heart transplantation may be required for hypertrophic cardiomyopathy.

Restrictive cardiomyopathy

For the patient with restrictive cardiomyopathy, treatment may involve:
• management of the underlying cause—for example, administering deferoxamine (Desferal) to bind iron in restrictive cardiomyopathy due to hemochromatosis
• digoxin, diuretics, and a restricted sodium diet to ease the symptoms of heart failure (although no therapy exists for patients with restricted ventricular filling)
• oral vasodilators to control intractable heart failure.

What to do

• Collaborate care with a skilled team, which may include a cardiologist, a cardiothoracic surgeon, a nutritionist, physical and occupational therapists, and a cardiac rehabilitation team.
• Administer drugs, as ordered, to promote adequate heart function.
• Assess hemodynamic status every 2 hours or more frequently, if necessary.

Ins and outs

• Monitor intake and output closely and obtain daily weights; institute fluid restrictions as ordered.

• Institute continuous cardiac monitoring to evaluate for arrhythmias.
• Assess the patient for possible adverse drug reactions, such as orthostatic hypotension with vasodilators, diuretics, or ACE inhibitors.

No quick moves

• Urge the patient to change positions slowly.
• Auscultate heart and lung sounds, being alert for S_3 heart sounds or murmurs or crackles, rhonchi, and wheezes indicating heart failure. Monitor vital signs for changes, especially a heart rate greater than 100 beats/minute, a respiratory rate greater than 20 breaths/minute, and a systolic blood pressure less than 90 mm Hg, all of which suggest heart failure.
• Assist the patient with activities of daily living (ADLs) to decrease oxygen demand.

When to call

• Teach the patient about his diagnosis, diagnostic tests, and treatment. Be sure to cover the patient's medications, administration, and potential adverse effects. Also, tell the patient about when to notify the doctor.
• Review dietary and fluid restrictions.
• Teach the patient about the signs and symptoms of heart failure.
• Document cardiac and respiratory status, vital signs, and daily weight. Note the patient's response to treatment. Document the patient's understanding of the teaching.

Oxygen orders

• Administer supplemental oxygen as ordered. Assess for changes in level of consciousness, such as restlessness or decreased responsiveness, indicating diminished cerebral perfusion. If the patient has a PA catheter in place, evaluate mixed venous oxygen saturation levels; if not, monitor oxygen saturation levels using pulse oximetry.
• Organize care to promote periods of rest for the patient.
• Prepare the patient, as indicated, for insertion of a pacemaker, implantable cardioverter-defibrillator, or an intra-aortic balloon pump or for heart transplantation.

Heart failure occurs when the myocardium can't pump hard enough to meet the body's needs.

Heart failure

When the myocardium can't pump effectively enough to meet the body's metabolic needs, heart failure oc-

(Text continues on page 260.)

Now I get it!

Understanding left- and right-sided heart failure

These illustrations show how myocardial damage leads to heart failure.

Left-sided heart failure

✌ Increased workload and end-diastolic volume enlarge the left ventricle (see illustration at right). Because of lack of oxygen, the ventricle enlarges with stretched tissue rather than functional tissue. The patient may experience increased heart rate, pale and cool skin, tingling in the extremities, decreased cardiac output, and arrhythmias.

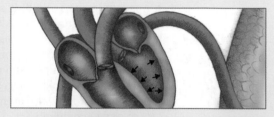

✌ Diminished left ventricular function allows blood to pool in the ventricle and the atrium and eventually back up into the pulmonary veins and capillaries (as shown at right). At this stage, the patient may experience dyspnea on exertion, confusion, dizziness, orthostatic hypotension, decreased peripheral pulses and pulse pressure, cyanosis, and an S_3 gallop.

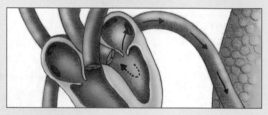

✋ As the pulmonary circulation becomes engorged, rising capillary pressure pushes sodium (Na) and water (H_2O) into the interstitial space (as shown at right), causing pulmonary edema. You'll note coughing, subclavian retractions, crackles, tachypnea, elevated pulmonary artery pressure, diminished pulmonary compliance, and increased partial pressure of carbon dioxide.

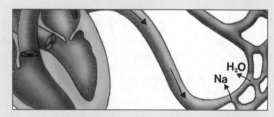

🖐 When the patient lies down, fluid in the extremities moves into the systemic circulation. Because the left ventricle can't handle the increased venous return, fluid pools in the pulmonary circulation, worsening pulmonary edema (see illustration at right). You may note decreased breath sounds, dullness on percussion, crackles, and orthopnea.

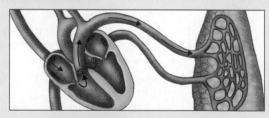

🖐 The right ventricle may now become stressed because it's pumping against greater pulmonary vascular resistance and left ventricular pressure (see illustration at right). When this occurs, the patient's symptoms worsen.

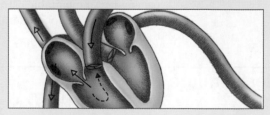

Right-sided heart failure

The stressed right ventricle enlarges with the formation of stretched tissue (see illustration at right). Increasing conduction time and deviation of the heart from its normal axis can cause arrhythmias. If the patient doesn't already have left-sided heart failure, he may experience increased heart rate, cool skin, cyanosis, decreased cardiac output, palpitations, and dyspnea.

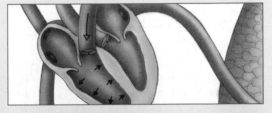

Blood pools in the right ventricle and right atrium. The backed-up blood causes pressure and congestion in the vena cava and systemic circulation (see illustration at right). The patient will have elevated central venous pressure, jugular vein distention, and hepatojugular reflux.

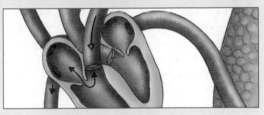

Backed-up blood also distends the visceral veins, especially the hepatic vein. As the liver and spleen become engorged (see illustration at right), their function is impaired. The patient may develop anorexia, nausea, abdominal pain, palpable liver and spleen, weakness, and dyspnea secondary to abdominal distention.

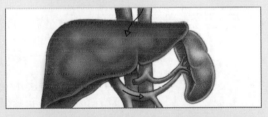

Rising capillary pressure forces excess fluid from the capillaries into the interstitial space (see illustration at right). This causes tissue edema, especially in the lower extremities and abdomen. The patient may experience weight gain, pitting edema, and nocturia.

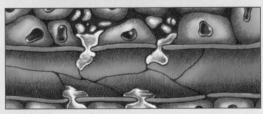

Classifying heart failure

Heart failure is classified according to its pathophysiology. It may be left- or right-sided, systolic or diastolic, and acute or chronic.

Right-sided or left-sided

Right-sided heart failure is the result of ineffective right ventricular contraction. It may be caused by an acute right ventricular infarction or pulmonary embolus. However, the most common cause is profound backward flow due to left-sided heart failure.

Left-sided heart failure is the result of ineffective left ventricular contraction. It may lead to pulmonary congestion or pulmonary edema and decreased cardiac output. Left ventricular myocardial infarction, hypertension, and aortic and mitral valve stenosis or insufficiency are common causes. As the decreased pumping ability of the left ventricle persists, fluid accumulates, backing up into the left atrium and then into the lungs. If this fluid accumulation worsens, pulmonary edema and right-sided heart failure may also result.

Systolic or diastolic

In systolic heart failure, the left ventricle can't pump enough blood out to the systemic circulation during systole and the ejection fraction falls. Consequently, blood backs up into the pulmonary circulation, pressure rises in the pulmonary venous system, and cardiac output falls.

In diastolic heart failure, the left ventricle can't relax and fill properly during diastole and the stroke volume falls. Therefore, larger ventricular volumes are needed to maintain cardiac output.

Acute or chronic

The term *acute* refers to the timing of the onset of symptoms and whether compensatory mechanisms kick in. Typically, in acute heart failure, fluid status is normal or low, and sodium and water retention don't occur.

In chronic heart failure, signs and symptoms have been present for some time, compensatory mechanisms have taken effect, and fluid volume overload persists. Drugs, diet changes, and activity restrictions usually control symptoms.

---

curs. Pump failure usually occurs in a damaged left ventricle but may also happen in the right ventricle. Usually, left-sided heart failure develops first. Heart failure is classified as:
- acute or chronic
- left-sided or right-sided (see *Understanding left- and right-sided heart failure*, pages 258 and 259)
- systolic or diastolic (see *Classifying heart failure*).

Quality time

Symptoms of heart failure may restrict a person's ability to perform ADLs and may severely affect quality of life. Advances in diagnostic and therapeutic techniques have greatly improved outcomes for these patients. However, prognosis still depends on the underlying cause and its response to treatment.

Daunting difficulties

Complications of heart failure include arrhythmias, valvular dysfunction, mental status changes, exercise intolerance, MODS and, possibly, death.

What causes it

Cardiovascular disorders that lead to heart failure include:
- atherosclerotic heart disease

- MI
- hypertension
- rheumatic heart disease
- congenital heart disease
- ischemic heart disease
- cardiomyopathy
- valvular diseases
- arrhythmias.

It's not all heart

Noncardiovascular causes of heart failure include:
- pregnancy and childbirth
- increased environmental temperature or humidity
- severe physical or mental stress
- thyrotoxicosis
- acute blood loss
- pulmonary embolism
- severe infection
- chronic obstructive pulmonary disease (COPD)
- hypervolemia
- sepsis.

How it happens

The patient's underlying condition determines whether heart failure is acute or insidious. Heart failure is commonly associated with systolic or diastolic overloading and myocardial weakness. As stress on the heart muscle reaches a critical level, the muscle's contractility is reduced and cardiac output declines. Venous input to the ventricle remains the same, however.

The body's responses to decreased cardiac output include:
- reflex increase in sympathetic nervous system activity
- release of renin from the juxtaglomerular cells of the kidney
- anaerobic metabolism by affected cells
- increased extraction of oxygen by the peripheral cells.

Adept at adaptation

When blood in the ventricles increases, the heart compensates, or adapts. Compensation may occur for long periods before signs and symptoms develop. Adaptations may be:
- *short-term*—As the end-diastolic fiber length increases, the ventricular muscle responds by dilating and increasing the force of contractions. (This is called the *Frank-Starling curve.*)
- *long-term*—Ventricular hypertrophy increases the heart muscle's ability to contract and push its volume of blood into the circulation.

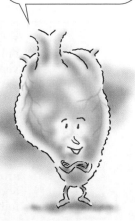

I can sometimes compensate for the increased workload, delaying symptoms for a long time.

What to look for

Clinical signs of left-sided heart failure include:
- dyspnea, initially on exertion
- paroxysmal nocturnal dyspnea
- Cheyne-Stokes respirations
- cough
- orthopnea
- tachycardia
- fatigue
- muscle weakness
- edema and weight gain
- irritability
- restlessness
- shortened attention span
- ventricular gallop (heard over the apex)
- bibasilar crackles.

Less to look for

The patient with right-sided heart failure may develop:
- edema, initially dependent
- jugular vein distention
- hepatomegaly
- ascites.

What tests tell you

- Blood tests may show elevated blood urea nitrogen (BUN) and creatinine levels, elevated serum norepinephrine levels, and elevated transaminase and bilirubin levels if hepatic function is impaired.
- Elevated blood levels of BNP may correctly identify heart failure in as much as 83% of patients.
- ECG reflects heart strain or ventricular enlargement (ischemia). It may also reveal atrial enlargement, tachycardia, and extrasystoles, suggesting heart failure.
- Chest X-ray shows increased pulmonary vascular markings, interstitial edema, or pleural effusion and cardiomegaly.
- Multiple-gated acquisition scanning shows a decreased ejection fraction in left-sided heart failure.
- Cardiac catheterization may show ventricular dilation, coronary artery occlusion, and valvular disorders (such as aortic stenosis and mitral valve insufficiency) in both left- and right-sided heart failure.

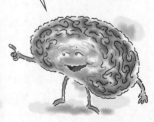

What are you doing here?

Hey! Elevated levels of a certain brain peptide can identify heart failure in 83% of patients.

• Echocardiography and transesophageal echocardiography may show ventricular hypertrophy, decreased contractility, and valvular disorders in both left- and right-sided heart failure. Serial echocardiograms may help assess the patient's response to therapy.

• Cardiopulmonary exercise testing to evaluate the patient's ventricular performance during exercise may show decreased oxygen uptake.

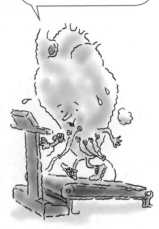

With heart failure, cardiopulmonary exercise testing may show decreased oxygen uptake.

How it's treated

Treatment for heart failure may involve using the New York Heart Association classification system and the American College of Cardiology/American Heart Association guidelines. (See *Classifying signs and symptoms to determine treatment*, page 264.)

Measures include diuretics that reduce preload by decreasing total blood volume and circulatory congestion. ACE inhibitors dilate blood vessels and decrease systemic vascular resistance, thereby reducing the workload of the heart. Vasodilators may be given to the patient who can't tolerate ACE inhibitors. Vasodilators increase cardiac output by reducing impedance to ventricular outflow, thereby decreasing afterload.

Strengthening medicine

Digoxin may help strengthen myocardial contractility. Beta-adrenergic blockers may prevent cardiac remodeling (left ventricular dilation and hypertrophy). Nesiritide (Natrecor), a human BNP, may be administered to augment diuresis and to decrease afterload. Positive inotropic agents, such as I.V. dopamine or dobutamine, are reserved for those with end-stage heart failure or those awaiting a VAD or heart transplantation.

Stop and go

The patient must alternate periods of rest with periods of activity and follow a sodium-restricted diet with smaller, more frequent meals. He may have to wear antiembolism stockings to prevent venostasis and possible thromboembolism formation. The doctor may also order oxygen therapy.

Surgery isn't a sure thing

Although controversial, surgery may be performed if the patient's heart failure doesn't improve after therapy and lifestyle modifications. If the patient with valve dysfunction has recurrent acute heart failure, he may undergo surgical valve replacement. CABG, PTCA, or stenting may be performed in a patient with heart failure caused by ischemia.

The Dor procedure, also called *partial left ventriculectomy* or *ventricular remodeling*, involves the removal of nonviable heart

Classifying signs and symptoms to determine treatment

Two sets of guidelines are available to help direct treatment of the patient with heart failure. The New York Heart Association (NYHA) classification is based on functional capacity. The American College of Cardiology/American Heart Association (ACC/AHA) guidelines are based on objective assessment. These guidelines are compared side-by-side below.

NYHA classification	ACC/AHA 2005 guidelines	Recommendations
	Stage A. Patient at high risk for developing heart failure but without structural heart disease or signs and symptoms of heart failure	• Treatment of hypertension, lipid disorders, and diabetes • Smoking cessation and regular exercise • Discouraged use of alcohol and illicit drugs • Angiotensin-converting enzyme (ACE) inhibitor, if indicated
Class I. Ordinary physical activity doesn't cause undue fatigue, palpitations, dyspnea, or angina.	*Stage B.* Structural heart disease without signs and symptoms of heart failure	• All stage A therapies • ACE inhibitor (unless contraindicated) • Beta-adrenergic blocker (unless contraindicated)
Class II. Patient has slight limitation of physical activity but is asymptomatic at rest. Ordinary physical activity causes fatigue, palpitations, dyspnea, or anginal pain. *Class III.* Patient has marked limitation of physical activity but is typically asymptomatic at rest. Less than ordinary physical activity causes fatigue, palpitations, dyspnea, or angina.	*Stage C.* Structural heart disease with prior or current signs and symptoms of heart failure	• All stage A and B therapies • Sodium-restricted diet • Diuretics • ACE inhibitors • Beta-adrenergic blockers • Avoiding or withdrawing antiarrhythmic agents, most calcium channel blockers, and nonsteroidal anti-inflammatory drugs • Aldosterone antagonists, angiotensin receptor blockers, hydralazine (Apresoline), nitrates, and digoxin (Lanoxin) • Biventricular pacing or implantable defibrillators (in selected patients)
Class IV. Patient is unable to perform any physical activity without discomfort; symptoms may be present at rest. Discomfort increases with physical activity.	*Stage D.* End-stage disease requiring specialized treatment strategies, such as mechanical circulatory support, continuous inotropic infusion, or heart transplantation	• All therapies for stages A, B, and C • Hospice care • Extraordinary measures: heart transplantation, chronic ionotropic therapy, permanent mechanical support, and experimental surgery or drugs

muscle to reduce the size of the hypertrophied ventricle, thereby allowing the heart to pump more efficiently. Patients with severe heart failure may benefit from a mechanical VAD or heart transplantation. An internal cardioverter-defibrillator may be implanted to treat life-threatening arrhythmias. A biventricular pacemaker may be placed to control ventricular dyssynchrony.

What to do

• Collaborate care with a skilled team, which may include a cardiologist, a cardiovascular surgeon, a nutritionist, physical and occupational therapists, a cardiac rehabilitation team, and social services.
• Frequently monitor BUN, serum creatinine, potassium, sodium, chloride, magnesium, and BNP levels.
• Reinforce the importance of adhering to the prescribed diet. If fluid restrictions have been ordered, arrange a mutually acceptable schedule for allowable fluids.
• Weigh the patient daily to assess for fluid overload.
• To prevent deep vein thrombosis from venous stasis, assist the patient with range-of-motion exercises. Enforce bed rest, and apply antiembolism stockings. Watch for calf pain and tenderness. Organize activities to provide periods of rest.
• Evaluate the patient. Successful recovery should reveal clear lungs, normal heart sounds, adequate blood pressure, and absence of dyspnea and edema. The patient should be able to perform ADLs and maintain his normal weight.

Sodium down, potassium up

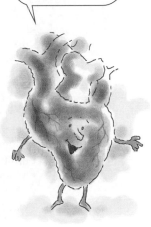

High-potassium foods help fight heart failure.

• Teach the patient about lifestyle changes. Advise him to avoid foods high in sodium to help curb fluid overload. Explain that the potassium he loses through diuretic therapy must be replaced by a prescribed potassium supplement and eating high-potassium foods. Stress the need for regular checkups and the benefits of balancing activity and rest.
• Stress the importance of taking cardiac glycosides exactly as prescribed. Tell him to watch for and report signs of toxicity.
• Tell him to notify the doctor if his pulse is unusually irregular or less than 60 beats/minute; if he experiences dizziness, blurred vision, shortness of breath, paroxysmal nocturnal dyspnea, swollen ankles, or decreased urine output; or if he gains 3 to 5 lb (1.5 to 2.5 kg) in 1 week.
• Document vital signs, intake and output, and daily weight. Note cardiac and respiratory status and response to treatment. Document patient teaching and the patient's understanding of the information.

Hypertension

Hypertension refers to intermittent or sustained elevation in diastolic or systolic blood pressure. Essential (idiopathic) hypertension is the most common form. Secondary hypertension results from a number of disorders. Malignant hypertension is a severe, fulminant form of hypertension common to both types.

Blood pressure classifications

This table classifies blood pressure according to systolic blood pressure (SBP) and diastolic blood pressure (DBP).

BP classification	Normal	Prehypertension	Stage 1	Stage 2
SBP (mm Hg)	< 120	120 to 139	140 to 159	≥ 160
	and	or	or	or
DBP (mm Hg)	< 80	80 to 89	90 to 99	≥ 100

Blood pressure is classified as normal, prehypertension, stage 1, or stage 2. The severity of hypertension helps to guide treatment. (See *Blood pressure classifications.*)

One thing leads to another

Uncontrolled hypertension may lead to stroke, MI, heart failure, peripheral arterial disease, retinopathy, and renal failure. Detecting and treating it before complications develop greatly improves the patient's prognosis. Severely elevated blood pressure may become fatal.

What causes it

Scientists haven't been able to identify a single cause for essential hypertension. The disorder probably reflects an interaction of multiple homeostatic forces, including changes in renal regulation of sodium and extracellular fluids, aldosterone secretion and metabolism, norepinephrine secretion and metabolism, and arterial walls.

Secondary hypertension may be caused by renal vascular disease, pheochromocytoma, primary hyperaldosteronism, Cushing's syndrome, or dysfunction of the thyroid, pituitary, or parathyroid glands. It may also result from coarctation of the aorta, pregnancy, and neurologic disorders.

Risky business

Certain risk factors appear to increase the likelihood of hypertension. These include:
- family history of hypertension
- race (more common in blacks)
- sex (men have a higher risk than premenopausal women initially)
- diabetes mellitus
- stress
- obesity
- high dietary intake of saturated fats or sodium

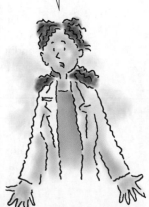

There are many risk factors for hypertension—one of them is stress.

- tobacco use
- hormonal contraceptive use
- sedentary lifestyle
- aging.

How it happens

Essential hypertension usually begins insidiously as a benign disease, slowly progressing to a malignant state. If left untreated, even mild cases can cause major complications and death.

Why? Why? Why?

Several theories help to explain the development of hypertension (see *Blood vessel damage*). It's thought to arise from:
- changes in the arteriolar bed, causing increased resistance.
- abnormally increased tone in the sensory nervous system that originates in the vasomotor system centers, causing increased peripheral vascular resistance.
- increased blood volume resulting from renal or hormonal dysfunction.
- increased arteriolar thickening caused by genetic factors, leading to increased peripheral vascular resistance.

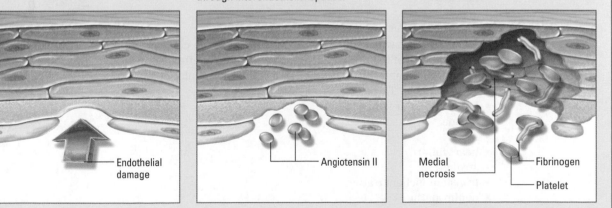

Blood vessel damage

Sustained hypertension damages blood vessels. Vascular injury begins with alternating areas of dilation and constriction in the arterioles. The illustrations below show how damage occurs.

Increased intra-arterial pressure damages the endothelium.

Angiotensin II induces endothelial wall contraction, allowing plasma to leak through interendothelial spaces.

Plasma constituents deposited in the vessel wall cause medial necrosis.

Endothelial damage

Angiotensin II

Medial necrosis — Fibrinogen

Platelet

• abnormal renin release resulting in the formation of angiotensin II, which constricts the arterioles and increases blood volume.

Secondary isn't small

The pathophysiology of secondary hypertension is related to the underlying disease. For example, consider these points:
• The most common cause of secondary hypertension is chronic renal disease. Insult to the kidney from chronic glomerulonephritis or renal artery stenosis interferes with sodium excretion, the renin-angiotensin-aldosterone system, or renal perfusion. This disruption causes blood pressure to rise.
• In Cushing's syndrome, increased cortisol levels raise blood pressure by increasing renal sodium retention, angiotensin II levels, and vascular response to norepinephrine.
• In primary aldosteronism, increased intravascular volume, altered sodium concentrations in vessel walls, or very high aldosterone levels cause vasoconstriction (increased resistance).
• Pheochromocytoma is a secreting tumor of chromaffin cells, usually of the adrenal medulla. It causes hypertension due to increased secretion of epinephrine and norepinephrine. Epinephrine functions mainly to increase cardiac contractility and rate; norepinephrine, to increase peripheral vascular resistance.

What to look for

Signs and symptoms may include:
• increased blood pressure measurements on two or more readings taken at two or more visits after an initial screening
• throbbing occipital headaches (especially upon waking)
• drowsiness
• confusion
• vision problems
• nausea.

Problems plus

Expect a patient with secondary hypertension to have clinical manifestations of the primary disease. Other clinical effects don't appear until complications develop as a result of vascular changes in target organs. These effects include:
• left ventricular hypertrophy
• angina
• MI
• heart failure
• stroke
• transient ischemic attack
• nephropathy

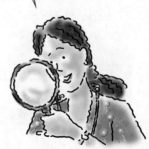

With secondary hypertension, you'll need to look for manifestations of the primary disease.

- peripheral arterial disease
- retinopathy.

What tests tell you

Along with patient history, these tests may show predisposing factors and help identify an underlying cause:
- Protein, red blood cells, and white blood cells in urinalysis may indicate glomerulonephritis.
- Elevated blood glucose levels may indicate diabetes.
- Anemia may cause a high-output state resulting in hypertension. Polycythemia I increases the risk of hypertension and stroke.
- Elevated total cholesterol and low-density lipoprotein levels increase the risk of atherosclerosis.
- Renal atrophy found during excretory urography indicates chronic renal disease; one kidney more than $\frac{5}{8}$" (1.5 cm) shorter than the other suggests unilateral renal disease.
- Serum potassium level less than 3.5 mEq/L may indicate adrenal dysfunction (primary hyperaldosteronism).
- A BUN level that's normal or elevated to more than 20 mg/dl and a creatinine level that's normal or elevated to more than 1.5 mg/dl suggest renal disease.

Detecting heart damage

Other tests help detect cardiovascular damage and other complications:
- ECG may show left ventricular hypertrophy or ischemia.
- Echocardiography may show left ventricular hypertrophy.
- Chest X-ray may show cardiomegaly.

How it's treated

Treatment of secondary hypertension includes correcting the underlying cause and controlling hypertensive effects. Although essential hypertension has no cure, lifestyle modifications and drug therapy can help to control it.

Time for a change

Prehypertension signals the need for teaching about lifestyle modifications and the prevention of developing hypertension. Lifestyle modifications, initiated in all patients, may include changes in diet, adoption of relaxation techniques, regular exercise, smoking cessation, limited intake of alcohol, and restriction of sodium and saturated fat intake.

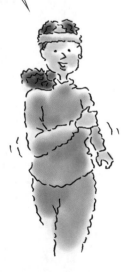

In early stages, lifestyle changes such as regular exercise may prevent hypertension from developing.

Pharming out therapy

The need for drug therapy is determined by blood pressure and the presence of target organ damage or risk factors. Drug therapy for uncomplicated hypertension usually begins with a thiazide diuretic, an ACE inhibitor, or a beta-adrenergic blocker. Other antihypertensive drugs include angiotensin II receptor blockers, alpha-receptor blockers, direct arteriole dilators, and calcium channel blockers. (See *Managing antihypertensive therapy.*)

What to do

• Collaborate care with a skilled team, which may include a cardiologist, a nutritionist, and a cardiac rehabilitation team.
• If a patient with hypertension is admitted to your facility, find out if he was taking prescribed medication. If not, help him identify reasons for noncompliance. If the patient can't afford the medication, refer him to an appropriate social service agency. If he has suffered severe adverse effects, he may need different medication.
• Routinely screen all patients for hypertension, especially those at high risk.
• Evaluate the patient. After successful treatment for hypertension, the patient will demonstrate blood pressure less than 140/90 mm Hg at rest, ability to tolerate activity, and absence of enlargement of the left ventricle (as revealed by ECG or chest X-ray).
• Teach the patient to use a self-monitoring blood pressure cuff and to record readings at the same time of the day at least twice weekly to review with his primary health care provider.
• Warn the patient that uncontrolled hypertension may cause a stroke, MI, or kidney failure.
• To encourage compliance with antihypertensive therapy, suggest that the patient establish a daily routine for taking medication. Tell him to report adverse drug effects and to keep a record of the effectiveness of drugs. Advise him to avoid high-sodium antacids and over-the-counter cold and sinus medications, which contain harmful vasoconstrictors.
• Help the patient examine and modify his lifestyle, and encourage necessary diet changes.
• If the patient smokes, encourage cessation and refer him to a smoking-cessation program.
• Document vital signs and intake and output. Note cardiac and respiratory status and response to treatment. Document patient teaching and the patient's understanding of the information.

Managing antihypertensive therapy

This flowchart is based on the approach to antihypertensive therapy endorsed by the Joint National Committee on Detection, Evaluation, and Treatment of High Blood Pressure.

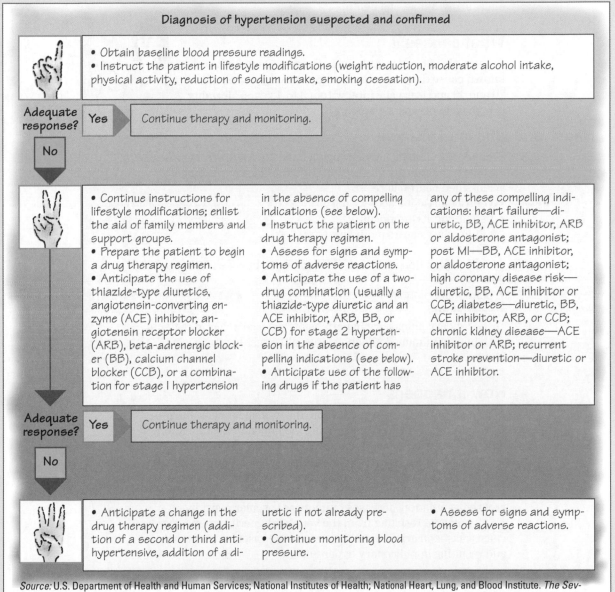

Diagnosis of hypertension suspected and confirmed

- Obtain baseline blood pressure readings.
- Instruct the patient in lifestyle modifications (weight reduction, moderate alcohol intake, physical activity, reduction of sodium intake, smoking cessation).

Adequate response? Yes → Continue therapy and monitoring.

No

- Continue instructions for lifestyle modifications; enlist the aid of family members and support groups.
- Prepare the patient to begin a drug therapy regimen.
- Anticipate the use of thiazide-type diuretics, angiotensin-converting enzyme (ACE) inhibitor, angiotensin receptor blocker (ARB), beta-adrenergic blocker (BB), calcium channel blocker (CCB), or a combination for stage I hypertension in the absence of compelling indications (see below).
- Instruct the patient on the drug therapy regimen.
- Assess for signs and symptoms of adverse reactions.
- Anticipate the use of a two-drug combination (usually a thiazide-type diuretic and an ACE inhibitor, ARB, BB, or CCB) for stage 2 hypertension in the absence of compelling indications (see below).
- Anticipate use of the following drugs if the patient has any of these compelling indications: heart failure—diuretic, BB, ACE inhibitor, ARB or aldosterone antagonist; post MI—BB, ACE inhibitor, or aldosterone antagonist; high coronary disease risk—diuretic, BB, ACE inhibitor or CCB; diabetes—diuretic, BB, ACE inhibitor, ARB, or CCB; chronic kidney disease—ACE inhibitor or ARB; recurrent stroke prevention—diuretic or ACE inhibitor.

Adequate response? Yes → Continue therapy and monitoring.

No

- Anticipate a change in the drug therapy regimen (addition of a second or third antihypertensive, addition of a diuretic if not already prescribed).
- Continue monitoring blood pressure.
- Assess for signs and symptoms of adverse reactions.

Source: U.S. Department of Health and Human Services; National Institutes of Health; National Heart, Lung, and Blood Institute. *The Seventh Report of the Joint National Committee on Detection, Evaluation, and Treatment of High Blood Pressure (JNC 7)*. Washington D.C.: Government Printing Office, 2003.

Pulmonary hypertension

Pulmonary hypertension refers to chronically elevated PAP (over 25 mm Hg). Complications of pulmonary hypertension include right- and left-sided heart failure, valvular dysfunction, hypoxemia, arrhythmias, and death.

Pulmonary hypertension is particularly dangerous during pregnancy.

What causes it

Primary, or idiopathic, pulmonary hypertension has no known cause. It's most common in women between ages 20 and 40 and is usually fatal within 3 to 4 years. Mortality is highest in pregnant women.

Heart and lung lead the way

Secondary pulmonary hypertension typically results from existing cardiac or pulmonary disease, or both. Cardiac causes include:
- left-sided heart failure
- ventricular septal defect
- patent ductus arteriosus.
    Pulmonary causes include:
- COPD
- vasoconstriction of the arterial bed due to hypoxemia and acidosis
- pulmonary emboli
- scleroderma.

Secondary pulmonary hypertension can also occur in patients with human immunodeficiency virus, although the cause is unknown.

How it happens

In primary pulmonary hypertension, the intimal lining of the pulmonary arteries thickens, narrowing the lumen of the artery, impairing distensibility, and increasing vascular resistance.

Alveolar hypoventilation can result from diseases causing alveolar destruction or diseases that prevent the chest wall from expanding sufficiently to allow air into the alveoli. The resulting decreased ventilation increases pulmonary vascular resistance.

Hypoxemia resulting from the ventilation-perfusion mismatch causes vasoconstriction, further increasing vascular resistance and resulting in pulmonary hypertension.

Sans treatment

If a patient with pulmonary hypertension doesn't receive treatment, here's what happens:

• Hypertrophy occurs in the medial smooth-muscle layer of the arterioles, worsening nondistensibility.
• Increased pressure in the lungs is transmitted to the right ventricle (which supplies the pulmonary artery).
• The ventricle becomes hypertrophic and eventually fails (cor pulmonale).
• Impaired distensibility due to hypertrophy can cause arrhythmias.

What to look for

Patients with pulmonary hypertension typically report increasing dyspnea on exertion, weakness, syncope, and fatigue.

Look, touch, and listen

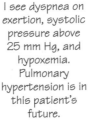

I see dyspnea on exertion, systolic pressure above 25 mm Hg, and hypoxemia. Pulmonary hypertension is in this patient's future.

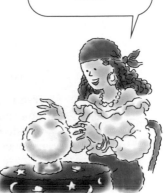

Signs of pulmonary hypertension include:
• tachycardia
• tachypnea with mild exertion
• decreased blood pressure
• changes in mental status, from restlessness to agitation or confusion
• signs of right-sided heart failure, such as ascites and jugular vein distention
• an easily palpable right ventricular lift and a reduced carotid pulse
• possible peripheral edema
• decreased diaphragmatic excursion and respiration
• point of maximal impulse displaced beyond the midclavicular line.
• systolic ejection murmur, a widely split S_2 and an S_3 or S_4 sound, or decreased breath sounds and loud, turbulent sounds heard on auscultation.

What tests tell you

• Arterial blood gas analysis reveals hypoxemia.
• ECG changes correspond with those of right ventricular hypertrophy and include right axis deviation and tall or peaked P waves in inferior leads.
• PA catheterization reveals increased PAP, with systolic pressure above 25 mm Hg. It may also show an increased PAWP if the underlying cause is left atrial myxoma, mitral stenosis, or left-sided heart failure; otherwise, PAWP is normal.
• Pulmonary angiography is used to detect filling defects in pulmonary vasculature.
• Pulmonary function studies may show decreased flow rates and increased residual volume in underlying obstructive disease. In

underlying restrictive disease, they may show reduced total lung capacity.
• Radionuclide imaging reveals abnormal right and left ventricular function.
• Echocardiography allows assessment of ventricular wall motion and possible valvular dysfunction. It's also used to identify right ventricular enlargement, abnormal septal configuration, and reduced left ventricular cavity size.
• Perfusion lung scanning may yield normal results or multiple patchy and diffuse filling defects not consistent with pulmonary embolism.

How it's treated

Treatment measures include oxygen therapy to correct hypoxemia, and fluid restriction to decrease preload and minimize workload of the right ventricle. In severe cases with irreversible changes, heart-lung transplantation may be necessary.

Diverse drugs

A patient with pulmonary hypertension may receive:
• inotropic medications, such as digoxin, to increase cardiac output
• diuretics to decrease intravascular volume and venous return
• calcium channel blockers and other vasodilators (possibly including continuous vasodilator infusion therapy) to reduce myocardial workload and oxygen consumption
• bronchodilators to relax smooth muscles and increase airway patency
• beta-adrenergic blockers to reduce cardiac workload and improve oxygenation
• anticoagulant therapy in case of concurrent hypercoagulability.

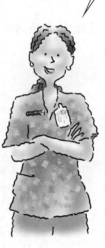

Medications can increase cardiac output, reduce workload, relax muscles, and help in other ways.

What to do

• Collaborate care with a skilled team, which may include a cardiologist, a nutritionist, and a cardiac rehabilitation team.
• Assess cardiopulmonary status. Auscultate heart and breath sounds, being alert for S_3 heart sounds, murmurs, or crackles indicating heart failure. Monitor vital signs, oxygen saturation, and heart rhythm.
• Assess hemodynamic status, including PAP and PAWP, every 2 hours, or more often depending on the patient's condition, and report any changes.
• Monitor intake and output closely and obtain daily weights. Institute fluid restriction as ordered.

- Administer medications as ordered to promote adequate heart and lung function. Assess for potential adverse reactions, such as orthostatic hypotension with diuretics and beta-adrenergic blockers.
- Administer supplemental oxygen as ordered, and organize care to allow rest periods.
- Teach the patient about his diagnosis, diagnostic tests, and treatment.
- Be sure to cover the patient's medications, administration, and potential adverse effects. Tell the patient about when to notify the doctor.
- Review dietary and fluid restrictions.
- Teach the patient about signs and symptoms of heart failure.
- Document cardiac and respiratory status, vital signs, and daily weight. Note the patient's response to treatment, and document the patient's understanding of the teaching.

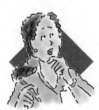

Quick quiz

1. Three risk factors involved with acute coronary syndromes include:
- A. smoking, family history of heart disease, and diabetes.
- B. family history, diabetes, and active lifestyle.
- C. smoking, diabetes, and high high-density lipoprotein level.
- D. weight loss, smoking, and low high-density lipoprotein level.

Answer: A. Risk factors for developing acute coronary syndromes include family history of heart disease, obesity, smoking, a high-fat and high-carbohydrate diet, sedentary lifestyle, menopause, stress, diabetes, hypertension, and hyperlipoproteinemia.

2. The most common direct cause of sudden death is:
- A. cardiomyopathy.
- B. pulmonary hypertension.
- C. heart failure.
- D. coronary artery disease.

Answer: D. Coronary artery disease is the most common direct cause of sudden death; cardiomyopathy is second.

3. Clinical signs of left-sided heart failure include:

A.   dyspnea and bradycardia.

B.   tachycardia and restlessness.

C.   dyspnea and tachycardia.

D.   restlessness and cough.

Answer: C. Clinical signs of left-sided heart failure include dyspnea, initially on exertion; paroxysmal nocturnal dyspnea; Cheyne-Stokes respirations; cough; orthopnea; tachycardia; fatigue; and muscle weakness.

4. Prehypertension is usually treated with:

A.   diuretics.

B.   lifestyle modification instructions.

C.   beta-adrenergic blockers.

D.   ACE inhibitors.

Answer: B. Prehypertension signals the need for teaching about lifestyle modifications and the prevention of developing hypertension. Lifestyle modifications may include changes in diet, adoption of relaxation techniques, regular exercise, smoking cessation, limited intake of alcohol, and restriction of sodium and saturated fat intake.

Scoring

☆☆☆ If you answered all four questions correctly, marvelous! You've mastered the MI info.

☆☆ If you answered three questions correctly, hooray! You're hanging in with hypertension.

☆ If you answered fewer than three questions correctly, don't sweat it. From heart failure to pulmonary hypertension, there's a lot to learn.

Vascular disorders

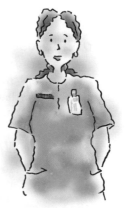

Just the facts

In this chapter, you'll learn:

♦ disorders that affect the vessels of the circulatory system

♦ pathophysiology and treatments related to these disorders

♦ diagnostic tests, assessment findings, and nursing interventions for each disorder.

A look at vascular disorders

Vascular disorders can affect arteries, veins, or both types of vessels. Arterial disorders include aneurysms, which result from weakening of the arterial wall, and arterial occlusive disease, which commonly results from atherosclerotic narrowing of the artery's lumen. Thrombophlebitis results from inflammation or occlusion of the veins.

When the wall of the aorta loses its strength, an aneurysm can occur.

Aortic aneurysm

An aortic aneurysm is an abnormal dilation in a weakened arterial wall. Aortic aneurysms typically occur in the abdominal aorta between the renal arteries and the iliac branches, but the thoracic aorta may also be affected.

Bumpy road ahead

Major complications of aortic aneurysm include hemorrhage, myocardial infarction (MI), renal failure, embolus, cerebrovascular insufficiency, circulatory collapse, and death.

What causes it

The exact cause of an aortic aneurysm is unclear, but several factors place a person at risk, including:

- age older than 55
- history of hypertension
- smoking
- atherosclerosis
- connective tissue disorders
- diabetes mellitus
- trauma
- heredity
- male sex.

How it happens

Aneurysms arise from a defect in the middle layer of the arterial wall (tunica media, or medial layer). When the elastic fibers and collagen in the middle layer are damaged, stretching and segmental dilation occur. As a result, the medial layer loses some of its elasticity, and it fragments. Smooth-muscle cells are lost, and the wall thins.

Thin and thinner

The thinned wall may contain calcium deposits and atherosclerotic plaque, making the wall brittle. As a person ages, the elastin in the wall decreases, further weakening the vessel. If hypertension is present, dilation of the arterial wall occurs more quickly, resulting in additional weakening.

Wide vessel, slow flow

When an aneurysm begins to develop, lateral pressure increases, causing the vessel lumen to widen and blood flow to slow. A thrombus may form within the dilated area. Over time, mechanical stressors contribute to elongation of the aneurysm.

Blood forces

Hemodynamic forces may also play a role, causing pulsatile stresses on the weakened wall and pressing on the small vessels that supply nutrients to the arterial wall. In aortic aneurysms, this causes the aorta to become bowed and tortuous.

What to look for

Most patients with aortic aneurysms are asymptomatic until the aneurysms enlarge and compress surrounding tissue. A large aneurysm may produce signs and symptoms that mimic those of MI, renal calculi, lumbar disk disease, and duodenal compression.

> An aneurysm generally produces no symptoms, at least in the beginning. If it ruptures, however, immediate treatment is necessary.

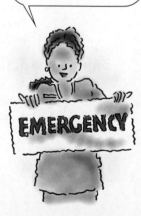

When symptoms arise

Usually, if the patient exhibits symptoms, it's because of rupture, expansion, embolization, thrombosis, or pressure from the mass on surrounding structures. Rupture is more common if the patient also has poorly controlled hypertension or if the aneurysm is 6 cm or larger. A patient with a leaking or ruptured aneurysm may report sharp, severe, and tearing pain.

Abdominal aortic aneurysm

The patient with an abdominal aortic aneurysm may experience:
• generalized, steady abdominal pain
• lower back pain that's unaffected by movement
• gastric or abdominal fullness
• palpable, pulsating mass in the periumbilical area (if the patient isn't obese)
• systolic bruit over the aorta on auscultation of the abdomen
• bruit over the femoral arteries
• hypotension (with aneurysm rupture).

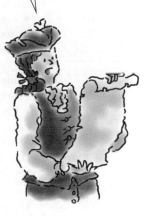

Hear ye! Hear ye! Let it be known that lower back pain that's unaffected by movement is a sign of abdominal aortic aneurysm.

Thoracic aortic aneurysm

If the patient has a suspected thoracic aortic aneurysm, assess for:
• complaints of substernal pain, possibly radiating to the neck, back, abdomen, or shoulders
• hoarseness or coughing
• difficulty swallowing
• difficulty breathing
• hemoptysis
• hematemesis
• unequal blood pressure and pulse when measured in both arms
• aortic insufficiency murmur.

Acute expansion

When acute expansion of a thoracic aortic aneurysm exists, assess for:
• severe hypertension
• neurologic changes
• a new murmur of aortic sufficiency
• right sternoclavicular lift
• jugular vein distention
• tracheal deviation
• acute onset of heart failure
• sharp, tearing pain in the chest or upper back.

What tests tell you

Most aneurysms are found incidentally during a physical examination or during testing for other medical problems. No specific laboratory test to diagnose an aortic aneurysm exists. However, these tests may be helpful:

• If blood is leaking from the aneurysm, a complete blood count (CBC) may reveal leukocytosis and a decrease in hemoglobin level and hematocrit.

• Abdominal ultrasonography or echocardiography may be used to determine the size, shape, length, location, and blood flow patterns of the aneurysm.

Telltale TEE

• Transesophageal echocardiography (TEE) allows visualization of the thoracic aorta. It's commonly combined with Doppler flow studies to provide information about blood flow.

• Anteroposterior and lateral X-rays of the chest or abdomen can be used to detect aortic calcification, and widened areas of the aorta may be visualized.

• Computed tomography (CT) scan and magnetic resonance imaging (MRI) can disclose the aneurysm's size and effect on nearby organs.

• Serial duplex ultrasonography at 6- to 12-month intervals reveals growth of small aneurysms.

• Aortography is used in determining the aneurysm's approximate size along with the patency of and the aneurysm's proximity to the visceral vessels.

How it's treated

Aneurysm treatment usually involves surgery and appropriate medical management.

Aortic aneurysms usually require open surgical resection and replacement of the aortic section using a vascular or Dacron graft. However, keep these points in mind:

• If the aneurysm is small and produces no symptoms, surgery may be delayed, with regular physical examination and duplex ultrasonography performed to monitor its progression.

• Large aneurysms and those that produce symptoms in the patient are at risk for rupture and need immediate repair.

• Endovascular grafting may be an option for a patient with an abdominal aortic aneurysm. (See *Endovascular grafting repair for AAA*.)

• Medications to control blood pressure and dyslipidemia, relieve anxiety, and control pain are also prescribed.

Rush to respond to rupture

Rupture of an aortic aneurysm is a medical emergency requiring prompt treatment, including:

• resuscitation with fluid and blood replacement

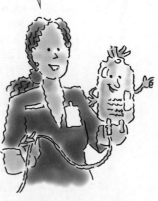

Treatment for a ruptured aortic aneurysm includes fluid resuscitation, blood replacement, and I.V. drugs.

Endovascular grafting repair for AAA

Endovascular grafting, shown at right, is an invasive procedure in which the walls of the aorta are reinforced to prevent expansion and rupture of an abdominal aortic aneurysm (AAA). The stent graft is threaded through the femoral artery and placed within the AAA. Blood flow is then routed through the graft and doesn't enter the aneursym sac. The procedure can be done using local or regional anesthesia. Because the procedure is performed percutaneously, it's less invasive than open surgical repair.

The patient is instructed to walk the first day after surgery and is discharged from the hospital in 1 to 3 days.

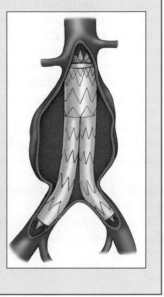

• I.V. propranolol to reduce myocardial contractility
• I.V. nitroprusside (Nitropress) to reduce blood pressure and maintain it at 90 to 100 mm Hg systolic
• analgesics to relieve pain
• an arterial line and indwelling urinary catheter to monitor the patient's condition preoperatively.

What to do

• Collaborate care with a skilled team, which may include emergency medical personnel, a vascular surgeon, cardiologist, and nutritional and physical therapists.
• Assess the patient's vital signs, especially blood pressure, every 2 to 4 hours or more frequently, depending on the severity of his condition. Monitor blood pressure and all pulses in the extremities and compare findings bilaterally. If the difference in systolic blood pressure exceeds 10 mm Hg, notify the doctor immediately.
• Assess cardiovascular status frequently, including heart rate, rhythm, electrocardiogram, and cardiac enzyme levels. MI is one of the most common complications.
• Obtain blood samples to evaluate kidney function by assessing blood urea nitrogen, creatinine, and electrolyte levels. Measure intake and output, hourly if necessary, depending on the patient's condition.

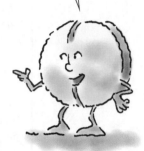

Analgesics can help relieve pain.

• Monitor CBC for evidence of blood loss, including decreased hemoglobin level, hematocrit, and red blood cell (RBC) count.
• If the patient's condition changes acutely, obtain an arterial blood sample for arterial blood gas analysis, as ordered, and monitor cardiac rhythm. Assist with arterial line insertion to allow for continuous blood pressure monitoring. Assist with insertion of a pulmonary artery catheter to assess hemodynamic balance.
• Administer ordered medications to control hypertension. Provide analgesics to relieve pain, if present.
• Observe the patient for signs of rupture, which may be immediately fatal. Watch closely for any signs of acute blood loss: decreasing blood pressure; increasing pulse and respiratory rates; cool, clammy skin; restlessness; and decreased level of consciousness.
• Explain the surgical procedure and the expected postoperative care to the patient.
• Reinforce instructions for controlling blood pressure. Stress the importance of medications and diet therapy and the need for smoking cessation.

Rupture response

• If rupture occurs, insert a large-bore I.V. catheter, begin fluid resuscitation, and administer nitroprusside I.V. as ordered, usually to maintain a mean arterial pressure of 70 to 80 mm Hg. Also administer propranolol I.V. as ordered until the heart rate ranges from 60 to 80 beats per minute. Expect to administer additional doses every 4 to 6 hours until oral medications can be used.
• If the patient is experiencing acute pain, administer morphine 2 to 10 mg I.V. as ordered.
• Prepare the patient for emergency surgery.

After surgery

• Administer nitroprusside or nitroglycerin and titrate to maintain a normotensive state.
• Perform meticulous pulmonary hygiene measures, including suctioning, chest physiotherapy, and deep breathing.
• Provide continuous cardiac monitoring.
• Assess urine output hourly.
• Maintain nasogastric tube patency to ensure gastric decompression.
• Assist with serial Doppler examination of all extremities to evaluate the adequacy of blood flow and to detect embolization.
• Assess for signs of poor arterial perfusion, such as pain, paresthesia, pallor, pulselessness, paralysis, and poikilothermy (coldness).

• Advise the patient about activity restrictions, such as no pushing, pulling, or lifting heavy objects until the doctor allows him to do so.

• Document cardiac, respiratory, and neurovascular statuses; wound appearance and care; intake and output; and vital signs or hemodynamic parameters. Document patient teaching provided as well as the patient's understanding of the instructions.

Arterial occlusive disease

Arterial occlusive disease is a common complication of atherosclerosis and inflammation. It may affect large vessels, such as the aorta and its branches, or the vertebral, innominate, subclavian, mesenteric, renal, or peripheral vessels. It may be acute or chronic. Men are more likely to suffer from arterial occlusive disease than women. (See *Possible sites of major artery occlusion*, page 284.)

Major complications of arterial occlusive disease include limb paralysis, gangrene, limb loss, infection, and death.

What causes it

Risk factors for arterial occlusive disease include smoking, aging, hypertension, hyperlipidemia, diabetes mellitus, and family history of vascular disorders, MI, or stroke.

Causes include:
• emboli formation
• thrombosis
• atherosclerotic lesions of the arterial wall.

How it happens

In arterial occlusive disease, obstruction or narrowing of the lumen of the aorta or its major branches causes an interruption of blood flow, usually to the legs and feet.

Location and timing

Prognosis depends on the location of the occlusion, the development of collateral circulation to counteract reduced blood flow and, in acute disease, the time elapsed between formation of the occlusion and restoration of adequate blood flow.

What to look for

Signs and symptoms depend on the severity and site of the arterial occlusion. (See *Types of arterial occlusive disease*, page 285.)

(Text continues on page 286.)

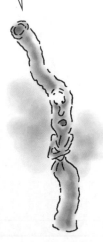

An occluded artery slows blood flow, usually to the legs and feet.

Possible sites of major artery occlusion

This illustration points out the possible sites of major artery occlusion.

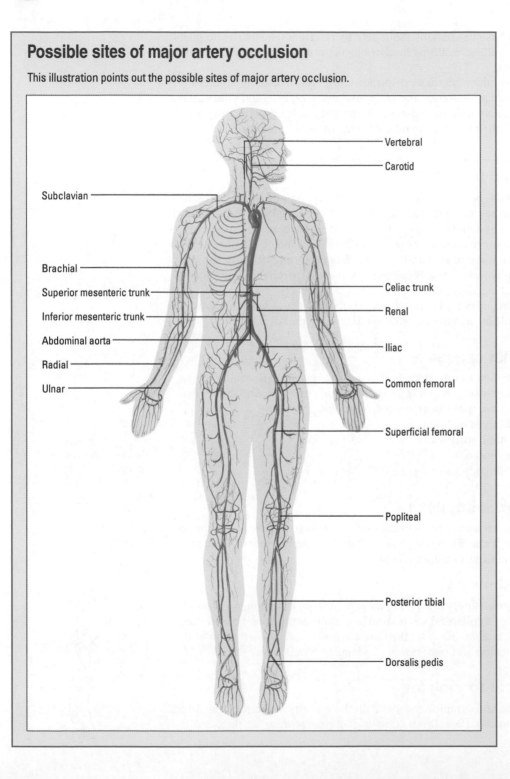

Types of arterial occlusive disease

The signs and symptoms of arterial occlusive disease depend on the location of the occlusion. Use this chart to help determine the site of your patient's occlusion.

Site of occlusion	Signs and symptoms
Carotid arterial system • Internal carotids • External carotids	Neurologic dysfunction: transient ischemic attacks (TIAs) due to reduced cerebral circulation produce unilateral sensory or motor dysfunction (transient monocular blindness, hemiparesis), possible aphasia or dysarthria, confusion, decreased mentation and, rarely, headache. These recurrent clinical features may last 5 to 10 minutes but may persist up to 24 hours and may herald a stroke. Decreased pulsation may be palpated or a bruit may be heard over the affected vessels.
Vertebrobasilar system • Vertebral arteries • Basilar arteries	Neurologic dysfunction: TIAs of the brain stem and cerebellum produce binocular visual disturbances, vertigo, dysarthria, and "drop attacks" (falling down without loss of consciousness.) Less common than carotid territory TIA.
Innominate • Brachiocephalic artery	Neurologic dysfunction: signs and symptoms of vertebrobasilar insufficiency. Decreased right arm pulses with claudication symptoms; possible bruit over lower right side of neck.
Subclavian artery	Subclavian steal syndrome (characterized by reversed blood flow from the brain through the vertebral artery on the same side as the occlusion, into the subclavian artery distal to the occlusion); clinical effects of vertebrobasilar insufficiency and exercise-induced arm claudication. Rarely, gangrene, usually limited to the digits.
Mesenteric artery • Superior (most commonly affected) • Celiac axis • Inferior	Bowel ischemia, infarct necrosis, and gangrene; sudden severe acute abdominal pain; nausea and vomiting; diarrhea; leukocytosis; and shock due to massive intraluminal fluid shifts.
Aortic bifurcation (saddle block occlusion; if acute, a medical emergency associated with cardiac embolization)	Sensory and motor deficits (muscle weakness, numbness, paresthesias, paralysis) and signs of ischemia (sudden pain; cold, pale legs with markedly decreased or absent peripheral pulses) and minimal to absent Doppler signals in both legs.
Iliac artery (Leriche's syndrome)	Exercise-induced claudication of lower back, buttocks, and thighs, relieved by rest; absent or reduced femoral or distal pulses; erectile dysfunction in males.
Femoral and popliteal artery (may be associated with aneurysm formation)	Intermittent claudication of the calves or thighs on exertion; pain in feet at rest; pretrophic pain (heralds necrosis and ulceration); leg pallor and coolness; blanching of feet on elevation and dependent rubor; gangrene; no palpable pulses in ankles and feet; absent to minimal Doppler signals.

Back to the classics

Acute arterial occlusion may produce the six classic Ps:

🤟 pain

✋ pallor

🖖 pulselessness

🖐 paresthesia

🖐 paralysis

🖐✌ poikilothermy.

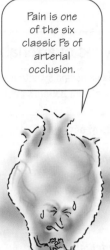

Pain is one of the six classic Ps of arterial occlusion.

Let's not forget the rest

Other signs and symptoms include:
• intermittent claudication
• severe burning pain in the feet (aggravated by elevating the extremity and sometimes relieved by keeping the extremity in a dependent position)
• ulcers, gangrene
• pallor on elevation, followed by redness with dependency
• delayed capillary filling, hair loss, or dry skin with trophic nail changes
• diminished or absent pulses.

What tests tell you

Pertinent supportive diagnostic tests include:
• arteriography, which demonstrates the type (thrombus or embolus), location, and degree of obstruction, and helps evaluate the collateral circulation (it's particularly useful for diagnosing chronic forms of the disease and evaluating candidates for reconstructive surgery)
• Doppler duplex ultrasonography and plethysmography, which show the speed, direction, and pattern of blood flow through the arteries and quantify the blood flow to the extremities.

How it's treated

Treatment for arterial occlusive disease depends on the cause, location, and degree of the obstruction. For patients with mild chronic disease, it usually consists of supportive measures, such as smoking cessation and controlling hypertension, dyslipidemia, and blood glucose level. Walking exercise promotes collateral blood flow.

Better blood

Drug therapy includes antiplatelet and hemorheologic drugs, such as aspirin, ticlopidine (Ticlid), pentoxifylline (Trental), and cilostazol (Pletal). Thrombolytic therapy may be used to treat an acute arterial thrombosis. Patients with hyperlipidemia may be treated with antilipemic drugs.

Embolectomy, grafting, amputation—oh, my!

Appropriate surgical procedures may include embolectomy, thromboendarterectomy, patch arterioplasty, bypass grafting, and lumbar sympathectomy. Amputation becomes necessary with failure of arterial interventions or with the development of nonhealing wounds or untreatable infections.

Lower the risk

Invasive endovascular techniques carry less risk than surgery and may include balloon angioplasty, atherectomy, and stenting. Other appropriate therapy includes anticoagulants to prevent emboli (for embolic occlusion) and bowel resection after restoration of blood flow (for mesenteric artery occlusion).

What to do

• Collaborate care with a skilled team, which may include a vascular surgeon, cardiologist, and nutritional and physical therapists.
• Following treatment, evaluate the patient's condition. He should be able to increase exercise tolerance without developing pain, and peripheral pulses should be normal. In addition, the extremities should maintain good skin color and temperature.
• Teach proper foot care or other appropriate measures, depending on the affected area.

Patient precautions

• Caution the patient against wearing constrictive clothing or crossing his legs while sitting.
• Instruct the patient about signs of recurrence (pain, pallor, numbness, paralysis, absence of pulse) that can result from a graft occlusion or occlusion at another site. Teach the patient to palpate his pulses and immediately report changes to his doctor.
• Advise the patient to stop smoking and refer him to a smoking-cessation program, if appropriate.
• Encourage the patient to follow his prescribed medication regimen closely.
• Advise the patient to avoid temperature extremes.
• Help the patient adjust to lifestyle constraints.

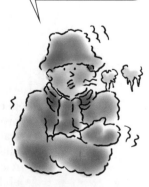

Patients with occluded arteries need to avoid temperature extremes.

• Document cardiac and neurovascular status, along with vital signs and wound condition and care, if appropriate. Document the patient's response to treatment and pain control. Document patient teaching provided and the patient's understanding of instructions.

Thrombophlebitis

An acute condition characterized by inflammation and thrombus formation, thrombophlebitis may occur in deep (intermuscular or intramuscular) or superficial (subcutaneous) veins. (See *Understanding thrombophlebitis*.)

Deep vein, deep trouble

Deep vein thrombophlebitis can affect small veins, such as the soleal venous sinuses, as well as large veins, such as the vena cava and the femoral, iliac, and subclavian veins. Usually progressive, this disorder may lead to pulmonary embolism, a potentially fatal condition. Superficial thrombophlebitis is usually self-limiting and rarely leads to pulmonary embolism.

Even more trouble

Other complications of thrombophlebitis include respiratory failure, right-sided heart failure, and postphlebitic syndrome (chronic edema, pain, venous stasis, ulcerations, and recurrent episodes of thrombophlebitis).

What causes it

Although deep vein thrombophlebitis may be idiopathic, it usually results from endothelial damage, accelerated blood clotting, or reduced blood flow.

Superficial thrombophlebitis may occur after:
• trauma
• infection
• I.V. drug abuse
• chemical irritation caused by extensive I.V. use.

Risk on the rise

Certain risk factors appear to increase the risk of developing deep vein or superficial thrombophlebitis. These factors include:
• prolonged immobility
• trauma
• childbirth
• use of hormonal contraceptives
• abdominal surgery
• major joint replacement surgery.

> Deep vein thrombophlebitis can affect small veins, such as the soleal venous sinuses, and large veins, such as the vena cava.

Understanding thrombophlebitis

Thrombophlebitis can occur in any vein as a result of thrombus formation with inflammation. It most commonly occurs at valve sites, as shown below.

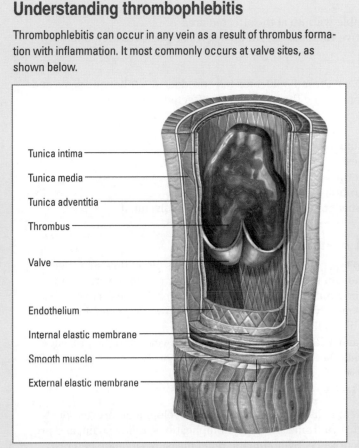

Tunica intima

Tunica media

Tunica adventitia

Thrombus

Valve

Endothelium

Internal elastic membrane

Smooth muscle

External elastic membrane

How it happens

Alteration in the epithelial lining causes platelet aggregation and fibrin entrapment of RBCs, white blood cells, and additional platelets. The thrombus initiates a chemical inflammatory process in the vessel epithelium that leads to fibrosis, which may occlude the vessel lumen or embolize.

What to look for

Clinical features vary with the site and length of the affected vein. Deep vein thrombophlebitis may produce:

• severe pain
• malaise

- nonpitting edema and cyanosis (late sign) of the affected arm or leg
- possible warmth at the affected area
- positive Homans' sign of the leg (false-positives are common).

Superficial swell

Superficial thrombophlebitis may produce the following signs and symptoms along the length of the affected vein:
- heat
- pain
- swelling
- redness
- tenderness
- induration
- lymphadenitis (with extensive vein involvement).

What tests tell you

- Doppler duplex ultrasonography shows blood flow in a specific area and can reveal the cause of any obstruction to venous flow.
- Phlebography (also called *venography*), which uses dye, is used less frequently than any other tests. It shows filling defects and diverted blood flow.
- CTs and MRIs provide visual images of veins and the presence of thrombus.

How it's treated

Treatment aims to control thrombus development, prevent postphlebitic syndrome and other complications, relieve pain, and prevent recurrence. Symptomatic relief measures include bed rest, with elevation of the affected arm or leg; warm, moist soaks to the affected area; and analgesics as ordered. After an acute episode of deep vein thrombophlebitis subsides, the patient may begin to walk while wearing antiembolism stockings (applied before getting out of bed).

Drugs and surgery

Treatment for thrombophlebitis includes anticoagulants (initially I.V., unfractionated or low-molecular-weight heparin; later, heparin and warfarin [Coumadin]) to prolong clotting time. Before any surgical procedure, discontinue the full anticoagulant dose, as ordered, to reduce the risk of hemorrhage. After some types of surgery, especially major abdominal or pelvic operations, prophylactic doses of anticoagulants may reduce the risk of deep vein thrombophlebitis and pulmonary embolism.

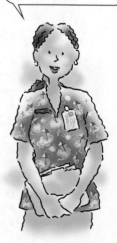

Your goals?
To control thrombus development and prevent complications.

Pardon the interruption

For lysis of acute, extensive deep vein thrombophlebitis, treatment may include thrombolytics (such as streptokinase). In rare cases, deep vein thrombophlebitis may cause complete venous occlusion, which necessitates venous interruption that may be achieved through simple ligation to vein plication, or clipping. Embolectomy may also be performed. Insertion of a vena cava filter may be necessary to prevent pulmonary embolism.

Stockings, soaks, and elevation

Therapy for severe superficial thrombophlebitis may include an anti-inflammatory drug, such as indomethacin (Indocin SR), along with antiembolism stockings, warm soaks, elevation of the patient's leg and, occasionally, anticoagulants.

What to do

• Collaborate care with a skilled team, which may include a vascular surgeon and nutritional and physical therapists.
• To prevent thrombophlebitis in high-risk patients, perform range-of-motion exercises while the patient is on bed rest. Use intermittent external compression antithrombic pumps during lengthy surgical or diagnostic procedures. Apply antiembolism stockings postoperatively, and encourage early ambulation.
• Remain alert for signs of pulmonary emboli, such as crackles, dyspnea, hemoptysis, restlessness, hypotension, and chest pain on inspiration.
• Closely monitor anticoagulant therapy to prevent serious complications such as hemorrhage. Watch for signs of bleeding, such as dark, tarry stools, coffee-ground vomitus, hematuria, and ecchymoses. Encourage the patient to use an electric razor and to avoid medications that contain aspirin.

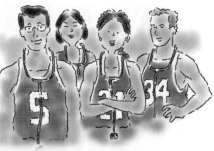

Be sure to collaborate your care with a skilled team.

Make veno go

To prevent venostasis in patients with thrombophlebitis, take these steps:
• Enforce bed rest, as ordered, and elevate the patient's affected arm or leg. If you plan to use pillows for elevating the leg, place them to support the entire length of the affected extremity and to prevent possible compression of the popliteal space.
• Apply warm soaks to improve circulation to the affected area and to relieve pain and inflammation. Also give analgesics to relieve pain as ordered.
• Measure and record the circumference of the affected arm or leg daily. Compare this with the circumference of the other arm or

leg. To ensure accuracy and consistency of serial measurements, mark the skin over the area and measure at the same spot daily.

• Administer anticoagulants as ordered.

• Evaluate the patient. After successful therapy, the patient shouldn't feel pain in the affected area. Edema should decrease.

• To prepare the patient with thrombophlebitis for discharge, emphasize the importance of follow-up blood studies to monitor anticoagulant therapy.

• Tell the patient to avoid prolonged sitting or standing to help prevent recurrence.

• Teach him how to apply and use antiembolism stockings properly.

• Document neurovascular status and vital signs. Note any respiratory difficulties. Document the patient's response to treatment and pain control. Document patient teaching provided and the patient's understanding of the instructions.

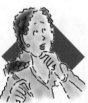

Quick quiz

1. Suspect an abdominal aortic aneurysm in a patient who complains of generalized, steady abdominal pain and has:

    A.   pulsating mass in the periumbilical area (if the patient isn't obese).

    B.   elevated cardiac enzymes.

    C.   positive Babinski's sign.

    D.   pink, frothy sputum.

Answer: A. Signs of an abdominal aortic aneurysm include generalized, steady abdominal pain; lower back pain that's unaffected by movement; gastric or abdominal fullness; palpable, pulsating mass in the periumbilical area (if the patient isn't obese); systolic bruit over the aorta on auscultation of the abdomen; bruit over the femoral arteries; and hypotension (with aneurysm rupture).

2. An important diagnostic test used to identify an arterial occlusion is:

    A.   electrocardiography.

    B.   EEG.

    C.   arteriography.

    D.   cardiac catheterization.

Answer: C. Arteriography can demonstrate the type (thrombus or embolus), location, and degree of obstruction and can help evaluate collateral circulation.

3. What are the key signs of recurrence of an arterial occlusion?
  A. Severe, substernal chest pain; diaphoresis; and hypotension
  B. Cyanosis, dyspnea, and cough
  C. Pain, pallor, numbness, paralysis, coldness, and absence of pulse
  D. Chills, fever, fatigue, and cough

Answer: C. Signs of recurrence of an arterial occlusion include pain, pallor, numbness, paralysis, coldness, and absence of pulse. These signs result from a graft occlusion or occlusion at another site.

4. A complication of deep vein thrombophlebitis may be:
  A. pulmonary embolism.
  B. acute renal failure.
  C. diabetes.
  D. liver failure.

Answer: A. Deep vein thrombophlebitis may lead to pulmonary embolism, a potentially fatal condition. Superficial thrombophlebitis is usually self-limiting and rarely leads to pulmonary embolism.

5. Which sign would lead you to suspect rupture of an aortic aneurysm?
  A. Increased urine output
  B. Increased blood pressure
  C. Decreased blood pressure
  D. Decreased pulse rate

Answer: C. Because rupture of an aortic aneurysm is an emergency, watch the patient closely for decreased blood pressure as well as increased pulse and respiratory rates; cool, clammy skin; restlessness; and decreased level of consciousness.

6. Which interventions are important when caring for a patient with thrombophlebitis?
  A. Apply cool soaks and keep the patient's legs lower than the level of the heart.
  B. Increase the patient's activity level and administer vasoconstrictors.
  C. Apply cool soaks and administer nitroglycerin.
  D. Apply warm soaks and elevate the patient's legs higher than the level of the heart.

Answer: D. To help treat thrombophlebitis, it's important to aim interventions at preventing venostasis. Such measures may include application of warm soaks and elevation of the patient's legs.

Scoring

☆☆☆   If you answered all six questions correctly, cool! You've caught all the clues about occlusions.

☆☆   If you answered four or five questions correctly, way to go! You've earned an A in aortic aneurysms.

☆   If you answered fewer than four questions correctly, keep it mellow. Remember, avoid ruptures at all costs.

10

Emergencies and complications

Just the facts

In this chapter, you'll learn:

♦ cardiac complications that require emergency measures
♦ pathophysiology and treatments related to these complications
♦ diagnostic tests, assessment findings, and nursing interventions for each complication.

A look at cardiac emergencies

Cardiac emergencies, which can result as a complication of another condition, require immediate assessment and treatment. They include cardiac trauma, cardiac tamponade, cardiogenic shock, and hypovolemic shock.

Cardiac trauma

Cardiac trauma, commonly dramatic in presentation, is usually associated with other thoracic injuries; it can occur as a result of blunt or penetrating trauma. Thoracic injuries—cardiac trauma included—account for about 25% of all trauma deaths.

Not always obvious

Although cardiac trauma can be severe, not all injuries are apparent on admission to the emergency department or intensive care unit, especially when the patient exhibits no external signs of chest wall damage. It may be several hours before signs are noticeable, and several days before complications are evident. As a result, keen observation and assess-

> Car accidents are a leading cause of cardiac trauma.

ment are essential for the early identification of cardiac injuries and potential complications.

The prognosis for a patient with cardiac trauma largely depends on the extent of the cardiac damage and his other injuries. Age and preexisting conditions also affect the prognosis.

What causes it

Cardiac trauma is a result of a blunt or penetrating chest injury.

How it happens

Blunt trauma typically results from vehicular accidents or falls. Rapid deceleration may result in shearing forces that tear cardiac structures and cause great-vessel disruption. Falls may cause a rapid increase in intra-abdominal and intrathoracic pressures, which can result in myocardial rupture, valvular rupture, or both. Crushing and compression forces may result in contusion or rupture as the heart becomes compressed between the sternum and vertebral column.

Cardiac concussion, a less severe form of blunt trauma, occurs when rapid deceleration causes the heart to strike the anterior chest wall and sternum, thereby resulting in myocardial contusion. (See *Understanding myocardial contusion.*)

Penetrating truths

Penetrating trauma to the heart, typically resulting from knife or gunshot wounds or foreign bodies in the heart, carries a high risk of mortality and usually requires immediate thoracotomy and surgical repair. This type of cardiac trauma commonly leads to cardiac tamponade. In 94% of cases involving penetrating cardiac trauma, death occurs before the patient reaches the hospital.

What to look for

Cardiac trauma may initially be overlooked as other life-threatening and more apparent injuries are treated. In addition, signs and symptoms of myocardial contusion or cardiac tamponade may not occur for several hours. Therefore, astute assessment skills are needed for early detection and prompt treatment.

Accident report

Typically, the patient with cardiac trauma is in pain and feels apprehensive. Attempt to ascertain the following information:
• mechanism of injury (for example, in an automobile accident, include how the accident occurred,

> In the rush to treat other injuries, cardiac trauma is sometimes overlooked.

Now I get it!

Understanding myocardial contusion

A myocardial contusion (bruising to the myocardium) is the most common type of injury sustained from blunt trauma. You should suspect it whenever a blow to the chest occurs. The contusion usually results from a fall or from impact with a steering wheel or other object. The right ventricle is the most common site of injury because of its location directly behind the sternum.

Here's what happens:
• During deceleration injuries, the myocardium strikes the sternum as the heart and aorta move forward.
• In addition, the aorta may be lacerated by shearing forces.
• Direct force also may be applied to the sternum, causing injury.

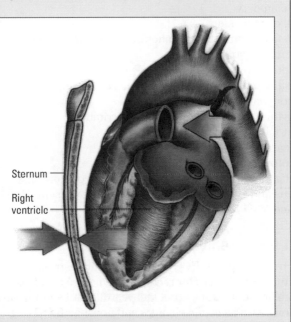

Sternum

Right ventricle

patient location and use of seat belts, and extent of internal car damage; for a fall, include how far the patient fell, onto what type of surface, and how he landed; for a gunshot wound, include the gun caliber and distance from which the patient was shot; for a stab wound, include the size and type of the weapon)
• history of cardiac or pulmonary problems
• pain location, onset, character, and severity
• presence of dyspnea.

Look for more

Other signs and symptoms associated with blunt trauma are:
• precordial chest pain
• bradycardia or tachycardia
• dyspnea
• contusion marks on the chest
• flail chest
• murmurs.

If the patient experienced penetrating trauma, look for:
- tachycardia
- shortness of breath
- weakness
- diaphoresis
- acute anxiety
- cool, clammy skin
- evidence of an external puncture wound or protrusion of the penetrating instrument
- symptoms of cardiac tamponade.

For the patient who has a cardiac contusion, look for:
- hemodynamic instability
- arrhythmias caused by ventricular irritability
- heart failure or cardiogenic shock
- pericardial friction rub
- symptoms of cardiac tamponade.

If the patient is experiencing a cardiac concussion, many of the signs and symptoms listed above will be present. However, evidence of cellular injury is absent.

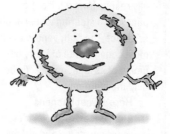

Evidence of cellular injury is absent in cases of cardiac concussion.

What tests tell you

- Electrocardiogram (ECG) reveals rhythm disturbances, such as premature ventricular contractions, premature atrial contractions, ventricular tachycardia, atrial tachycardia, and ventricular fibrillation along with ischemic changes and nonspecific ST-segment or T-wave changes (with cardiac contusion) occurring within 48 hours after the injury.
- Chest X-ray shows widened mediastinum (with cardiac tamponade) and pulmonary edema (with septal defect).
- An echocardiogram shows evidence of cardiac tamponade and valvular abnormalities, abnormal ventricular wall movement, and decreased ejection fraction (with myocardial contusion).
- Transesophageal echocardiogram shows evidence of aortic disruptions, cardiac tamponade, and atrial and septal defects.
- A multiple-gated acquisition scan detects decreased ability of effective heart pumping (with cardiac contusion).
- Cardiac enzyme levels show elevated CK-MB to greater than 8% of total creatine kinase (CK) within 4 hours after the injury (in conjunction with ECG changes suggestive of cardiac contusion).
- Cardiac troponin I shows elevations 24 hours after the injury (suggestive of cardiac injury).

How it's treated

Maintaining hemodynamic stability is crucial to the patient's care. Penetrating trauma may be associated with massive hemorrhage leading to acute hypotension and shock. In addition, cardiac output is affected if the patient develops cardiac tamponade or arrhythmias occurring with myocardial contusion. Hemodynamic monitoring is key to evaluating the patient's status and maintaining its adequacy. I.V. fluid therapy, including blood component therapy, may be necessary. Continuous ECG monitoring is important to detect possible arrhythmias. Amiodarone (Cordarone) may be used to treat ventricular arrhythmias. Digoxin (Lanoxin) may be given for pump failure. Inotropic agents may be used to assist with improving cardiac output and ejection fraction.

> There's a lot to juggle when treating cardiac trauma—but it's all designed to maintain hemodynamic stability.

Look out for the lungs

The patient with cardiac trauma must be monitored closely for signs and symptoms of cardiopulmonary compromise because cardiac trauma is commonly associated with pulmonary trauma. Supplemental oxygen administration and assessment of oxygen saturation are important. If the degree of associated pulmonary trauma is great, endotracheal (ET) intubation and mechanical ventilation may be warranted to maintain adequate oxygenation.

Meds and other measures

If the patient is experiencing severe pain, I.V. morphine is administered in small amounts to the well-hydrated patient, unless the patient is hypotensive (in which case, other less potent analgesics are used). In addition, corrective surgery may be indicated to correct septal or valvular defects, penetrating injuries, or rupture. Emergency pericardiocentesis is used to treat acute cardiac tamponade.

What to do

• Collaborate care with a skilled team, which may include emergency medical services personnel, a surgeon, a respiratory therapist, and social services.

Cardiac check-in

• Assess the patient's cardiopulmonary status at least every 4 hours—or more frequently, if indicated—to detect signs and symptoms of possible injury. Evaluate peripheral pulses and capillary refill to detect decreased peripheral tissue perfusion.
• Auscultate breath sounds at least every 4 hours, reporting signs of congestion or fluid accumulation.

• Monitor heart rate and rhythm, heart sounds, and blood pressure every hour for changes; institute hemodynamic monitoring—which may include right ventricular ejection fraction, right ventricular end-diastolic volume index (RVEDVI), mixed venous oxygen saturation, central venous pressure (CVP), pulmonary artery wedge pressure (PAWP), and continuous cardiac output as indicated—at least every 2 hours.
• Institute continuous cardiac monitoring for the first 48 to 72 hours to detect arrhythmias or conduction defects. If arrhythmias occur, administer antiarrhythmic agents as ordered and monitor electrolyte levels.

Fluids in and out

• Administer fluid replacement therapy, including blood component therapy as prescribed, typically to maintain systolic blood pressure above 90 mm Hg.
• Monitor urine output every hour, notifying the doctor if output is less than 30 ml/hour.
• Assess the patient's degree of pain and administer analgesic therapy as ordered, monitoring for effectiveness. Position the patient comfortably, usually with the head of the bed elevated 30 to 45 degrees.
• Encourage coughing and deep breathing, splinting the chest as necessary.
• If the patient has undergone surgery, monitor and assess chest tubes for patency, volume and color of drainage, and presence of an air leak.
• Assess vital signs postoperatively, especially temperature.
• Inspect the surgical site for evidence of infection or bleeding at least every 4 hours, noting redness, drainage, warmth, edema, or localized pain at the site.

Outside help

• Arrange for possible social service consultation depending on the cause of the injury—for example, alcohol-related automobile accident or gang-related gunshot injury.
• Provide brief explanations about the patient's condition and why it's occurring. Inform the patient and his family about how the condition will be treated, being sure to explain new procedures before beginning them.
• Review signs and symptoms of a worsening condition, stressing the importance of alerting the nurse if any occur.
• Teach the patient about signs and symptoms of complications and the need for follow-up.
• Document vital signs and assessment findings. Document the patient's response to treatment.

Cardiac tamponade

Cardiac tamponade is a rapid, unchecked increase in pressure in the pericardial sac. This pressure compresses the heart, impairs diastolic filling, and reduces cardiac output.

The increase in pressure usually results from blood or fluid accumulation in the pericardial sac. Even a small amount of fluid (50 to 100 ml) can cause a serious tamponade if it accumulates rapidly.

Quick fill, quick response

If fluid accumulates rapidly, cardiac tamponade requires emergency lifesaving measures to prevent death. A slow accumulation and increase in pressure may not produce immediate symptoms because the fibrous wall of the pericardial sac can gradually stretch to accommodate as much as 1 to 2 L of fluid.

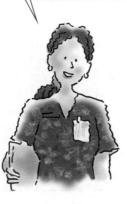

Cardiac tamponade occurs when pressure in the pericardial sac shoots up quickly.

What causes it

Cardiac tamponade may result from:
• idiopathic causes (such as Dressler's syndrome)
• effusion (from cancer, bacterial infections, tuberculosis and, rarely, acute rheumatic fever)
• hemorrhage caused by trauma (such as gunshot or stab wounds of the chest)
• hemorrhage caused by nontraumatic causes (such as anticoagulant therapy in patients with pericarditis or rupture of the heart or great vessels)
• viral or postirradiation pericarditis
• chronic renal failure requiring dialysis
• drug reaction from procainamide, hydralazine, minoxidil, isoniazid, penicillin, or daunorubicin
• connective tissue disorders (such as rheumatoid arthritis, systemic lupus erythematosus, rheumatic fever, and scleroderma)
• acute myocardial infarction (MI).

How it happens

In cardiac tamponade, accumulation of fluid in the pericardial sac causes compression of the heart chambers. This compression obstructs blood flow into the ventricles and reduces the amount of blood that can be pumped out of the heart with each contraction. (See *Understanding cardiac tamponade*, page 302.)

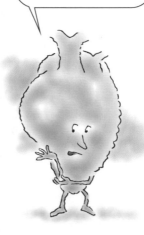

Compression of the heart chambers obstructs blood flow into the ventricles and reduces the amount of blood that can be pumped out of the heart with each contraction.

Now I get it!

Understanding cardiac tamponade

The pericardial sac, which surrounds and protects the heart, is composed of several layers:
• The fibrous pericardium is the tough outermost membrane.
• The inner membrane, called the *serous membrane,* consists of the visceral and parietal layers.
• The visceral layer clings to the heart and is also known as the *epicardial layer* of the heart.
• The parietal layer lies between the visceral layer and the fibrous pericardium.

• The pericardial space—between the visceral and parietal layers—contains 10 to to 50 ml of pericardial fluid. This fluid lubricates the layers and minimizes friction when the heart contracts.

In cardiac tamponade, shown below right, blood or fluid fills the pericardial space, compressing the heart chambers, increasing intracardiac pressure, and obstructing venous return. As blood flow into the ventricles decreases, so does cardiac output. Without prompt treatment, low cardiac output can be fatal.

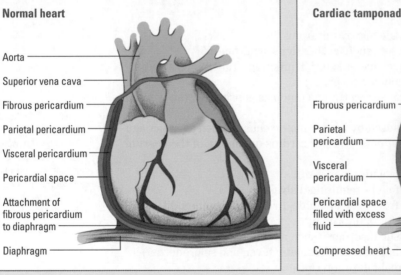

Normal heart

- Aorta
- Superior vena cava
- Fibrous pericardium
- Parietal pericardium
- Visceral pericardium
- Pericardial space
- Attachment of fibrous pericardium to diaphragm
- Diaphragm

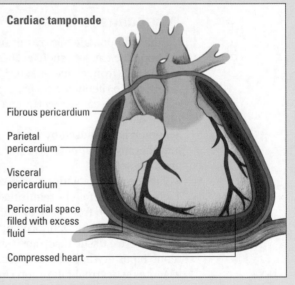

Cardiac tamponade

- Fibrous pericardium
- Parietal pericardium
- Visceral pericardium
- Pericardial space filled with excess fluid
- Compressed heart

What to look for

Cardiac tamponade has three classic features, which are known as *Beck's triad:*

   elevated central venous pressure (CVP) with jugular vein distention

   muffled heart sounds

pulsus paradoxus (inspiratory drop in systemic blood pressure greater than 10 mm Hg).

That's not all

Other signs include:
- narrowed pulse pressure
- orthopnea
- diaphoresis
- anxiety
- restlessness
- cyanosis
- weak, rapid peripheral pulse.

What tests tell you

- Chest X-ray shows a slightly widened mediastinum and an enlarged cardiac silhouette.
- ECG may show a low-amplitude QRS complex and electrical alternans, an alternating beat-to-beat change in amplitude of the P wave, QRS complex, and T wave. Generalized ST-segment elevation is noted in all leads. An ECG is used to rule out other cardiac disorders; it may reveal changes produced by acute pericarditis.
- Pulmonary artery catheterization discloses increased right atrial pressure, right ventricular diastolic pressure, and CVP.
- Echocardiography may reveal pericardial effusion with signs of right ventricular and atrial compression.
- Computed tomography scanning or magnetic resonance imaging can be used to identify pericardial effusions or pericardial thickening caused by constrictive pericarditis.

How it's treated

The goal of treatment is to relieve intrapericardial pressure and cardiac compression by removing accumulated blood or fluid. This removal can be done three different ways:
- pericardiocentesis (needle aspiration of the pericardial cavity)
- surgical creation of an opening, called a *pericardial window*
- insertion of a drain into the pericardial sac to drain the effusion.

When pressure is low

If the patient is hypotensive, trial volume loading with crystalloids, such as I.V. normal saline solution, may be used to maintain systolic blood pressure. An inotropic drug, such as dopamine, may be necessary to improve myocardial contractility until fluid in the pericardial sac can be removed.

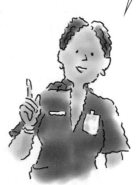

The goals of treatment for cardiac tamponade are to drain fluid and relieve pressure.

More to do

Additional treatment may be necessary, depending on the cause. Examples of such causes and treatments are:
• traumatic injury—blood transfusion or a thoracotomy to drain reaccumulating fluid or to repair bleeding sites
• heparin-induced tamponade—administration of the heparin antagonist protamine sulfate
• warfarin-induced tamponade (rare)—vitamin K administration.

What to do

• Collaborate care with a skilled team, which may include emergency medical personnel, a cardiovascular surgeon, and critical care personnel.
• Monitor the patient's cardiovascular status frequently, at least every hour, noting the extent of jugular vein distention, the quality of heart sounds, and blood pressure.
• Assess hemodynamic status, including CVP, right atrial pressure, and pulmonary artery pressure (PAP), and determine cardiac output.

It's a paradox

• Monitor for pulsus paradoxus (pulse that rapidly decreases during inspiration).
• Be alert for ST-segment and T-wave changes on the ECG. Note rate and rhythm, and report evidence of any arrhythmias.
• Watch closely for signs of increasing tamponade or dyspnea, and report them immediately.
• Infuse I.V. solutions and inotropic drugs, such as dopamine, as ordered to maintain the patient's blood pressure.
• Administer oxygen therapy as needed, and assess oxygen saturation levels. Monitor the patient's respiratory status for signs of respiratory distress, such as severe tachypnea and changes in the patient's level of consciousness (LOC). Anticipate the need for ET intubation and mechanical ventilation if the patient's respiratory status deteriorates.
• Prepare the patient for pericardiocentesis or thoracotomy.
• If the patient has trauma-induced tamponade, assess for other signs of trauma and institute appropriate care, including the use of colloids, crystalloids, and blood component therapy under pressure or by rapid volume infuser, if massive fluid replacement is needed; administration of protamine sulfate for heparin-induced tamponade; and vitamin K administration for warfarin-induced tamponade.

Don't forget me! Be sure to monitor for signs of respiratory distress.

- Assess renal function status closely, monitoring urine output every hour and notifying the doctor if output is less than 30 ml/hour.
- Monitor capillary refill time, LOC, peripheral pulses, and skin temperature for evidence of diminished tissue perfusion.
- Explain the patient's condition and why it's occurring. Inform the patient and his family how the condition will be treated, being sure to explain new procedures before beginning them.
- Review signs and symptoms of a worsening condition, stressing the importance of alerting the nurse if such signs occur.
- Document the patient's vital signs, cardiac and respiratory status, and response to treatment.

Cardiogenic shock

Cardiogenic shock is a condition of diminished cardiac output that severely impairs tissue perfusion. It's sometimes called *pump failure*.

Shocking stats

Cardiogenic shock is a serious complication in 6% to 7% of all patients hospitalized with acute MI. It typically affects patients whose area of infarction involves 40% or more of left ventricular muscle mass; in such patients the overall in-hospital mortality rate is 57%.

What causes it

Cardiogenic shock can result from any condition that causes significant left ventricular dysfunction with reduced cardiac output, such as:
- MI (most common)
- myocardial ischemia
- papillary muscle dysfunction
- end-stage cardiomyopathy
- myocardial wall rupture.

Other offenders

Other causes include myocarditis, pericarditis, and depression of myocardial contractility after cardiac arrest and prolonged cardiac surgery. Mechanical abnormalities of the ventricle, such as acute mitral or aortic insufficiency or an acutely acquired ventricular septal defect or ventricular aneurysm, may also result in cardiogenic shock.

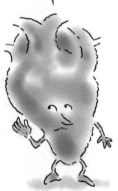

Did I hear that right? Cardiogenic shock occurs in 6% to 7% of patients with acute MI.

How it happens

Regardless of the cause, here's what happens:
• Left ventricular dysfunction initiates a series of compensatory mechanisms that attempt to increase cardiac output and, in turn, maintain vital organ function.
• If cardiogenic shock results from an acute MI, a systemic inflammatory response syndrome may occur, possibly resulting in delayed pumping recovery (stunned myocardium).
• As cardiac output falls, baroreceptors in the aorta and carotid arteries initiate responses in the sympathetic nervous system. These responses, in turn, increase heart rate, left ventricular filling pressure, and peripheral resistance to flow to enhance venous return to the heart.
• These compensatory responses initially stabilize the patient but later cause him to deteriorate as the oxygen demands of the already compromised heart increase.

Lower and lower output

The events involved in cardiogenic shock comprise a vicious cycle of low cardiac output, sympathetic compensation, myocardial ischemia, and even lower cardiac output.

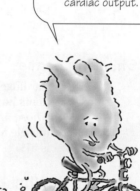

Cardiogenic shock begins a cycle that increasingly lowers cardiac output.

What to look for

Cardiogenic shock produces signs of poor tissue perfusion, such as:
• cold, pale, clammy skin
• drop in systolic blood pressure to 30 mm Hg below baseline or a sustained reading below 90 mm Hg that isn't attributable to medication
• tachycardia
• rapid, shallow respirations
• oliguria (urine output less than 20 ml/hour)
• restlessness and anxiety
• confusion
• narrowing pulse pressure
• cyanosis
• gallop murmur, faint heart sounds and, possibly, a holosystolic murmur.

What tests tell you

• Hemodynamic pressure monitoring reveals increased PAP, PAWP, and RVEDVI reflecting an increase in left ventricular end-diastolic pressure (preload) and heightened resistance to left ventricular emptying (afterload) caused by ineffective pumping and increased peripheral vascular resistance. Thermodilution

Interpreting hemodynamic parameters in cardiogenic shock

This chart can help you quickly determine hemodynamic parameters associated with cardiogenic shock.

Parameter	Values associated with cardiogenic shock
Right atrial pressure	6 to 10 mm Hg
Right ventricular pressure	40 to 50/6 to 15 mm Hg
Pulmonary artery pressure	50/25 to 30 mm Hg
Pulmonary artery wedge pressure	25 to 40 mm Hg
Systemic vascular resistance	>1,200 dynes/sec/cm^5
Mixed venous oxygen saturation	50%
Cardiac output	<4 L/minute
Cardiac index	<1.5 L/minute/m^2

catheterization reveals a reduced cardiac index. (See *Interpreting hemodynamic parameters in cardiogenic shock.*)

• Invasive arterial pressure monitoring shows systolic arterial pressure less than 90 mm Hg caused by impaired ventricular ejection.

• Arterial blood gas (ABG) analysis may show metabolic and respiratory acidosis and hypoxemia.

• ECG demonstrates possible evidence of acute MI, ischemia, or ventricular aneurysm.

• Echocardiography is used to determine left ventricular function and reveals valvular abnormalities.

• Serum enzyme measurements display elevated levels of cardiac tropinin I and T, CK, aspartate aminotransferase, and alanine aminotransferase, which indicate MI or ischemia and suggest heart failure or shock. CK-MB (an isoenzyme of CK that occurs in cardiac tissue) may confirm acute MI. An increased brain natriuretic peptide level may indicate heart failure and help predict survival.

• Cardiac catheterization and echocardiography may reveal other conditions that can lead to pump dysfunction and failure, such as cardiac tamponade, papillary muscle infarct or rupture, ventricular septal rupture, pulmonary emboli, venous pooling (associated with vasodilators and continuous or intermittent positive-pressure breathing), and hypovolemia.

How it's treated

The goal of treatment is to enhance cardiovascular status by increasing cardiac output, improving myocardial perfusion, and decreasing cardiac workload. Treatment consists of administering a combination of cardiovascular drugs and mechanical-assist techniques.

Treatment ABCs

Treatment begins with these measures:
• maintaining a patent airway, including preparing for intubation and mechanical ventilation if the patient develops respiratory distress
• administering supplemental oxygen to increase oxygenation
• continuous cardiac monitoring to detect changes in heart rate and rhythm; administration of antiarrhythmics as necessary
• initiating and maintaining at least two I.V. lines with large-gauge needles for fluid and drug administration
• administering I.V. fluids, crystalloids, colloids, or blood products, as necessary, to maintain intravascular volume.

Increase flow

Drug therapy may include I.V. dopamine, phenylephrine, or norepinephrine (Levophed) to increase blood pressure and blood flow to kidneys. Inamrinone (Amrinone) or dobutamine—inotropic agents that increase myocardial contractility and cardiac output—are commonly used.

Decrease resistance and pressure

A vasodilator—nitroglycerin or nitroprusside (Nitropress)—may be used with a vasopressor to further improve cardiac output by decreasing peripheral vascular resistance (afterload) and reducing left ventricular end-diastolic pressure (preload). However, the patient's blood pressure must be adequate to support nitroprusside therapy and must be monitored closely. Diuretics also may be used to reduce preload in patients with fluid volume overload. Nesiritide (Natrecor) dilates veins and arteries, reduces PAWP, and improves dyspnea.

Bring in the hardware

Treatment may also include mechanical assistance by intra-aortic balloon pump (IABP) to improve coronary artery perfusion and decrease cardiac workload. The IABP is inserted through the femoral artery into the descending thoracic aorta. The balloon in-

A combo of cardio drugs and mechanical assistance gets me pumped up again.

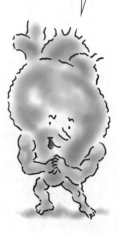

flates during diastole to increase coronary artery perfusion pressure and deflates before systole (before the aortic valve opens) to reduce resistance to ejection (afterload) and therefore reduce cardiac workload.

Improved ventricular ejection significantly improves cardiac output. Subsequent vasodilation in the peripheral vessels leads to lower preload volume and reduced workload of the left ventricle because of decreasing systemic vascular resistance.

End-stage effort

When drug therapy and IABP insertion fail, a ventricular assist device may be inserted to assist the pumping action of the heart. When all other medical and surgical therapies fail, heart transplantation may be considered.

Even more

Additional treatment measures for cardiogenic shock may include:
- thrombolytic therapy or coronary artery revascularization to restore coronary artery blood flow, if cardiogenic shock is due to acute MI
- emergency surgery to repair papillary muscle rupture or ventricular septal defect, if either is the cause of cardiogenic shock.

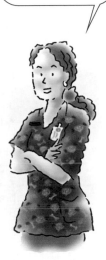

Heart transplantation is the last resort for treatment of cardiogenic shock.

What to do

- Collaborate care with a skilled team, which may include emergency medical personnel, a cardiologist, a nutritional therapist, and a cardiac rehabilitation team.
- Begin I.V. infusions of normal saline solution or lactated Ringer's solution, using a large-bore (16G to 18G) catheter, which allows easier administration of later blood transfusions.
- Administer oxygen by face mask or artificial airway to ensure adequate oxygenation of tissues. Adjust the oxygen flow rate to a higher or lower level, as ABG measurements indicate. Many patients need 100% oxygen, and some require 5 to 15 cm H_2O of positive end-expiratory pressure or continuous positive airway pressure ventilation.

Monitor, record, and then monitor more

- Monitor and record blood pressure, pulse, respiratory rate, and peripheral pulses every 1 to 5 minutes until the patient's condition stabilizes. Monitor cardiac rhythm continuously. Systolic blood pressure less than 90 mm Hg usually results in inadequate coronary artery blood flow, cardiac ischemia, arrhythmias, and further complications of low cardiac output.

• Using a thermodilution catheter, closely monitor PAP, PAWP, RVEDVI, and cardiac output. High PAWP indicates heart failure, increased systemic vascular resistance, decreased cardiac output, and decreased cardiac index and should be reported immediately.
• Determine how much fluid to give by checking blood pressure, urine output, CVP, or PAWP. (To increase accuracy, measure CVP at the level of the right atrium, using the same reference point on the chest each time.) Whenever the fluid infusion rate is increased, watch for signs of fluid overload, such as an increase in PAWP. If the patient is hypovolemic, preload may need to be increased; this is typically accomplished with I.V. fluids. However, I.V. fluids must be given cautiously, increasing them gradually while hemodynamic parameters are closely monitored. In this situation, diuretics aren't given.
• Insert an indwelling urinary catheter to measure hourly urine output. If output is less than 30 ml/hour in adults, increase the fluid infusion rate but watch for signs of fluid overload such as an increase in PAWP. Notify the doctor if urine output doesn't improve.
• Administer a diuretic, such as furosemide (Lasix) or bumetanide (Bumex), as ordered, to decrease preload and improve stroke volume and cardiac output.
• Monitor ABG values, complete blood count, and electrolyte levels. Expect to administer sodium bicarbonate by I.V. push if the patient is acidotic. Administer electrolyte replacement therapy as ordered.
• During therapy, assess skin color and temperature and note any changes. Cold, clammy skin may be a sign of continuing peripheral vascular constriction, indicating progressive shock.

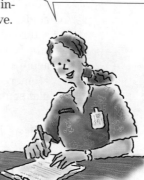

Report high PAWP readings, which may indicate complications such as heart failure and fluid overload.

Minimize movement

• During use of the IABP, move the patient as little as possible. Never flex the "ballooned" leg at the hip because this may displace or kink the catheter. Never place the patient in a sitting position for any reason (including chest X-rays) while the balloon is inflated because the balloon will tear through the aorta and result in immediate death.
• Also during use of the IABP, assess leg pulses and skin temperature and color to ensure adequate peripheral circulation. Check the dressing over the insertion site frequently for bleeding, and change it according to facility protocol. Also check the site for hematoma or signs of infection, and culture any drainage.
• If the patient becomes hemodynamically stable, gradually reduce the frequency of balloon inflation to wean him from the IABP.

• When weaning the patient from the IABP, watch for ECG changes, chest pain, decreased cardiac output, and other signs of recurring cardiac ischemia as well as for shock.
• Prepare the patient for possible emergency cardiac catheterization to determine eligibility for percutaneous transluminal coronary angioplasty or coronary artery bypass grafting to restore blood flow to areas with reversible injury patterns.

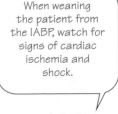

When weaning the patient from the IABP, watch for signs of cardiac ischemia and shock.

Provide regular rest and support

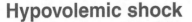

• To ease emotional stress, plan care measures to allow frequent rest periods and provide as much privacy as possible. Allow family members to visit, and comfort the patient as much as possible.
• Because the patient and his family may be anxious about the intensive care unit and about the IABP and other devices, offer explanations and reassurance.
• Prepare the patient and his family for a possible fatal outcome, and help them find effective coping strategies. Assist in discussing end-of-life issues.
• Document vital signs, hemodynamic parameters, and assessment findings. Document the patient's response to treatment and patient and family wishes associated with patient care.

Hypovolemic shock

Hypovolemic shock most commonly results from acute blood loss—about 20% of total volume. Without sufficient blood or fluid replacement, hypovolemic shock may lead to irreversible damage to organs and systems.

Acute blood loss can lead to hypovolemic shock.

What causes it

Massive volume loss may result from:
• GI bleeding, internal or external hemorrhage, or any condition that reduces circulating intravascular volume or other body fluids
• intestinal obstruction
• peritonitis
• acute pancreatitis
• ascites
• dehydration from excessive perspiration, severe diarrhea or protracted vomiting, diabetes insipidus, diuresis, or inadequate fluid intake.

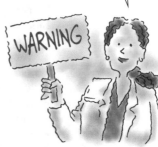

WARNING

How it happens

Potentially life-threatening, hypovolemic shock stems from reduced intravascular blood volume, which leads to decreased cardiac output and inadequate tissue perfusion. The subsequent tissue anoxia prompts a shift in cellular metabolism from aerobic to anaerobic pathways. This results in an accumulation of lactic acid, which produces metabolic acidosis.

The road to shockville

When compensatory mechanisms fail, hypovolemic shock occurs in this sequence:

☝ decreased intravascular fluid volume

✌ diminished venous return, which reduces preload and decreases stroke volume

🖐 reduced cardiac output

🖐 decreased mean arterial pressure (MAP)

🖐 impaired tissue perfusion

🖐 👋 decreased oxygen and nutrient delivery to cells

🖐 👋 multiple-organ-dysfunction syndrome.

What to look for

The specific signs and symptoms exhibited by the patient depend on the amount of fluid loss. (See *Estimating fluid loss.*)

Where, oh where, has the blood volume gone?

Typically, the patient's history includes conditions that reduce blood volume, such as GI hemorrhage, trauma, and severe diarrhea and vomiting.

Assessment findings may include:
• pale skin
• decreased sensorium
• rapid, shallow respirations
• urine output below 25 ml/hour
• rapid, thready peripheral pulses
• cold, clammy skin
• MAP below 60 mm Hg and a narrowing pulse pressure
• decreased CVP, right atrial pressure, PAWP, and cardiac output.

Advice from the experts

Estimating fluid loss

Use the following assessment parameters to determine the severity of fluid loss.

Minimal fluid loss

Signs and symptoms of minimal fluid loss include:
- slight tachycardia
- normal supine blood pressure
- positive postural vital signs, including a decrease in systolic blood pressure > 10 mm Hg or an increase in pulse rate > 20 beats/minute
- increased capillary refill time > 3 seconds

- urine output > 30 ml/hour
- cool, pale skin on arms and legs
- anxiety.

Moderate fluid loss

Signs and symptoms of moderate fluid loss include:
- rapid, thready pulse
- supine hypotension
- cool truncal skin
- urine output of 10 to 30 ml/hour
- severe thirst
- restlessness, confusion, or irritability.

Severe fluid loss

Signs and symptoms of severe fluid loss include:
- marked tachycardia
- marked hypotension
- weak or absent peripheral pulses
- cold, mottled, or cyanotic skin
- urine output < 10 ml/hour
- unconsciousness.

What tests tell you

No single diagnostic test confirms hypovolemic shock, but these test results help to support the diagnosis:
- decreased hemoglobin (Hb) level
- low hematocrit (HCT)
- decreased red blood cell and platelet counts
- coagulation studies for coagulopathy from disseminated intravascular coagulation
- elevated serum potassium, sodium, LD, creatinine, and blood urea nitrogen levels
- increased urine specific gravity (greater than 1.020) and urine osmolality
- urine sodium levels less than 50 mEq/L
- decreased urine creatinine levels
- decreased pH and partial pressure of arterial oxygen and increased partial pressure of arterial carbon dioxide
- gastroscopy, X-rays, aspiration of gastric contents through a nasogastric tube, and tests for occult blood.

How it's treated

Emergency treatment relies on prompt and adequate fluid and blood replacement to restore intravascular volume and to raise blood pressure and maintain it above 90 mm Hg. Rapid infusion of normal saline or lactated Ringer's solution and, possibly, albumin or other plasma expanders may expand volume adequately until whole blood can be matched. (See *When blood pressure drops.*)

Fashion forward

Treatment may also include application of a pneumatic anti-shock garment (although controversial), oxygen administration, control of bleeding, dopamine or another inotropic drug, and surgery, if appropriate.

What to do

• Collaborate care with a skilled team, which may include emergency medical personnel, a doctor, and nutritional and physical therapists.
• Assess the patient for the extent of fluid loss, and begin fluid replacement as ordered. Obtain a type and crossmatch for blood component therapy.

ABCs and ABGs

• Assess airway, breathing, and circulation (ABCs). If the patient experiences cardiac or respiratory arrest, start cardiopulmonary resuscitation.
• Administer supplemental oxygen as ordered. Monitor oxygen saturation and ABG studies for evidence of hypoxemia, and

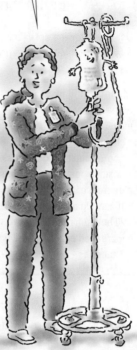

Fluid and blood replacement is the first step in treating hypovolemic shock.

Advice from the experts

When blood pressure drops

A drop below 90 mm Hg in systolic blood pressure usually signals inadequate cardiac output from reduced intravascular volume. Such a drop usually results in inadequate coronary artery blood flow, cardiac ischemia, arrhythmias, and other complications of low cardiac output.

Increase flow and go
If systolic blood pressure drops below 90 mm Hg and the patient's pulse is thready, increase the oxygen flow rate and notify the doctor immediately.

anticipate the need for ET intubation and mechanical ventilation should the patient's respiratory status deteriorate. Place the patient in semi-Fowler's position to maximize chest expansion. Keep the patient as quiet and comfortable as possible to minimize oxygen demands.

• Monitor vital signs, neurologic status, and cardiac rhythm continuously for such changes as cardiac arrhythmias or myocardial ischemia. Observe skin color and check capillary refill. Notify the doctor if capillary refill is greater than 2 seconds.

• Monitor hemodynamic parameters, including CVP, PAWP, and cardiac output, frequently—as often as every 15 minutes—to evaluate the patient's status and response to treatment.

• Monitor intake and output closely. Insert an indwelling urinary catheter and assess urine output hourly. If bleeding from the GI tract is the suspected cause, check all stools, emesis, and gastric drainage for occult blood. If output falls below 30 ml/hour in an adult, expect to increase the I.V. fluid infusion rate, but watch for signs of fluid overload, such as elevated PAWP. Notify the doctor if urine output doesn't increase.

• Administer blood component therapy as ordered; monitor serial Hb values and HCT to evaluate the effects of treatment.

• Administer dopamine or norepinephrine I.V., as ordered, to increase cardiac contractility and renal perfusion.

Clot concerns

• Watch for signs of impending coagulopathy (such as petechiae, bruising, and bleeding or oozing from the gums or venipuncture sites), and report them immediately.

• Provide emotional support and reassurance appropriately in the wake of massive fluid losses.

• Prepare the patient for surgery as appropriate. Explain the treatment needed as well as expectations for the patient's condition after surgery.

• Document vital signs and assessment findings. Note the patient's response to treatment.

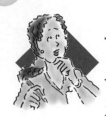

Quick quiz

See if you can hit the mark with this Quick quiz!

1. What's the most common site of injury from blunt chest trauma?
    A.   Aorta
    B.   Left ventricle
    C.   Superior vena cava
    D.   Right ventricle

Answer: D. Because of its location directly behind the sternum, the right ventricle is the most common site of injury from a blunt chest trauma.

2. What's the immediate goal of treatment for cardiac tamponade?
    A.   Relieving pain
    B.   Alleviating anxiety
    C.   Improving mobility
    D.   Relieving intrapericardial pressure

Answer: D. The goal of treatment is to relieve intrapericardial pressure and cardiac compression by removing accumulated blood or fluid.

3. Emergency treatment of hypovolemic shock includes:
    A.   administration of antibiotics.
    B.   administration of I.V. fluid or blood products.
    C.   relief of pain.
    D.   administration of vasodilators.

Answer: B. Emergency treatment relies on prompt and adequate fluid and blood replacement to restore intravascular volume and to raise systolic blood pressure and maintain it above 90 mm Hg. Rapid infusion of normal saline or lactated Ringer's solution and, possibly, albumin or other plasma expanders may expand volume adequately until whole blood can be matched.

Scoring

★★★   If you answered all three questions correctly, perfect! To be blunt, your response to this chapter is penetrating.

★★   If you answered two questions correctly, terrific! You've suffered no traumas learning this chapter.

★   If you answered only one question correctly, it's no emergency. Rereading the chapter will keep complications to a minimum.

Appendices and index

Practice makes perfect

1. The nurse is developing a teaching plan that describes the events involved with the cardiac cycle. Order the events in the correct sequence of occurrence beginning with systole. Use all of the options.

1.	Atrial kick

2.	Isovolumetric relaxation

3.	Ventricular filling

4.	Isovolumetric ventricular contraction

5.	Ventricular ejection

2. The nurse is assessing a client's arterial pulses using a head-to-toe approach. Which pulse would the nurse palpate first?
  1. Radial
  2. Popliteal
  3   Femoral
  4. Brachial

3. Which symptoms would the nurse be most likely to find in a client with arterial insufficiency? Select all that apply.
  1. Pitting edema
  2. Diminished pulses
  3. Cool and pale skin
  4. Thickened, ridged toenails

4. The nurse is preparing to auscultate a client's heart sounds. Identify the area where the nurse should place the stethoscope to hear S_2 at its loudest.

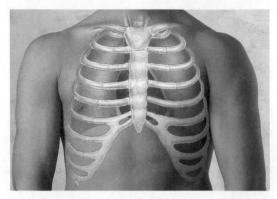

5. When providing care for a client who has had an acute myocardial infarction (MI), the nurse reviews the client's laboratory tests results. Which test results would be most useful for the nurse to review? Select all that apply.
    1. CK-MB
    2. Creatinine
    3. Homocysteine
    4. Myoglobin
    5. Troponin I
    6. B-type natriuretic peptide

6. A client is receiving warfarin (Coumadin) therapy for treatment and prevention of deep vein thrombophlebitis after having received heparin therapy. On which day would the nurse first identify that a therapeutic level of warfarin has been achieved?

LAB RESULTS		
Daily coagulation times		
Day	**Prothrombin time**	**Partial thromboplastin time**
1	10 seconds	52.5 seconds
2	12 seconds	42.5 seconds
3	16 seconds	35 seconds
4	18 seconds	30 seconds
5	20 seconds	22 seconds

    1. Day 1
    2. Day 2
    3. Day 3
    4. Day 4

7. A client is to receive cardiac monitoring via telemetry using the lead MCL_1. Identify the area where the nurse would apply the ground electrode when using three electrodes.

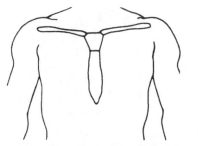

8. The client has a cardiac output of 6.5 L/minute and a body surface area of 1.6 m^2. The client's heart rate is 78 beats/minute. What would the nurse record as the client's cardiac index? Record your answer to one decimal place.

_____ L/minute/m^2

9. A client at risk for developing deep vein thrombophlebitis is to receive prophylactic intermittent heparin therapy. The physician orders 5,000 units subcutaneously every 12 hours. The label on the heparin vial from the pharmacy reads: 10,000 units/ml. How many milliliters would the nurse prepare to administer each dose? Record your answer to one decimal place.

_____ ml

10. When evaluating the rhythm strip of a client, the nurse determines that the client is experiencing premature atrial contractions (PACs). Which findings would support the nurse's interpretation? Select all that apply.
1. Absent QRS complexes
2. Irregular atrial and ventricular rates
3. Abnormally shaped P waves
4. Premature P waves
5. Progressive shortening of the P-P interval

11. When defibrillating a client, the paddles are placed anterolaterally. One of the paddles is positioned to the right of the upper sternum. Where would the nurse place the other paddle?
1. Over the fifth or sixth intercostal space at the left anterior axillary line
2. Directly over the heart at the precordium to the left of the lower sternal border
3. Under the client's body beneath the heart and immediately below the scapulae
4. On the right side of the chest on the same level as the nipple line

12. The physician determines that a client who's critically ill and recently admitted to the emergency department requires a pacemaker. The nurse would assist in preparing the client for which type of pacemaker?
1. Permanent
2. Transcutaneous
3. Transvenous
4. Epicardial

13. When reviewing the medical record of a client diagnosed with ventricular tachycardia, what would the nurse expect to be the most likely cause associated with the client's condition?

1. History of rheumatic heart disease
2. Frequent ingestion of large amounts of tea
3. Report of a highly stressful employment environment
4. Cocaine drug intoxication

14. While auscultating a client's chest, the nurse notes a high-pitched blowing murmur occurring throughout systole that's heard best at the apex. The murmur doesn't become louder when the client inhales. The nurse interprets this as:

1. tricuspid insufficiency.
2. mitral insufficiency.
3. aortic stenosis.
4. pulmonic stenosis.

15. While interviewing a client with acute pericarditis, the client describes his complaint of chest pain. Which statement would most likely reflect the pain the client is experiencing?

1. "It feels like someone is putting a huge weight on my chest and I can't breathe."
2. "I feel this burning sensation that happens not long after I eat."
3. "It's the worst pain I've ever felt, like something is tearing inside."
4. "It's sharp and stabbing and gets much worse when I breathe deeply."

16. The nurse is teaching a client diagnosed with prehypertension about ways to modify his lifestyle. Which client statement indicates that the teaching has been effective?

1. "I guess I can eat more steak and less fish, now."
2. "I'll be sure to have two glasses of wine with dinner each night."
3. "I just joined the local health club so that I can exercise at least three times a week."
4. "I can drink water but I need to watch exactly how much I actually drink."

17. A client who's undergoing an exercise stress test develops chest pain and dyspnea. What should the nurse do next?

1. Have the client slow down.
2. Stop the test immediately.
3. Encourage the client to take deep breaths.
4. Administer dipyridamole (Persantine) as ordered.

18. The son of a client who has had a heart transplant asks the nurse, "Why do I have to wear all this stuff, like the gown, when I visit my father?" Which explanation by the nurse would be most appropriate?

1. "You need to be protected from any infections that your father might have developed after the surgery."
2. "Don't worry. These are all just routine procedures after any transplant-type surgery."
3. "Your father is at risk for infection because of the drugs he's receiving to prevent rejection."
4. "You should be more concerned about your father than about what you have to put on to see him."

19. The nurse has just reviewed discharge instructions with a client who has undergone a minimally invasive direct coronary artery bypass. Which statement made by the client indicates the need for further instructions?

1. "I'm so glad that now I don't have to watch what I eat anymore."
2. "I won't lift anything over 10 lb for at least the next 4 weeks."
3. "I should check my incision every day for changes such as redness or swelling."
4. "I'll continue with the exercise program that I was taught to do here."

20. The nurse is participating in a local health fair and is preparing a poster about chest pain in women. Which statement would the nurse include on the poster?

1. The pain is consistently associated with activity.
2. Arm or shoulder pain is more common.
3. The pain is usually crushing in nature.
4. Diarrhea commonly accompanies the pain.

21. Which nursing intervention would be the priority when caring for a client who's experiencing a ruptured aortic aneurysm?

1. Administering analgesics for pain
2. Inserting an indwelling catheter
3. Ensuring a patent airway
4. Administering fluid replacement

22. A client is receiving a digoxin (Lanoxin) as treatment of heart failure. When teaching the client about this medication, the nurse explains that the drug achieves it effects by:

1. reducing total blood volume.
2. dilating the blood vessels.
3. strengthening myocardial contractility.
4. decreasing systemic vascular resistance.

23. A nurse is conducting a staff in-service education program about aortic aneurysms, including the different types. Upon the completion of the program, the nurse asks the group to identify the type of aortic aneurysm that involves an outpouching of the arterial wall. The nurse determines that the teaching has been effective when the group correctly identifies the aneurysm as:

1. fusiform.
2. dissecting.
3. false.
4. saccular.

24. Which assessment finding would lead the nurse to suspect that a client is developing cardiac tamponade?

1. Widening pulse pressure
2. Decreased central venous pressure
3. Pulsus paradoxus
4. Decreased right atrial pressure

25. Assessment of a client with left-sided heart failure reveals dyspnea on exertion, fatigue, weight gain of 5 lb over the last 4 days, swollen ankles, and cough. When developing the care plan for this client, which nursing diagnosis would be the priority?
  1. Imbalanced nutrition: More than body requirements
  2. Excess fluid volume
  3. Deficient knowledge
  4. Activity intolerance

26. A client develops acute atrial fibrillation and is symptomatic. Which intervention would be the priority?
  1. Synchronized cardioversion
  2. Administration of digoxin
  3. Radiofrequency ablation therapy
  4. Atrial overdrive pacing

27. When reviewing a client's electrocardiogram (ECG), the nurse counts the number of small squares between two P waves and divides this number into 1,500. The nurse is determining which parameter?
  1. Atrial rhythm
  2. Duration of PR interval
  3. Ventricular rate
  4. Atrial rate

28. The nurse is assessing a client who has had a pulmonary artery catheter inserted. Which result would lead the nurse to notify the physician?
  1. Pulmonary artery wedge pressure (PAWP) of 9 mm Hg
  2. Right atrial pressure (RAP) of 4 mm Hg
  3. Systolic pulmonary artery pressure (PAP) of 38 mm Hg
  4. Mean PAP of 16 mm Hg

29. What would the nurse expect to administer as the first-line treatment for a client with dilated cardiomyopathy?
  1. Angiotensin-converting enzyme (ACE) inhibitor
  2. Beta-adrenergic blocker
  3. Cardiac glycoside
  4. Antiarrhythmic

30. When developing the care plan for a client with cardiovascular disease who has a nursing diagnosis of *Activity intolerance*, which intervention would be most appropriate for the nurse to include?
  1. Have the client complete all aspects of care at one time.
  2. Urge the client to consume foods high in calories.
  3. Teach the client about energy conservation measures.
  4. Encourage activity immediately after eating.

31. After teaching a client diagnosed with valvular heart disease about the valves of the heart, the nurse determines that the teaching has been successful when the client identifies which valve as responsible for preventing the backflow of blood into the left ventricle?
  1. Aortic semilunar
  2. Pulmonic semilunar
  3. Tricuspid
  4. Mitral

32. Which client would be at greatest risk for digoxin toxicity?
    1. A client who's experiencing atrial tachycardia
    2. A client who's receiving furosemide (Lasix)
    3. A client who has a history of prehypertension
    4. A client who's receiving simvastatin (Zocor)

33. When assessing the capillary refill of a client, which finding would the nurse document as normal?
    1. 6 seconds
    2. 5 seconds
    3. 4 seconds
    4. 3 seconds

34. While assessing a client's arterial pulses, the nurse notes that the amplitude increases and decreases with the client's inspiration and expiration. The nurse documents this finding as:
    1. pulsus alternans.
    2. pulsus bigeminus.
    3. pulsus paradoxus.
    4. pulsus biferiens.

35. A client has just returned after undergoing insertion of an intra-aortic balloon pump (IABP) for counterpulsation. Which intervention would be most appropriate?
    1. Elevating the head of the client's bed to at least 45 degrees
    2. Monitoring pulses every 2 hours
    3. Encouraging active range-of-motion (ROM) exercises of all joints of the four extremities every hour
    4. Applying direct pressure to catheter insertion site if bleeding occurs

36. A client comes to the health care facility for a follow-up visit because his blood pressure was 132/84 mm Hg. On this visit, his blood pressure is 138/88 mm Hg. He states, "When I saw the doctor a couple of months ago, my blood pressure was 122/80 mm Hg." The nurse interprets this finding to suggest that the client is experiencing:
    1. normal blood pressure.
    2. prehypertension.
    3. stage 1 hypertension.
    4. stage 2 hypertension.

37. When planning the care for a client with left-sided heart failure, which outcome would be most appropriate to include as part of the care plan?
    1. Client exhibits a weight gain of 2 to 3 lb per week.
    2. Client verbalizes understanding about the need for strict bed rest.
    3. Client demonstrates the ability to monitor pulse rate and rhythm.
    4. Client describes the need for ingestion of high-fiber foods.

38. When teaching a class on health promotion and cardiovascular disease prevention to a local community group, the nurse focuses on ways to address the common causes of sudden death. What would the nurse include as the most common cause?
    1. Cardiomyopathy
    2. Hypertension
    3. Cardiogenic shock
    4. Coronary artery disease (CAD)

39. The nurse is preparing a client for an echocardiogram. Which statement indicates that the client has understood the nurse's teaching?

1. "I'll have to lie really still during the test and will probably hear a banging noise."
2. "A device placed on my chest picks up sound waves that are recorded."
3. "A radioactive substance will be injected into my vein to show the injured area."
4. "A device attached to a scope is inserted into my esophagus to take pictures of my heart."

40. Which client would the nurse expect to be discharged first?

1. A client who has had a percutaneous transluminal coronary angioplasty (PTCA)
2. A client who has undergone a minimally invasive direct coronary artery bypass
3. A client who has had an aortic valve replacement
4. A client who has undergone repair of an aortic aneurysm

41. The nurse would be especially alert for which adverse effects in a client receiving carotid sinus massage?

1. Atrial arrhythmias
2. Signs of vasoconstriction
3. Decreased heart rate
4. Hypertension

42. The rhythm strip of a client reveals that the atrial rate is greater than the ventricular rate, the P wave appears saw-toothed in shape, the T wave can't be identified, and the QT interval can't be measured. The nurse interprets this waveform as:

1. atrial fibrillation.
2. atrial flutter.
3. ventricular tachycardia.
4. ventricular fibrillation.

43. Which nursing diagnosis would be the priority for a client who develops cardiogenic shock?

1. Activity intolerance related to increased metabolic demands
2. Risk for injury related to invasive treatment methods
3. Deficient knowledge related to complication development
4. Decreased cardiac output related to pump failure

44. A 36-year-old client is brought to the emergency department after being stabbed in the upper chest near the sternum. The client is diagnosed with cardiac trauma. The nurse would continuously monitor the client for signs and symptoms of:

1. infection.
2. cardiomyopathy.
3. cardiac tamponade.
4. cardiogenic shock.

45. The nurse is preparing a presentation about risk reduction and coronary artery disease (CAD) for a health fair at a local facility. The nurse is planning to discuss the role of lipids in contributing to a person's risk. Which statement would be most appropriate for the nurse to include in the presentation?

1. Elevated high-density lipoprotein (HDL) levels are associated with an increased risk for developing CAD.
2. Triglycerides are the key to determining a person's risk for CAD.
3. Total cholesterol levels greater than 240 mg/dl are considered normal for adults.
4. Elevated low-density lipoprotein (LDL) levels are associated with an increased risk for developing CAD.

46. A client's electrocardiogram strip reveals asystole. Which action would be initiated first?

1. Administration of epinephrine I.V. push
2. Cardiopulmonary resuscitation (CPR)
3. Administration of atropine I.V.
4. Endotracheal (ET) intubation

47. The nurse is auscultating a client's heart sounds and places the stethoscope at the mitral valve area. What best describes this location?

1. Third intercostal space at the left sternal border
2. Second intercostal space at the right sternal border
3. Second intercostal space at the left sternal border
4. Fifth intercostal space near the midclavicular line

48. A client in asystole is receiving atropine 1 mg I.V. that's being repeated every 3 to 5 minutes to a maximum dose of 0.04 mg/kg. The client weighs 154 lb. How many milligrams could the client receive as his maximum dose? Record your answer to one decimal place.

_____ mg

49. A client is to receive heparin 1,000 units/hour via an I.V. infusion as treatment for deep vein thrombophlebitis. The pharmacy supplies a 500-ml bag containing 50,000 units of heparin. The nurse is using an infusion pump. The nurse would set the infusion pump to administer how many milliliters per hour?

1. 150
2. 100
3. 50
4. 10

50. What would alert the nurse to a possible arterial occlusion in a client who has undergone a vascular repair of an aneurysm?

1. Decreased urine output
2. Severely diminished or absent peripheral pulses
3. Tachycardia
4. Shallow respirations

Answers

1.

4.	Isovolumetric ventricular contraction

5.	Ventricular ejection

2.	Isovolumetric relaxation

3.	Ventricular filling

1.	Atrial kick

The cardiac cycle consists of five events occurring in sequence: isovolumetric ventricular contraction (in response to ventricular depolarization leading to closure of the mitral and tricuspid valves); ventricular ejection (increased ventricular pressure exceeds aortic and pulmonary arterial pressure leading to the opening of the aortic and pulmonic valves with the ventricles ejecting blood); isovolumetric relaxation (in response to falling pressure leading to closure of the aortic and pulmonic valves and blood filling the atria); ventricular filling (increased atrial pressure exceeding ventricular pressure leading to the opening of the mitral and tricuspid valves with passive blood flow into the ventricles); and atrial kick (or systole, which supplies the ventricles with the remaining blood for each heartbeat).

> Client needs category: Physiological integrity
> Client needs subcategory: Physiological adaptation
> Cognitive level: Comprehension

2. 4. When assessing a client's pulses using a head-to-toe approach, the nurse would first palpate the brachial pulse (at the biceps tendon) and then radial pulse (at the wrist). Next, the nurse would assess the femoral pulse (groin area), followed by the popliteal pulse (at the back of the knee).

> Client needs category: Health promotion and maintenance
> Client needs subcategory: None
> Cognitive level: Application

3. 2, 3, 4. Typical findings associated with arterial insufficiency include diminished or absent pulses; cool, pale shiny skin; pain in legs and feet; ulcerations usually around the toes; and thick, ridged nails. Pitting edema is most commonly associated with chronic venous insufficiency.

> Client needs category: Physiological integrity
> Client needs subcategory: Physiological adaptation
> Cognitive level: Application

4.

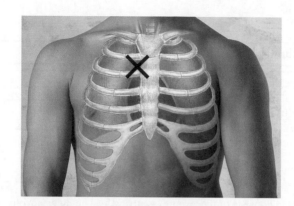

S_2 is loudest at the aortic area, which is located at the second intercostal space to the right of the client's sternum.

 Client needs category: Health promotion and maintenance
 Client needs subcategory: None
 Cognitive level: Application

5.　1, 4, 5. CK-MB is an isoenzyme found specifically in heart muscle that, if increased, reliably indicates an acute MI. Rising myoglobin levels may be the first marker of cardiac injury after an acute MI. Troponin I, an isotope of the protein troponin, is found only in the myocardium and is a highly specific indicator of myocardial damage. Creatinine levels assess renal glomerular filtration and screen for renal damage. Homocysteine is an amino acid produced by the body and, when elevated, can irritate blood vessels leading to atherosclerosis and increase coagulation, which increases the risk of vessel blockages. However, it isn't a reliable indicator of myocardial damage. B-type natriuretic peptide is a hormone secreted by ventricular tissue as a response to increased ventricular volume and pressure that occurs with heart failure.

 Client needs category: Physiological integrity
 Client needs subcategory: Reduction of risk potential
 Cognitive level: Analysis

6.　3. To evaluate the therapeutic effect of warfarin, the nurse would monitor the client's prothrombin time (PT). Normally, PT ranges from 10 to 14 seconds. In a client receiving warfarin therapy, the goal is to achieve a PT level of 1.5 to 2 times the normal value, or a level of 15 to 20. Day 3 was the first day in which the PT level was within the therapeutic range. Partial thromboplastin time is used to monitor the effectiveness of heparin therapy and isn't affected by warfarin.

 Client needs category: Physiological integrity
 Client needs subcategory: Reduction of risk potential
 Cognitive level: Application

7.

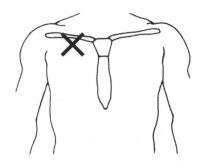

The ground electrode for a three-electrode system would be placed on the client's upper right chest below the clavicle for lead MCL_1. The positive electrode would be placed at the client's midchest just to the right of the sternum. The negative electrode would be placed on the client's upper left chest below the clavicle.

Client needs category: Physiological integrity
Client needs subcategory: Reduction of risk potential
Cognitive level: Application

8. 4.1. Cardiac index is calculated by dividing the client's cardiac output by his body surface area. In this case, 6.5 L/minute divided by 1.6 m², which yields 4.1 L/minute/m².

Client needs category: Physiological integrity
Client needs subcategory: Physiological adaptation
Cognitive level: Analysis

9. 0.5. The vial contains 10,000 units in 1 milliliter. The physician has ordered 5,000 units.

Setting up a proportion:

$$10,000/1 = 5,000/X$$
$$10,000X = 5,000$$

Solving for X:

$$X = 5,000/10,000$$
$$X = 5/10 \text{ or } 0.5 \text{ ml}$$

Client needs category: Physiological integrity
Client needs subcategory: Pharmacological and parenteral therapies
Cognitive level: Analysis

10. 2, 3, 4. The hallmark characteristic of a PAC is a premature P wave with an abnormal configuration; the P wave may be lost in the previous T wave. Atrial and ventricular rates are also irregular. Absent QRS complexes are associated with sinus arrest. Progressive shortening of the P-P interval is associated with second degree sinoatrial type 1 block.

Client needs category: Physiological integrity
Client needs subcategory: Reduction of risk potential
Cognitive level: Analysis

11. 1. For anterolateral placement, one paddle is placed to the right of the upper sternum just below the right clavicle and the other paddle is placed over the fifth or sixth intercostal space at the left anterior axillary line. For anteroposterior placement, the anterior paddle is placed directly over the heart at the precordium, to the left of the lower sternal border. The posterior paddle is placed under the client's body beneath the heart

and immediately below the scapula. Placing the paddle on the right side of the chest at the nipple line is inappropriate for either method of defibrillator paddle placement.

    Client needs category: Physiological integrity
    Client needs subcategory: Physiological adaptation
    Cognitive level: Comprehension

12. 2. In a life-threatening situation a transcutaneous pacemaker is the best choice because it's quick and effective. However, it's used only until transvenous or permanent pacing can be implemented. Epicardial pacing is used during cardiac surgery.

    Client needs category: Physiological integrity
    Client needs subcategory: Physiological adaptation
    Cognitive level: Application

13. 4. Drug intoxication, such as from cocaine, digoxin (Lanoxin), procainamide (Procanbid) or quinidine, can cause ventricular tachycardia. A history of rheumatic heart disease is associated with junctional arrhythmias. Use of coffee, alcohol or cigarettes, fatigue or stress, and use of such drugs as aminophylline and digoxin (Lanoxin) are causes associated with atrial fibrillation.

    Client needs category: Physiological integrity
    Client needs subcategory: Physiological adaptation
    Cognitive level: Comprehension

14. 2. With mitral insufficiency, blood regurgitates into the left atrium producing a high-pitched, blowing murmur throughout systole that's best heart at the apex. The murmur associated with tricuspid insufficiency causes a high-pitched, blowing murmur throughout systole in the tricuspid area that becomes louder when the client inhales. Aortic stenosis causes a midsystolic, low-pitched, harsh murmur that radiates from the valve to the carotid artery and shifts from crescendo to decrescendo and back. Pulmonic stenosis causes a medium-pitched, systolic, harsh murmur that shifts from crescendo to decrescendo and back.

    Client needs category: Physiological integrity
    Client needs subcategory: Physiological adaptation
    Cognitive level: Analysis

15. 4. The client with acute pericarditis typically complains of sharp, sudden pain usually starting over the sternum and radiating to the neck, shoulders, back, and arms. The pain is usually pleuritic and increases with deep inspiration and decreases when the client sits up and leans forward. Feelings of pressure, squeezing, heaviness or tightness are commonly associated with the pain of angina pectoris or acute myocardial infarction. A burning sensation soon after eating is typical of peptic ulcer disease. Excruciating, tearing pain is associated with a dissecting aortic aneurysm.

    Client needs category: Physiological integrity
    Client needs subcategory: Physiological adaptation
    Cognitive level: Application

16. 3. Lifestyle modifications include changes in diet, adoption of relaxation techniques, regular exercise, smoking cessation, limited alcohol intake, and restriction of sodium and saturated fats. The client's statement about exercising three times a week indicates that he has understood the nurse's instructions. Steak is a red meat that's high in saturated fats and should be limited. Wine is alcohol and should also be limited. Restricting the intake of water isn't appropriate; adequate water intake is necessary to maintain hydration and fluid balance.

Client needs category: Health promotion and maintenance
Client needs subcategory: None
Cognitive level: Analysis

17. 2. If the client experiences chest pain, fatigue, or other signs of exercise intolerance, such as dyspnea, claudication, weakness, dizziness, hypotension, pallor or vasoconstriction, disorientation, ataxia, or electrocardiogram changes indicating ischemia, disturbed rhythm, or heart block, the nurse must stop the test immediately to prevent further complications. Having the client slow down or encouraging him to take deep breaths is inappropriate. Dipyridamole is a coronary vasodilator used to stress a heart for a drug-induced stress test. Administration at this time would be contraindicated because it would further stress the heart.

Client needs category: Physiological integrity
Client needs subcategory: Reduction of risk potential
Cognitive level: Application

18. 3. A client who has had a heart transplant receives potent immunosuppressants to prevent rejection but that also increase his risk for infection. Therefore, use of protective equipment, such as gowns, is necessary to prevent exposing the client to potential sources of infection. The infection control precautions protect the client, not the client's son. Telling the client's son not to worry doesn't address the son's concern. Telling the son to be more concerned about his father is condescending and derogatory.

Client needs category: Safe, effective care environment
Client needs subcategory: Safety and infection control
Cognitive level: Application

19. 1. After a minimally invasive direct coronary artery bypass, clients need to continue to follow dietary restrictions, such as limiting their intake of sodium and cholesterol, to help reduce the risk of recurrent arterial occlusion. The client should refrain from lifting objects weighing over 10 lb for 4 to 6 weeks, check the incision site daily, and continue with the progressive exercises that he was taught.

Client needs category: Physiological integrity
Client needs subcategory: Reduction of risk potential
Cognitive level: Analysis

20. 2. Women are more likely to experience arm or shoulder pain in contrast to men, who tend to complain of crushing chest pain in the center of the chest. Women with coronary artery disease may experience classic chest pain that may occur without any relationship to activity or stress. However, they commonly experience atypical chest pain, vague chest pain, or no chest pain. Women may also complain of jaw, neck, or throat pain, toothache, back pain, or pain under the breastbone or in the stomach. Other symptoms women may experience include nausea, dizziness, shortness of breath, unexplained anxiety, weakness or fatigue, palpitations, cold sweat, or paleness. Diarrhea isn't typically associated with chest pain in women.

Client needs category: Health promotion and maintenance
Client needs subcategory: None
Cognitive level: Comprehension

21. 3. Rupture of an aortic aneurysm is a medical emergency requiring prompt treatment. The priority is to ensure that the client's airway is patent. Then other interventions, such as fluid replacement, analgesic administration for pain, and urinary catheter insertion can be initiated afterward.

> Client needs category: Safe, effective care environment
> Client needs subcategory: Management of care
> Cognitive level: Application

22. 3. Digoxin is a cardiac glycoside that acts to strengthen myocardial contractility. Diuretics reduce preload by decreasing total blood volume and circulatory congestion. Angiotensin-converting enzyme inhibitors dilate blood vessels and decrease systemic vascular resistance.

> Client needs category: Physiological integrity
> Client needs subcategory: Pharmacological and parenteral therapies
> Cognitive level: Comprehension

23. 4. A saccular aneurysm is one that involves an outpouching of the arterial wall. A fusiform aneurysm involves a spindle-shaped enlargement encompassing the entire aortic circumference. A dissecting aneurysm involves a hemorrhagic separation in the aortic wall usually within the medial layer. A false aneurysm occurs when the entire wall is injured, resulting in a break in all the layers of the arterial wall.

> Client needs category: Physiological integrity
> Client needs subcategory: Physiological adaptation
> Cognitive level: Analysis

24. 3. Cardiac tamponade has three classic features: pulsus paradoxus, muffled heart sounds, and elevated central venous pressure with jugular vein distention. In addition, right atrial pressure would be increased.

> Client needs category: Physiological integrity
> Client needs subcategory: Physiological adaptation
> Cognitive level: Application

25. 2. The client described has experienced a significant weight gain along with swelling of the ankles. The client is most likely experiencing fluid overload secondary to the left-sided heart failure. The priority nursing diagnosis would be *Excess fluid volume. Activity intolerance* and *Deficient knowledge* are appropriate nursing diagnoses for the client with heart failure, but aren't the priority. The client is experiencing weight gain due to the excess fluid, not excess intake. *Imbalanced nutrition* may be appropriate later in the course of the client's care if excessive caloric intake were an additional underlying problem.

> Client needs category: Physiological integrity
> Client needs subcategory: Physiological adaptation
> Cognitive level: Analysis

26. 1. If a client is symptomatic with acute atrial fibrillation, immediate synchronized cardioversion is necessary. Drugs such as digoxin, beta-adrenergic blockers, and calcium channel blockers can be given after successful cardioversion to maintain normal sinus rhythm and control the ventricular rate. Radiofrequency ablation therapy is used for symptom-producing atrial fibrillation that doesn't respond to routine treatment. Atrial overdrive pacing is appropriate therapy to stop atrial tachycardia.

> Client needs category: Physiological integrity
> Client needs subcategory: Reduction of risk potential
> Cognitive level: Comprehension

27. 4. The atrial rate is determined by counting the number of small squares between the two P waves using either the apex of the wave or the initial upstroke of the wave. (Each small square equals 0.04 second; 1,500 squares equal 1 minute). Then 1,500 is divided by the number of squares counted. Atrial rhythm is determined with calipers to measure the interval between P waves. This measurement is then compared in several ECG cycles to determine if it's regular (same distance) or irregular. The duration of the PR interval is determined by counting the number of small squares between the beginning of the P wave and the beginning of the QRS complex. Then this number is multiplied by 0.04 second. The ventricular rate is determined by counting the number of small squares between two R waves and then using this number divided into 1,500 to arrive at the ventricular rate.

    Client needs category: Physiological integrity
    Client needs subcategory: Reduction of risk potential
    Cognitive level: Comprehension

28. 3. Normal systolic PAP ranges from 20 to 30 mm Hg. A reading above or below this range would warrant notification of the physician. A PAWP of 9 mm Hg is within the normal range of 6 to 12 mm Hg. An RAP of 4 mm Hg is within the acceptable range of 1 to 6 mm Hg. A mean PAP of 16 mm Hg is in the normal range, which is less than 20 mm Hg.

    Client needs category: Physiological integrity
    Client needs subcategory: Reduction of risk potential
    Cognitive level: Analysis

29. 1. ACE inhibitors are considered first-line therapy for clients with dilated cardiomyopathy to help reduce afterload via vasodilation. Other agents may be used, but they aren't considered as first-line therapy. For example, beta-adrenergic blockers may be used to help treat clients who have mild to moderate heart failure. Cardiac glycosides such as digoxin may be used for clients who don't respond to ACE inhibitors and diuretics. Antiarrhythmics may be used cautiously to control arrhythmias.

    Client needs category: Physiological integrity
    Client needs subcategory: Pharmacological and parenteral therapies
    Cognitive level: Application

30. 3. A client with a nursing diagnosis of *Activity intolerance* would need to conserve energy to allow him to be able to perform activities as much as he's capable. Teaching the client about ways to conserve energy would be most helpful. Having the client complete all aspects of care at one time would require an increased expenditure of energy and be tiring. Rather, allowing the client to do some activities and then rest would be more appropriate. Consuming foods high in calories may be helpful to provide the client with energy. However, high-calorie foods can be high in fat and wouldn't be the best choice for a client with cardiovascular disease. Encouraging the client to be active after eating would be inappropriate because it would result in a greater expenditure of energy and oxygen consumption.

    Client needs category: Physiological integrity
    Client needs subcategory: Basic care and comfort
    Cognitive level: Application

31. 1. When closed, the aortic semilunar valve prevents the backflow of blood from the aorta into the left ventricle. The pulmonic semilunar valve prevents backflow of blood from the pulmonary artery into the right ventricle. The tricuspid valve prevents backflow of blood from the right ventricle into the right atrium. The mitral valve prevents backflow of blood from the left ventricle into the left atrium.

Client needs category: Physiological integrity
Client needs subcategory: Physiological adaptation
Cognitive level: Analysis

32. 2. The client taking digoxin in conjunction with furosemide would be at greatest risk for digoxin toxicity. Furosemide is a loop diuretic that also leads to the loss of potassium, predisposing the client to hypokalemia. The risk of digoxin toxicity is increased in a client who's taking digoxin and has hypokalemia. Atrial tachycardia is a common manifestation of digoxin toxicity. A client with a history of prehypertension probably wouldn't be at risk for digoxin toxicity because treatment primarily focuses on lifestyle changes. However, if the client required additional therapy, such as with thiazide-type diuretics, then the combination of digoxin and these agents may increase his risk for toxicity. Use of a lipid-lowering agent (simvastatin) isn't associated with an increased risk for digoxin toxicity.

Client needs category: Physiological integrity
Client needs subcategory: Pharmacological and parenteral therapies
Cognitive level: Application

33. 4. Capillary refill time should be no more than 3 seconds. Any time greater than 3 seconds would be considered abnormal and should be reported.

Client needs category: Physiological integrity
Client needs subcategory: Reduction of risk potential
Cognitive level: Comprehension

34. 3. Pulsus paradoxus has increases and decreases in amplitude associated with the respiratory cycle. Marked decreases occur when the client inhales. Pulsus alternans has a regular, alternating pattern of a weak and strong pulse. Pulsus bigeminus is similar to pulsus alternans but occurs at irregular intervals. Pulsus biferiens is manifested with an initial upstroke, subsequent downstroke, and then another upstroke during systole.

Client needs category: Physiological integrity
Client needs subcategory: Reduction of risk potential
Cognitive level: Comprehension

35. 4. After insertion of the catheter for IABP counterpulsation, the nurse should inspect the insertion site frequently and apply direct pressure to the site if bleeding is noted. The physician should also be notified. The client's head shouldn't be raised more than 30 degrees to prevent upward migration of the catheter and occlusion of the left subclavian artery. Distal pulses should be assessed frequently, such as every 15 minutes for the first 4 hours and then every hour. Active ROM exercises should be encouraged every 2 hours for the upper extremities, unaffected leg, and the ankle of the affected leg.

Client needs category: Physiological integrity
Client needs subcategory: Reduction of risk potential
Cognitive level: Application

36. 2. Blood pressure is classified as normal, prehypertension, or stage 1 or stage 2 hypertension. Classification of prehypertension or hypertension requires an increased blood pressure reading on two or more attempts during two or more visits following an initial screening. The client's blood pressure readings of 132/84 and 138/88 mm Hg fall within the range of prehypertension (systolic blood pressure of 120 to 139 mm Hg; diastolic blood pressure of 80 to 89 mm Hg). Normal systolic blood pressure readings fall below 120 mm Hg and normal diastolic readings fall below 80 mm Hg. Stage 1 hypertension is classified by systolic blood pressure between 140 to 159 mm Hg and diastolic blood pressure between 90 to 99 mm Hg. Stage 2 hypertension is classified by systolic blood pressure greater than or equal to 160 mm Hg and diastolic blood pressure greater than or equal to 100 mm Hg.

> Client needs category: Health promotion and maintenance
> Client needs subcategory: None
> Cognitive level: Application

37. 3. Care for the client with left-sided heart failure commonly involves the use of medications such as cardiac glycosides; for example, digoxin. Clients taking digoxin need to know how to monitor their pulse rate and rhythm and to report any unusually irregular pulse or pulse rate less than 60 beats per minute. The client's demonstration of pulse monitoring is important to ensure that he can perform this skill. A weight gain of 2 to 3 lb per week is inappropriate because the client already has fluid overload. The client needs to balance activity and rest, not remain on strict bed rest. Ingestion of foods high in potassium may be necessary if the client is prescribed a diuretic. Foods high in sodium should also be avoided. High-fiber foods would be important if the client were experiencing constipation.

> Client needs category: Physiological integrity
> Client needs subcategory: Reduction of risk potential
> Cognitive level: Application

38. 4. CAD is the most common cause of sudden death. Cardiomyopathy ranks as the second most common cause. Hypertension is commonly called the silent killer because of its insidious onset. If left untreated, it can cause major complications and death but it isn't typically associated with sudden death. Cardiogenic shock is a serious complication commonly associated with acute myocardial infarction (MI). When the MI involves 40% or more of the ventricular muscle mass, mortality is extremely high.

> Client needs category: Health promotion and maintenance
> Client needs subcategory: None
> Cognitive level: Comprehension

39. 2. An echocardiogram involves the placement of a transducer on the client's chest that directs sound waves toward cardiac structures. The transducer picks up the echoes, converts them to electrical impulses and relays them for display on a screen and for recording on a strip chart or videotape. Lying still and hearing a banging noise are commonly associated with magnetic resonance imaging. Injection of a radioactive substance to show the injured area may be used with hot spot imaging (^{99m}Tc pyrophosphate scanning) or cold spot imaging (thallium scanning). In transesophageal echocardiography, a small transducer is attached to the end of a gastroscope and inserted into the esophagus so that images of the heart's structure can be obtained.

> Client needs category: Physiological integrity
> Client needs subcategory: Reduction of risk potential
> Cognitive level: Analysis

40. 1. A client who has had a PTCA will usually be discharged within 6 to 12 hours after the procedure. After a minimally invasive direct coronary artery bypass, the client may be discharged within 48 hours. Discharge times vary for a client who has had an aortic valve replacement or who has undergone repair of an aortic aneurysm.

Client needs category: Safe, effective care environment
Client needs subcategory: Management of care
Cognitive level: Application

41. 3. Risks associated with carotid sinus massage include decreased heart rate, vasodilation (not vasoconstriction), ventricular (not atrial) arrhythmias, stroke, and cardiac standstill. Hypertension isn't associated with carotid sinus massage.

Client needs category: Physiological integrity
Client needs subcategory: Reduction of risk potential
Cognitive level: Comprehension

42. 2. Atrial flutter is characterized by abnormal P waves that produce a saw-toothed appearance. The atrial rate is greater than the ventricular rate and the QRS complex is usually normal. The T wave can't be identified and the QT interval can't be measured. Atrial fibrillation is characterized by an irregularly irregular rhythm, an indiscernible atrial rate, and absent P waves. Ventricular tachycardia is usually evidenced by absent P waves and wide, bizarre QRS complexes. Ventricular fibrillation is characterized by erratic baseline waves with no recognizable pattern. The rhythm is chaotic, P wave is absent, and T wave can't be identified.

Client needs category: Physiological integrity
Client needs subcategory: Physiological adaptation
Cognitive level: Application

43. 4. Cardiogenic shock is a condition of diminished cardiac output that severely impairs tissue perfusion. Thus, care focuses on restoring the client's cardiac output. Although *Activity intolerance*, *Risk for injury*, and *Deficient knowledge* are possible nursing diagnoses, they wouldn't take precedence over the decreased cardiac output.

Client needs category: Safe, effective care environment
Client needs subcategory: Management of care
Cognitive level: Application

44. 3. Penetrating cardiac trauma carries a high risk of mortality and commonly leads to cardiac tamponade, a condition in which blood or fluid fills the pericardial space, compressing the heart chambers, increasing intracardiac pressure, and obstructing venous return. It's a medical emergency and requires immediate treatment. Infection is possible but wouldn't be as life-threatening as the development of cardiac tamponade. Cardiomyopathy and cardiogenic shock aren't associated with penetrating cardiac trauma.

Client needs category: Physiological integrity
Client needs subcategory: Reduction of risk potential
Cognitive level: Comprehension

45. 4. LDL levels correlate closely with a person's risk for CAD, such that the higher the LDL level, the higher the incidence of CAD. HDL levels are inversely related to the risk of CAD, such that the higher the level of HDL, the lower the person's risk for CAD. Lipid studies including triglycerides, total cholesterol, and lipoprotein fractionation (HDL and LDL) are used to determine a person's overall risk for CAD. All levels are evaluated to obtain a total picture of the client's risk. Triglyceride levels are age- and gender-related and levels above or below normal suggest an abnormality and nothing more. These levels must be evaluated in light of other results. Total cholesterol levels are considered high if they are greater than 240 mg/dl. Typically, desirable total cholesterol levels are less than 200 mg/dl.

Client needs category: Health promotion and maintenance
Client needs subcategory: None
Cognitive level: Comprehension

46. 2. The immediate treatment for asystole is CPR. This is followed rapidly by ET intubation and administration of such drugs as epinephrine and atropine as appropriate.

Client needs category: Physiological integrity
Client needs subcategory: Reduction of risk potential
Cognitive level: Application

47. 4. The mitral area is located at the fifth intercostal space near the midclavicular line. Erb's point is located at the third intercostal space at the left sternal border. The aortic area is located at the second intercostal space at the right sternal border while the pulmonic area is located at the second intercostal space at the left sternal border.

Client needs category: Health promotion and maintenance
Client needs subcategory: None
Cognitive level: Application

48. 2.8. To solve, keep in mind that 1 kg = 2.2 lb. The client weighs 154 lb, which is equivalent to 70 kg. The maximum dose is 0.04 mg/kg.

$$X = 0.04 \times 70$$

$$X = 2.8$$

Client needs category: Physiological integrity
Client needs subcategory: Pharmacological and parenteral therapies
Cognitive level: Analysis

49. 4. The heparin solution contains 50,000 units in 500 milliliters. Therefore, 1 milliliter of the solution contains 100 units of heparin. The order is for 1,000 units/hour.

Setting up the proportion:

$$100/1,000 = 1/X$$

Cross multiplying:

$$100X = 1,000$$

Solving:

$$X = 10$$

Client needs category: Physiological integrity
Client needs subcategory: Pharmacological and parenteral therapies
Cognitive level: Analysis

50. 2. Arterial occlusion after vascular repair most likely would be manifested by severely diminished or absent peripheral pulses, paresthesia, severe pain, cyanosis, and cold extremities. Decreased urine output would most likely suggest renal dysfunction. Tachycardia and shallow respirations would suggest hemorrhage.

Client needs category: Physiological integrity
Client needs subcategory: Reduction of risk potential
Cognitive level: Application

Selected references

Almenar, L., et al. "Is There a Correlation Between Brain Na-turietic Peptide Levels and Echocardiographic and Hemody-namic Parameters in Heart Transplant Patients?" *Transplant Procedures* 38(8):2534-36, October 2006.

American College of Cardiology/American Heart Association. "Guideline Update for the Diagnosis and Management of Chronic Heart Failure in the Adult," *Circulation* 112(12):1825-52, September 2005.

Berra, K., et al. "Cardiovascular Disease Prevention and Dis-ease Management: A Critical Role for Nursing," *Journal of Cardiopulmonary Rehabilitation* 26(4):197-206, July-August 2006.

Bickley, L.S., and Szilagyi, P.G. *Bates' Guide to Physical Ex-amination and History Taking*, 9th ed. Philadelphia: Lippin-cott Williams & Wilkins, 2006.

Binanay, C., et al. "Evaluation Study of Congestive Heart Fail-ure and Pulmonary Artery Catheterization Effectiveness: The ESCAPE Trial," *JAMA* 294(13):1625-33, October 2005.

Dash Eating Plan. NIH Publication Number 06-4082, 2006. Bethesda, Md.: U.S. Department of Health and Human Ser-vices; National Institutes of Health; National Heart, Lung, and Blood Institute.

Diseases: A Nursing Process Approach to Excellent Care, 4th ed. Philadelphia: Lippincott Williams & Wilkins, 2006.

Dressler, D., et al. "Caring for Patients with Femoral Sheaths: After Percutaneous Coronary Intervention, Sheath Removal and Site Monitoring are the Nurse's Responsibility," *AJN* 106(5):64A-64H, May 2006.

Dumont, C.J. "Predictors of Vascular Complications Post Diag-nostic Cardiac Catheterization and Percutaneous Coronary In-terventions," *Dimensions in Critical Care Nursing* 25(3):137-42, May-June 2006.

Fox, F.I. *A Laboratory Guide to Human Physiology: Concepts and Clinical Applications*, 12th ed. New York: McGraw-Hill Book Co., 2007.

Goldstein, L.B., et al. "Primary Prevention of Ischemic Stroke: A Guideline from the American Heart Association/American Stroke Association Stroke Council: Cosponsored by the Ather-osclerotic Peripheral Vascular Disease Interdisciplinary Work-ing Group; Cardiovascular Nursing Council; Clinical Cardiolo-gy Council; Nutrition, Physical Activity, and Metabolism Coun-cil; and the Quality of Care and Outcomes Research Interdisciplinary Working Group: the American Academy of Neurology affirms the value of this guideline." *Stroke* 37(6):1583-633, June 2006.

Headley, J.M. "Arterial Pressure-Based Technologies: A New Trend in Cardiac Output Monitoring," *Critical Care Nursing Clinics of North America* 18(2):179-87, June 2006.

Hirsh, A.T., et al. "Peripheral Arterial Disease: ACC/AHA Guidelines for Management of Patients with Peripheral Arteri-al Disease (Lower Extremity, Renal, Mesenteric and Abdomi-nal Aortic): A Collaborative Report From The American Asso-ciation for Vascular Surgery/Society for Vascular Surgery, Soci-ety for Cardiovascular Angiography and Interventions, Society for Vascular Medicine and Biology, Society of Interventional Radiology and the ACC/AHA Task Force on Practice Guide-lines (Writing Committee to Develop Guidelines for the Man-agement of Patients With Peripheral Arterial Disease)," *Jour-nal of the American College of Cardiology* 47(6):1239-312, March 2006.

JNC Express, The Seventh Report of the Joint National Com-mittee on Prevention, Detection, Evaluation and Treatment of High Blood Pressure. NIH Publication Number 03-5233, 2003. Bethesda, Md.: National Institutes of Health; National Heart, Lung, and Blood Institute; National High Blood Pressure Education Program.

Karch, A.M. *2007 Lippincott's Nursing Drug Guide.* Philadel-phia: Lippincott Williams & Wilkins, 2007.

Lindsey, H. "Systolic Blood Pressure at Admission and Heart Failure Outcomes," *AJN* 107(3):72B, March 2007.

Moser, D.K., et al. "Reducing Delay in Seeking Treatment by Patients with Acute Coronary Syndrome and Stroke: A Scien-tific Statement from the American Heart Association Council on Cardiovascular Nursing and Stroke Council," *Circulation* 114(2):168-82, July 2006.

Phibb, B. *A Basic Guide to Heart Disease*, 2nd ed. Philadelphia: Lippincott Williams & Wilkins, 2007.

Porth, C.M. *Essentials of Pathophysiology: Concepts of Altered Health States*, 2nd ed. Philadelphia: Lippincott Williams & Wilkins, 2007.

Price, A.S., et al. "Impending Cardiac Tamponade: A Case Report Highlighting the Value of Bedside Echocardiography," *Journal of Emergency Medicine* 30(4):415-19, May 2006.

Sauerbeck, L. "Primary Stroke Prevention," *AJN* 106(11):40-49, November 2006.

Scheetz, L. "Aortic Dissection: This Uncommon but Dangerous Cardiac Condition Can Have Pronounced Symptoms," *AJN* 106(4):55-59, April 2006.

Segal, J., et al. "Review of the Evidence on Diagnosis of Deep Venous Thrombosis and Pulmonary Embolism," *Annals of Family Medicine* 5(1):63-73, January-February 2007.

Silly, L., ed. *Pathophysiology of Heart Disease*, 4th ed. Philadelphia: Lippincott Williams & Wilkins, 2007.

Index

i refers to an illustration; t refers to a table.

Atrioventricular block
  causes of, 201, 202
  classifying, 202
  first-degree. *See* First-degree atrioventric-
    ular block.
  high-grade, 207i
  second-degree. *See* Second-degree atri-
    oventricular block.
  third-degree. *See* Third-degree atrioven-
    tricular block.
Atrioventricular node, 6, 6i, 7
Atrioventricular valves, 4
Auscultation
  in heart assessment, 26, 27i, 28, 29, 30i
  in vascular system assessment, 33
Automated external defibrillators, 193
Automaticity, 5, 155

B

Bachmann's bundle, 6i
Balloon catheter treatments. *See specific
    procedure.*
Balloon pump, 118i
Balloon valvuloplasty, 240, 243
Beck's triad, 302
Bicuspid valve, 4, 5i
Bigeminy, 187i
Bile acid resins, 47
Blood flow, 9-15, 11i, 12i, 14i
Blood pool imaging, 85
Blood pressure
  classifying, 48, 266, 266t, 324, 334
  dropping, interventions for, 314
Blood vessels, 9-10, 11i, 12i
Body hair, absent, 33
Bounding pulse, 35i
Brachial pulse, 31, 32i
Brachiocephalic artery, 13
Bradycardia
  sinus. *See* Sinus bradycardia.
  symptom-producing, treating, 142, 143i
Bruits, 38
B-type natriuretic peptide, 58
Bundle-branch blocks. *See* Left bundle-
    branch block; Right bundle-branch
    block.
Bundle branches, 6i, 7
Bundle of His, 6i, 7
Burst pacing, 170
Bypass grafting, 102, 103i

C

Capillaries, 10, 13
Capillary pressure, 13
Capillary refill, 31, 40, 324, 334
Cardiac catheterization, 79-81
Cardiac concussion, 296, 298
Cardiac cycle, 7, 8i, 318, 327
Cardiac enzymes and proteins, 54-58, 55i, 90
Cardiac index, 320, 329
Cardiac output, 8, 9i
  altered, characteristics of, 33
  calculating, 78
Cardiac output monitoring, 77-78, 79, 320, 328
Cardiac rehab, 96
Cardiac tamponade, 301-305
  causes of, 301
  characteristics of, 302, 322, 332
  interventions for, 304
  pathophysiology of, 301, 302i
  testing for, 303
  treatment of, 303, 316
Cardiac trauma, 295-300
  causes of, 295, 296
  characteristics of, 296, 297i, 325, 336
  interventions for, 299
  pathophysiology of, 296, 316
  testing for, 298
  treatment of, 299
Cardiogenic shock, 305-311
  causes of, 305
  characteristics of, 306
  hemodynamic parameters in, 307, 307t
  interventions for, 309, 325, 336
  pathophysiology of, 306
  testing for, 306, 307t
  treatment of, 308
Cardiomyopathy, 251-257
  causes of, 252
  characteristics of, 253
  complications of, 251, 252
  interventions for, 256
  pathophysiology of, 252
  risk factors for, 252
  testing for, 255
  treatment of, 255, 323, 333
  types of, 251
Cardiovascular assessment, 17-40
  abnormal findings in, 33-38
  chief complaint in, 17-22
  health history in, 17-23

Cardiovascular assessment *(continued)*
  landmarks for, 24, 25i
  personal and family health in, 22-23
  physical, 23-33
Cardiovascular disease
  incidence of, 41
  modifiable risk factors for, 45-51
  nonmodifiable risk factors for, 44-45
  patient teaching for, 323, 333
  risk assessment in, 42, 43i
Cardiovascular landmarks, 24, 25i
Cardiovascular system
  anatomy and physiology of, 1-16
  blood flow and, 9-15, 11i, 12i, 14i
  conduction system and, 5-8, 6i, 8i
  heart structure and, 1-4, 2i, 5i
Cardioversion, 127-129
  in atrial fibrillation, 164
  choosing correct energy level for, 128
  patient teaching after, 129
  synchronized, 161
Carotid artery, 31
Carotid pulse, 31, 32i
Carotid sinus massage, 167, 171i, 325, 335
Catheterization, cardiac, 79-81
Chest pain
  anginal, 18t, 92, 94, 246, 247
  anxiety and, 19t
  assessing, 17, 18-19t
  in chest-wall syndrome, 19t
  in cholecystitis, 19t
  in esophageal spasm, 19t
  in hiatal hernia, 19t
  in myocardial infarction, 18t, 247
  in peptic ulcer, 19t
  in pericarditis, 18t, 321, 330
  pleuritic, 230, 243
  in pneumothorax, 18t
  in pulmonary embolus, 18t
  in women, 247, 322, 331
Chest-wall syndrome, chest pain in, 19t
Cholecystitis, chest pain in, 19t
Cholesterol levels, 46, 47, 59
Cholesterol Score Sheet, 43i
Chordae tendineae, 2i, 4
Circuit reentry, and atrial arrhythmias, 155
Circulation
  and blood flow, 10-15
  coronary, 14i, 15
  pulmonary, 10
  systemic, 13

i refers to an illustration; t refers to a table.

i refers to an illustration; t refers to a table.

i refers to an illustration; t refers to a table.

i refers to an illustration; t refers to a table.

i refers to an illustration; t refers to a table.